THE TOOTHWRIGHTS' TALE

To Andrew,

With grateful and fond memories of your father Tony.

Ted Grant

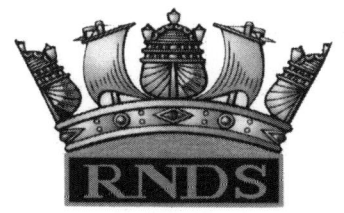

THE TOOTHWRIGHTS' TALE
A History of Dentistry in the
Royal Navy

1964 – 1995

By E J Grant

And the Officers and Ratings of
The Royal Naval Dental Services

CHAPLIN BOOKS
www.chaplinbooks.co.uk

First published in 2012 by Chaplin Books

Main text copyright © E J Grant 2012

Boxed texts and unattributed images copyright © Director Naval Dental Services

ISBN 978-0-9565595-9-3

Every effort has been made to trace the attribution or ownership of all images used in the book

All rights reserved

No part of this publication may be reproduced or transmitted in any form or by any means, electronic or mechanical, including photocopying, recording or any information storage or retrieval system, without prior permission in writing from the publishers

The views expressed in this book are those of the author and do not necessarily represent those of the UK Ministry of Defence, or any other department of Her Majesty's Government of the United Kingdom. Further, such views should not be considered as constituting an official endorsement of factual accuracy, opinion, conclusion or recommendation of the UK Ministry of Defence or any other department of Her Majesty's Government of the United Kingdom

A CIP catalogue record for this book is available from The British Library

Design by The Better Book Company

Printed in the UK by ImprintDigital.net

Chaplin Books
1 Eliza Place
Gosport
PO12 4UN
Tel: 023 9252 9020
www.chaplinbooks.co.uk

CONTENTS

List of illustrations .... *i*

Acknowledgements .... *iii*

Foreword by the Director of Naval Dental Services.. *vii*

Introduction .... *ix*

Prologue... *xi*

Chapter 1: 'MoDification' – Commencing the Cycle of Change – 1964-1969 1

Chapter 2; A Smaller World – 1970-1979 12

Chapter 3: Threats & Opportunities – 1980-1982 36

Chapter 4: Down South – The RNDS Contribution to the Falklands Conflict 53

Chapter 5: After the Storm – 1982-1985 78

Chapter 6: Changes and Challenges – 1985-1989.. 113

Chapter 7: "Change is Here to Stay" – 1990-1991 142

Chapter 8: Sand, Sea and Saddam – 1990-1991 162

Chapter 9: Options for Change – 1991-1993 180

Chapter 10: A Purple Dawn? – 1994-1995 212

Epilogue... 232

Appendix 1: A Brief History of the Evolution and Development
    of Hospital Dentistry Within the RNDS – By T J C Hall 235

Appendix 2: Recipients of the Harvey-Fletcher Medal and Prize........................ 270

Appendix 3: RN Dental Officers Deployed on Operation Corporate 271

References 272

Index... 278

LIST OF ILLUSTRATIONS

Front cover/title page – Emblem of the Royal Naval Dental Services

1. Surgeon Rear Admiral (D) W L Mountain CB QHDS 2
2. Frigate Portable Dental Unit. Circa 1964. Deployed with Royal Marines in Arctic Norway 4
3. Surgeon Lieutenant Commander (D) Peter Moorhouse. Hong Kong 'Penetration Squad' – 1967..5
4. Surgeon Rear Admiral (D) W I N Forrest CB QHDS................................10
5. The Soviet Kotlyn Class Destroyer cuts close under the stern of *HMS Ark Royal* 17
6. Surgeon Rear Admiral (D) John Hunter CB QHDS..................................21
7. Plan View of Alan Davies' Prime Mover 25
8. Surgeon Rear Admiral (D) A E Cadman CB QHDS..................................29
9. Mark II Frigate Portable Dental Unit with Lacon Box – Circa 1977 31
10. Surgeon Rear Admiral (D) B F Rogers CB QHDS 32
11. Wren DSA Rig 1950s and Wren DSA/DH Rig 1980s................................33
12. Surgeon Rear Admiral (D) P R J Duly CB QHDS..................................37
13. Combat Casualty Care Course. Dental Officers on New Forest Exercise in Arduous Conditions..43
14. Map Showing April 1982 Route of the Task Force to the Falkland Islands and South Georgia 55
15. Map of the Falkland Islands 58
16. Yomping! Iconic Photograph of the Royal Marines 'Yomping' into Port Stanley following the Surrender of the Argentinean Forces................70
17. Surgeon Captain (D) Brian Robinson receives the Harvey-Fletcher Medal from Surgeon Rear Admiral (D) Philip Duly.......83
18. Surgeon Rear Admiral (D) F R B Mathias OStJ QHDS..........................87
19. Surgeon Rear Admiral (D) David Coppock CB OStJ QHDS 103
20. Surgeon Commodore (D) Brian Robinson OStJ QHDS........................145

21.	*RFA Argus* Leaving Plymouth – October 1990	164
22.	PO Wren DH Mary Norris with a young Kurd Land Mine Victim	176
23.	Surgeon Commodore (D) T J C Hall OBE OStJ QHDS	198
24.	DNDS, Surgeon Commodore (D) T J C Hall greeting Rear Admiral Ron Morse DC USN, Chief of the US Navy Dental Corps – 9 June 1994	213
25.	Surgeon Commodore (D) E J Grant OStJ QHDS	221
26.	The Royal Naval Medical School – Later the Institute of Naval Medicine	248
27.	Tri-Service Oral Surgery Symposium – RNH Haslar – 1992	250
28.	The Royal Naval Hospital Haslar – From a watercolour by Kevin Holmes	251
29.	Royal Naval Hospital Bighi – Malta	263
30.	Royal Naval Hospital Gibraltar – Previously the British Military Hospital	265

Back Cover – The Harvey-Fletcher Medal

Acknowledgements

The writing of this History has been a labour of love. It has, however, taken me far longer than it should. It is well over ten years since Surgeon Commodore (D) John Hargraves, the then Director of Naval Dental Services, telephoned me to ask whether I would consider writing a continuation of the Branch History. After some thought, I agreed. At that time, Surgeon Captain (D) John Holland, co-author of Volume I, was the custodian of the Branch archive. This consisted of a number of large cardboard boxes full to the brim with loose papers, old files and photographs! John Holland was, himself, on the brink of retirement, and it was therefore with some relief (on his part) that he delivered them to my home.

The boxes sat for almost a year in our dining room until, under pressure from my wife, I found a new home for them at the Institute of Naval Medicine (INM). I had spent that year slowly sorting, but not cataloguing, the papers. I was therefore very grateful when Surgeon Captain (formerly Commodore) (D) Brian Robinson, agreed to tackle the job of Branch Archivist, sorting the papers chronologically and by subject and filing them in some filing cabinets acquired from various sources. Brian gave this task his usual level of meticulous care and thought, thus allowing me to start writing.

Through the good offices of John Hargraves and his successors as DNDS, a succession of Medical Officers in Charge at INM, granted me permission to use a desk and a computer in the attic of the White House (the main building at INM), by strange coincidence, the same room used for many years by Directors of Dental Training and Research. Here, I began my labours, spending around three or four mornings a month, researching, with the aid of Brian Robinson's archive and writing.

The research, initially, was easy. Surgeon Commander (D) Nick Daws was a gifted amateur naval historian. He was also co-author of Volume I of this History. Although the first volume had covered only up to the year 1964, Nick had written a meticulously referenced draft which covered up to the late 1980s. Although I did not use his text, his references I found invaluable. It was with huge sadness that I learned of Nick Daws' untimely death during the spring of 2010. I had very much hoped to seek his approval of this Volume.

At an early stage I discovered that there already existed a wealth of writing by the officers and ratings of the RNDS and it was not a difficult decision to incorporate many of these into the text. It seemed appropriate to let those who had made the History, tell their stories.

The main, but not the only sources of these have been the RNDS Newsletter, launched by Brian Robinson in 1980 and the Journal of the Royal Naval Medical Service (JRNMS). I have considered the content of the former to be the intellectual property of the RNDS and have therefore not sought the permission of the authors to reprint their work herein. 'Editor of JRNMS' is an additional hat worn by Medical Officers in Charge at INM and it is thanks to them that I am able to reproduce articles and passages from the Journal.

Whilst Brian Robinson was busy with the archive, Surgeon Captain (D) (formerly Commodore) Timothy Hall carried out another task. He undertook a 'trawl' through the issues of the JRNMS which covered the same period as this History, cataloguing all articles and other pieces relevant to the RNDS. This again has enormously eased my own research task. Timothy Hall, together with colleagues of the RNDS cadre of Oral and Maxillofacial Surgeons have also undertaken to research and write Appendix 1 to this History, which follows the main text and which tells the history of hospital dentistry in the Royal Navy. For this too, he and his colleagues earn my sincere gratitude.

The JRNMS continues in production but I am saddened and concerned that in recent years, the RNDS Newsletter seems to have 'died a death'. I hope that the reader will agree that the accounts of 'derring do' and life in general in the RNDS make fascinating and at times, gripping reading. My biggest vote of thanks is to the authors of these pieces who have helped in no small measure to bring the story of the RNDS alive. Members of the Branch, both senior and junior are still, perhaps more than ever, involved in both the continuously evolving political and managerial scenario and some increasingly demanding operational deployments. It is to be hoped that accounts of these are being recorded in some format which will enable someone else to pick up the baton and write the next volume of this History. As I have written in the Epilogue, it is a story worth telling.

I am acutely aware that there are many officers and ratings of the RNDS, senior and junior, who have all played a part in its History, but who have received no mention in these pages. This is in no way because I think that their contributions are any less than those, whose work and writings are chronicled herein. Any such omissions are due either to lack of space, or lack of written source material from which to tell their stories. I have had frequently to choose which accounts to include and which to omit. This has not always been easy, but the History of the RNDS is their History just as much as it is of those whose stories I have included or told.

Last, but not least, my thanks must go again to Brian Robinson, Timothy Hall and my wife Julia, each of whom has proof-read some or all of the draft chapters, giving me much apposite comment which has been invaluable in ensuring the accuracy and determining the structure of this History.

Author's Note

Having written this book around the many fascinating accounts of the experiences of officers and ratings of the Royal Naval Dental Services, during the period covered, I decided to use a 'Headline' title above the explanatory one: 'A History of Dentistry in the Royal Navy – 1964-1995'. A more illustrative title would, I felt, better arouse the interest of potential readers more than just the 'History' label. After a certain amount of trial and error, I decided upon THE TOOTHWRIGHTS' TALE. For those readers not familiar with Royal Navy jargon, 'Toothwright' is a familiar, even affectionate term, used by naval personnel for 'the Dentist'. Dental Officers are also often addressed, by their peers as 'Toothie'. The title has about it, I thought, a slightly Chaucerian ring and, indeed, writing this History, all of which has been within my own time as a dentist in the Royal Navy, has seemed at times something of a pilgrimage. The position of the apostrophe in 'TOOTHWRIGHTS'' is intentional. The word is pluralised in recognition of the fact that this is not just my story, but that of all those who served in the RNDS during that period.

Foreword

The first volume of *a History of Dentistry in the Royal Navy* by Nick Daws and John Holland covered the period 1905 to 1964, taking the reader on a fascinating trip that started with the birth of the Royal Naval Dental Services. It covered a period in History that saw, amongst many other challenges, two World Wars and the settling into the political, cultural, economic and military face-off between Western democracies and the Eastern Bloc. The emerging Cold War era was the context in which the Royal Navy operated as we left the first volume.

This second volume picks up the story at a time when technological advances were leading the world into a dangerous and uncertain era; nuclear proliferation, terrorism and interstate quarrels challenged policy makers and strategists. Born of such tensions, both political and economic, was the Falklands Conflict in which no less than 14 RN dental officers were deployed in the ships of the Task Force and with the Royal Marines. The reader will find herein a number of gripping eyewitness accounts of the experiences of those who were thus deployed.

The end of the Cold War gave momentary hope in 1989 for a more peaceful world but, within a couple of years, Operation Granby, the First Gulf War, introduced new military alliances and new military challenges. Like its predecessor, this History tells the story of its times through the eyes of those in the Naval Dental Services, drawing on firsthand accounts of deployed and headquarters' activity. For those who experienced the period, I'm sure that the stories and analysis of this book will bring back clear memories of the events and add some understanding to the whole. For those who were not part of the story, there may be a surprising resemblance to the objectives, challenges and successes of today's RNDS.

I congratulate and thank all those who have made this book possible. In particular, I acknowledge the tenacity and immense effort of Surgeon Commodore (D) Ted Grant. Without his dogged determination, this book would not have been possible.

Finally, I commend this book to all those who have dedicated their working lives to the dental care of Royal Navy and Royal Marines personnel. I also commend it to others, both within and outside the Service, whose curiosity may lead them to discover what it is which makes our people in the Royal Naval Dental Services so special! At the heart of our achievements and service is a deep-seated belief that we are a part of something immensely worthwhile.

R E Norris QHDS
Surgeon Captain (D)
Director of Naval Dental Services
February 2012

Introduction

The early years of the Royal Naval Dental Services from 1905 until 1964 have been recorded by Nick Daws and John Holland in the excellent first volume of this History, published in 1995. This book will continue to tell the story covering the following three decades.

It was now eighteen years since the end of World War II, a period which had seen firstly the rapid shrinkage of the Armed Forces, as 'hostilities only' personnel were demobbed. This was followed by a period of consolidation as the three Services adjusted to the threats and challenges of 'Peacetime'.

Sadly, there were still nations which did not seem to have acquired the knack of living at peace with their neighbours. The Cold War was now the driving force that dictated defence policy in the UK, with the protagonists confronting each other from both sides of Churchill's 'Iron Curtain'.

In June 1950, crisis had erupted in Korea, leading to an intense and at times bloody confrontation between the North Korean communist forces and the South Koreans. North Korea was supported principally by the Chinese, but also by the Soviet Union who supplied MIG 15 aircraft to the Chinese, as well as (covertly), the pilots to fly them. South Korea was supported by a large United Nations force, including the Armed Forces of the United Kingdom. By chance, it was a unit of the Royal Navy which was one of the first to see action in this conflict, when aircraft from the light fleet carrier *HMS Triumph,* which happened to be close to Korean waters at the outbreak of hostilities, engaged enemy targets. The Korean armistice was signed in July 1953, resulting in the partition of Korea at the 38th Parallel; a truce which exists uneasily until the present day.

The Korean War was the first 'hot' outbreak of the Cold War and was followed through the 1950s by a succession of 'bush fire' conflicts, some of which demanded the engagement of the UK through its membership of NATO and others which were symptomatic of the breakup of the British Empire, following World War II. They included the Chinese Communist Insurgency in Malaya, the Suez crisis and the heightening of tension along the Iron Curtain, following the suppression by the Soviet Union of liberal and freedom movements among its satellites, particularly in Czechoslovakia and Hungary. Following also an attempted incursion into Malaysia by Indonesian forces in 1963, British Armed Forces were involved in the three-year 'Indonesian Confrontation', during which a significant number of RNDS personnel were deployed, ashore and afloat, in support of the Fleet and the Royal Marines.

Thus the period between the end of the War in 1945 and 1963, where we take up once again the story of the Royal Naval Dental Services, had been an active and challenging time for the UK Armed Forces. Active because of the continuing conflicts around the world and challenging because of the post-war political instinct, which led to significant reduction in resources for the "Defence of the Realm". This, in turn had led to competition and in-fighting between the three Services for what each saw as its rightful slice of the Defence Budget cake.

In April 1964, a few months before losing a General Election to Harold Wilson's Labour Party, the Conservative Government of Sir Alec Douglas-Home abolished the single-Service Ministries combining them into an integrated Ministry of Defence with a Minister for each of the Armed Forces. This was the first step of many towards 'Rationalisation', which for the three Dental Branches of the Armed Forces was to lead ultimately to the Defence Dental Services of today.

This volume tells the story of that period, as it affected the Royal Naval Dental Services.

Prologue

At a time when the UK National Health Service was still young and general dental practitioners were enjoying a higher income and greater clinical freedom than most general medical practitioners, what induced new dental graduates to join the Armed Forces? Was it the pay? Almost certainly not. In 1963, the annual salary of a Surgeon Lieutenant (D) in the Royal Navy, which was a little over £900 per annum, was raised to £1500 in order to compete with the NHS, within which the new graduate 'on the high street' could expect to earn in excess of £2000. Was it the working conditions? Again, almost certainly not. Although these were to change very favourably over the years to come, greater stability and a free choice of where the graduate could practise were more readily available in civilian practice. Was it then the attraction of travel, adventure and the opportunity to acquire skills and experience outside clinical dental practice? The author of this volume has his own opinion on this, but let the reader judge for him or herself.

In order to illustrate some of the more interesting operational and extramural experiences of personnel in the Royal Naval Dental Services (RNDS), the central text of this History has been 'seasoned' with accounts of individual experiences and achievements of the men and women who are its most important assets. Almost invariably these were experiences which would not have been encountered in civilian practice. They were not always fun, as Surgeon Lieutenant Commander (D) F R B (Frank) Mathias, the Senior Dental Surgeon of the aircraft carrier *HMS Centaur* was to discover.

By the end of 1963, it was Government policy to maintain a continuous presence of two front-line aircraft carriers "East of Suez". *HMS Ark Royal* was one of these but had suffered serious mechanical problems and was limping back to the UK. Thus it was, in order to maintain that presence, *Centaur* sailed for the Far East, for a twelve month deployment, on 22 December 1963. Having missed Christmas at home by three days, morale on board was not good, but at mid-day on 23 December, when off Cape Finisterre, the ship was ordered at "best speed" to assist in the rescue of survivors of the Greek cruise liner *Lakonia*, which was on fire about 250 miles west of Casablanca. It took some 12 hours at 27 knots to reach the scene of the disaster. In the meantime, some assistance had already arrived.

Life rafts had been dropped by an American C-54 and the merchant ship *Montcalm*, the first on the scene, had taken on board over 900 survivors. By the time *Centaur* arrived on the scene and took command of the operation, 14 other ships were involved in the search and rescue.

An engineer officer from *Centaur* was winched by helicopter on to the deck of the *Lakonia*, which was by this time, a burning hulk. Sadly, he assessed that there could be no more survivors on board in such an inferno. While this evolution was taking place, the other ships were conducting a wide sweep, in unfavourable sea conditions, in the vain hope of finding more survivors.

It was decided that *Centaur* would take on board all bodies which had been recovered by the merchant ships during the day and these were embarked by helicopter. *Centaur*'s own boats and helicopters had recovered more bodies and the final total brought on board was 55. The casualties were mostly elderly but, distressingly, included a number of young children.

A medical team, consisting of one of the ship's three doctors and the dental officer, supported by sick birth and regulating staff, spent from dawn to dusk in a screened area on the flight deck examining the bodies and cataloguing personal effects. Many of the casualties were in their night attire and identification was thus a problem. By the end of the day, out of the 55 casualties, 39 had been positively identified. Frank Mathias had made a full dental chart of each one and these were to be of great value in the identification of the remaining 16 bodies at a later date. The bodies were disembarked at Gibraltar on Christmas Day!

Not all the experiences recounted in this book are as distressing as that described above, but there is little doubt that time spent in the RNDS, whether on a Short-Service Commission or as a Full Career, offered young dentists both the opportunity to hone their clinical skills and a lot more besides!

After the *Lakonia* disaster, *HMS Centaur* sailed on to Suez, to yet more trouble and into a new era for the Royal Navy, the RNDS and for Britain's Armed Forces. Read on!

Chapter 1

'MoDification'

Commencing the Cycle of Change

1964-1969

On 1 April 1964, the Royal Naval Dental Services (RNDS) found themselves together with all departments of the UK Armed Forces, subsumed within the newly established Ministry of Defence (MoD)[1]. This was the start of a process of rationalisation and downsizing, which would gradually draw together the three Services and with them their Dental Branches. This History will chronicle that process and the concurrent military events over the next three decades.

Whilst the single Services were now within the new, all-embracing organisation, Dentistry in the UK had been taking its first, faltering steps towards independence. The Dentists Act 1956, had set up the General Dental Council, the new governing body of the profession. Prior to this, the dental profession had been regulated by the Dental Board of the United Kingdom, itself responsible to the General Medical Council. It was the latter body, alone which had had the power to erase the names of dental practitioners from the Dental Register.

The General Dental Council was now responsible directly to the Privy Council and had direct responsibility for the registration and discipline of all UK dental practitioners. In order to reflect Dentistry's new found status, within the Ministry of Defence it was decided that the Head of the Dental Branch would now bear the title Director of Naval Dental Services (DNDS), rather than the Deputy Director General for Dental Services, within the organisation of the Medical Director General (Naval) (MDG(N)). DNDS would, nonetheless remain directly subordinate to the MDG, a situation which was to lead to some significant political manoeuvring in later years. Similar changes were made in the sister Dental Services of the Army and the Royal Air Force.

In his 'State of the Union' address at the annual dinner of the Royal Navy Medical Club, the MDG, Surgeon Vice Admiral D D Steele-Perkins commented that the Dental Branch was now fully complemented* and that there were more applicants than vacancies. He continued with a statement, which some may see as prescient, but which those who served

---

* At that time there were 120 dental officers in the Royal Naval Dental Services, including six Surgeon Sub Lieutenants (D), dental students entered under the recently introduced Dental Cadetship scheme.

through the last three or four decades of the Twentieth Century will recognise as 'business as usual'! He said: "The new position of our Service under the umbrella of the Ministry of Defence is bound to affect the development of the Medical Branch ... Its association with the other two Defence Medical Services will come under critical review. It is a situation which no planner could resist looking at again, ... although it will be the 3rd or 4th time since the war."[2]

On 13 November 1964, Surgeon Rear Admiral (D) P S (Titch) Turner was relieved as DNDS by Surgeon Rear Admiral (D) W L (Leonard) Mountain, who had joined the RNDS in 1933 and who had spent the war mostly at sea in battleships, cruisers and depot ships. During his years of service in the RNDS, Mountain had shown a particular interest in the design of dental surgeries, especially those in the ships.

With the post-war contraction of the Fleet, there were now less sea-going units which could reasonably offer space for a full-time dental officer. Thus, a greater proportion of naval personnel, at dental risk, had little or no access to either routine or emergency dental treatment.

It was something of a *coup*, therefore, that the design of the new County Class guided missile destroyers included space in which a dental surgery could be installed. Somewhat bizarrely, however, it was left to the individual commanding officers of these ships to choose whether they should carry a dental officer or a chaplain! Some admitted to having some difficulty over the decision 'Teeth or Souls?' Thus it was that the first of the class, *HMS Devonshire*, put to sea without dental support, but the next two, *HM Ships Hampshire* and *London*, were both equipped with dental surgeries, bearing, as permanent members of their ships' companies, their own dental officers; Surgeon Lieutenant (D) Mark Blake in the *HMS Hampshire* and Surgeon Lieutenant (D) Jonathan Bradbeer in the *HMS London*.

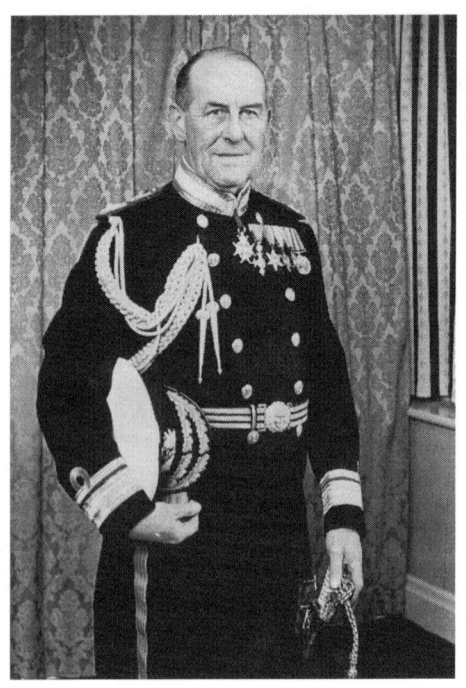

Surgeon Rear Admiral (D)
W L Mountain CB QHDS

Looking after a ship's company of around 440 men was not the most taxing job in the Dental Branch. With time to spare when at sea, many of the young dental officers deployed in these ships found themselves detailed off, not only for the more traditional tasks, such as Wardroom wine caterer or Public Relations Officer, but also as Ship's Diver and Flight Deck Officer, for which jobs they received the appropriate training. Jonathan Bradbeer took on both of these latter roles, as did several of his colleagues in *London's* sister ships. The County Class 'drafts' were much sought after by junior dental officers during the 1960s and 70s and were regarded as very much 'a nice number'!

In all of the smaller ships, each sickbay carried a Minor Dental Valise. It contained the basic instruments necessary to provide dental first aid, assuming that a member of the sickbay staff or, in the case of those very small ships which carried no medical staff (mine hunters, diesel submarines and patrol craft), the cox'n, had done the appropriate course and that they had the confidence to use it! Unfortunately, this was seldom so and, at best, the Valise was used to provide the occasional, poorly mixed zinc oxide/eugenol temporary filling!

A 'Bush Fire' War

By January 1964, *HMS Centaur* had found herself off the port of Dar-es-Salaam in Tanganyika, in company with the destroyer *HMS Cambrian*. She had been diverted there from her planned deployment to the Far East following a mutiny by the Tanganyikan Rifles and a request for assistance from President Julius Nyerere. In Aden, the ship had embarked 45 Commando, Royal Marines, together with two twin-rotored RAF Belvedere helicopters and their support staff and an element of the 16/5th Lancers, with their Ferret armoured cars.

After a bombardment of the landing beaches by the destroyer *HMS Cambrian*, the commandos were landed by helicopter and *Centaur* put to sea in order to launch her Sea-Vixen aircraft to provide close air support. The resistance was heavier than anticipated and the rebels sustained a number of casualties. About 35 of the more serious cases were embarked in *Centaur* for medical treatment.

After one day of such action, the mutiny collapsed and since the ship was to be relieved on station by another carrier, *HMS Victorious*, and in order to allow the continuation of her deployment, casualties incurred by the 'opposition' had to be treated as quickly as possible and disembarked.

Two surgical teams were set up, the dental officer, Surgeon Lieutenant Commander (D) Frank Mathias, being the anaesthetist for the second team. Fortunately, he had recently received some refresher training in anaesthetics, from the Eastman Dental Institute and the Royal Naval Hospital, Haslar, against just such an eventuality.

Under Mountain's guidance, development work continued on the Frigate Portable Dental Unit (FPDU), which in prototype had seen service in the late

1950s and early 1960s. It had been latterly trialled and further developed in the Persian Gulf by Surgeon Lieutenant (D) T J C (Timothy) Hall. Oversight of FPDU development was under the direction of Surgeon Captain (D) K A (Johnny) Johnson, who, in 1964, was serving as the Command Dental Surgeon in Plymouth. The FPDU Mk I was produced in Devonport Dockyard, using robust, metal-framed containers. It was also designed to be deployed operationally with the Royal Marines ashore, with the addition of a small, petrol-driven compressor.

It was exhibited at the British Dental Association Conference that year, in London, and was displayed in a mock-up of the sickbay in *HMS Leander*, the first of a new class of anti-submarine frigate.[3]

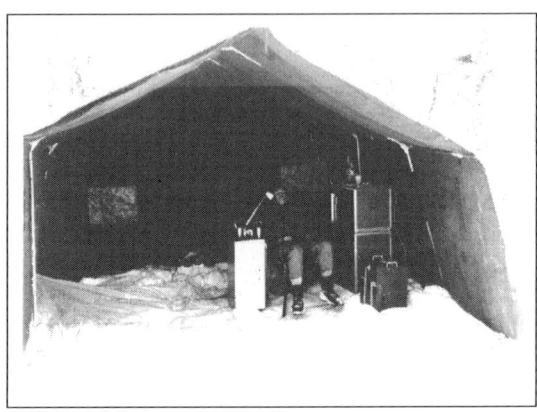

Frigate Portable Dental Unit – Circa 1964 Deployed with Royal Marines in Arctic Norway

The deployment of dental officers with their FPDUs in the small ships was well received in the Fleet and also by the MDG, who, in his speech at the RN Medical Club Dinner in 1966, declared, "I am delighted at the success of the Mobile Dental Service. It has done a great deal to raise the morale of ships' companies in the smaller ships on detached service".[4]

To underline this success, a short PR film was produced, *Small Ship's Dental Officer*. This showed the FPDU in use and included a sequence showing the dental officer, Surgeon Lieutenant (D) David James and his kit, being transferred by jackstay from *HMS Urchin* to *HMS Venus*.

Over the years, the Frigate Portable Dental Unit has evolved into the sophisticated outfit of today. It is in constant use in both small ships and in the field with Royal Marines units and has provided many young dental officers with the opportunity to experience life in the front line.

The dental officers working with FPDUs in small ships were working in model conditions compared with Surgeon Lieutenant (D) Frank Mathias, who, whilst serving at *HMS Tamar* in Hong Kong in the mid-1950s, had been called upon to practice dentistry of an altogether more primitive nature. To provide some form of medical and dental care to the more remote areas of the colony, the St. John's Ambulance Brigade set up 'penetration squads' of volunteers. In the best traditions of the Service, Mathias volunteered to work with the squads in his spare time.

In an article in the British Dental Journal which he wrote some years later[5], he explained that it was only possible to visit each location once a year, thus, of necessity; the treatment consisted mainly of emergency extractions. These were carried out at sites ranging from village squares, temples and, when their luck was in, village school rooms. The working conditions were nearly always hot, dusty and fly-ridden

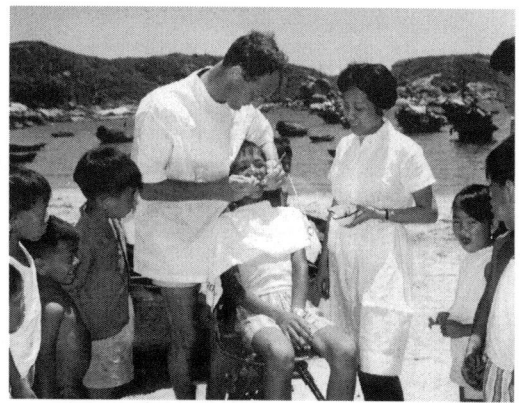

Surgeon Lieutenant Commander (D) Peter Moorhouse Hong Kong 'Penetration Squad' 1967

– a far cry from the conditions of cross-infection control, in which today's dental officers are obliged to work!

This voluntary service was expanded by successive dental officers serving in *HMS Tamar* and, during his time in Hong Kong in 1967, Surgeon Lieutenant Commander (D) P (Peter) Moorhouse described, in an article in the Journal of the Royal Naval Medical Service[6] how, as well as continuing to work with the 'Penetration Squads', he had also provided dental treatment for the boys of the Hong Kong Sea School, which taught basic seamanship to youths from the dreadful squatter colonies which were a feature of Hong Kong at that time. The students were aged 14 to 17 and the school provided training to fit them for service in the Merchant Navy as well as some health care to which they had had no previous access.

Until 1965, Specialists (in Oral Surgery) were appointed to the Naval Hospitals on the basis of experience only, although many had gained their Fellowship in Dental Surgery (FDS). That year saw the introduction of formal Specialist Selection Boards[7]. Candidates for selection were expected to have at least two years' hospital experience. For those graded Specialist, a further five years of experience and an appropriate higher qualification were required before they became eligible for selection to one of the limited number of Senior Specialist posts.*

In 1966, Wren Dental Surgery Assistants (DSAs) were still undergoing their basic professional training (Part II) in the Dental Training Department and Dental Clinic of the Royal Naval Barracks, Portsmouth. The DSAs were prepared for their subsequent advancement examinations within their own clinics, by their Senior Dental Surgeons (SDS). Not all SDSs showed a flair

---

* The History and development of the RNDS Oral and Maxillofacial Surgery Service is described in Appendix 1 to this Volume. It is compiled and written by Surgeon Captain (D) T J C Hall OBE, Royal Navy, together with contributions from other colleagues from the Oral Surgery cadre of the RNDS.

for this aspect of their duties and the standard of professional knowledge amongst advancement candidates was unacceptably variable. This problem was overcome by the introduction of a three-day Advancement Course in the Portsmouth training department, prior to sitting the exam [8].

It was also recognised, during the same year, that the problems of young dental officers serving with the Royal Marines required the appointment of a more experienced dental officer, preferably Commando trained.

He would act as a point of contact between this part of the RNDS, the Commands and the Directorate. Thus the then Staff Dental Surgeon to Major General Royal Marines, Surgeon Lieutenant Commander (D) P C (Peter) Wrigley, was appointed also as Royal Marines Dental Adviser to DNDS. Peter Wrigley was also the first dental officer to hold the coveted Commando Green Beret. Inspection of dental officers serving with the Royal Marines, remained in the hands of the Command and Fleet Dental Surgeons[9].

It was at this time, when the UK was undergoing a period of rapid inflation that discontent with military pay lead to a pay rise for the Armed Forces of an average of 18%, effective on 1 April 1966. Unfortunately, doctors and dentists were excluded from this rise, the government white paper explaining that the pay of these personnel was tied to that of civilian doctors and dentists working within the National Health Service, whose rates had not yet been agreed[10].

It was whilst civilian medical and dental rates of pay were under discussion, that the Government, fearful of losing control of the economy, introduced a general prices and incomes freeze. Six months later, doctors and dentists in the Armed Forces were awarded a 10% pay rise. This was significantly less than the awards to both their other military colleagues and the previously agreed NHS general practitioner analogue. This engendered further discontent with subsequent effect upon recruiting and retention within the Defence Medical Services[11].

September 1966 saw the death of Surgeon Captain (D) J T Wood at the age of 73. It was he who had succeeded Edward Fletcher as the second Head of Branch and who had sacrificed his chance of further promotion to Acting Surgeon Rear Admiral (D), in order to consolidate the status of the Branch and its Head during the post-war years[12]. His memory is honoured to this day by the triennial Wood Lecture and Clinical Day.

In June 1967, as a result of further belt tightening in the Royal Navy, the Far East Fleet and the Western (formerly Home) Fleets were brought under the operational control of the Commander-in-Chief Fleet in the new headquarters at Northwood, Middlesex. This move brought about the subsequent downgrading of the C-in-C posts in Plymouth and Portsmouth to that of Flag Officer, whilst the new Naval Home Command was established in Portsmouth in 1969, to oversee the non-operational tasks of the Navy – training, supply etc. With the demise of Plymouth Command, came the eventual loss, in 1973, of the post of Command Dental Surgeon, Plymouth, but a Surgeon Captain (D) billet was retained in the West Country for the time being in the newly established post of Fleet Dental Surgeon to C-in-C Fleet.*

In 1965, Surgeon Commander (D) Philip Duly had been appointed as the first Officer-in-Charge of the newly established Royal Naval Dental Training School at *HMS Nelson*. His task was, in addition to the continuation and development of existing training, to set up the first RN training course for Dental Hygienists, to a syllabus approved by the General Dental Council.

In this he was given invaluable support by Dr M N Naylor, a Surgeon Lieutenant Commander (D) in the Royal Naval Reserve and Head of Preventive Dentistry at Guy's Hospital Dental School in London. In setting up and running the first few courses, he was ably assisted by Flight Lieutenant Freda Rimini, a senior DH Tutor from the Institute of Dental Health and Training at RAF Halton. The school was established in the old *HMS Nelson* dental clinic and the former offices of the Command Dental Surgeon.

The clinic and the Command Dental Surgeon moved to new premises in the clinic's present location in *HMS Nelson*. The CDS later decamped to the Commander-in-Chief's offices in the Old Naval Academy, in the Dockyard.

The first batch of qualified Wren Dental Hygienists (DH) was drafted to dental clinics in April 1967[13].

In September 1968, a number of RN Dental Officers attended a course at Guy's Hospital to introduce them to the gentle art of how to employ a Dental Hygienist. It was not sufficient just to provide each RN dental clinic with a hygienist. The dental officers had to be educated in the capabilities and the correct employment of the new members of their teams.

The initial concept of the job of a Dental Hygienist in the RNDS and elsewhere, was that she (in the Navy, they were all Wrens at that time), was there to relieve the dental officer of the drudgery of the quick 'S&P' (Scale & Polish) at the end of each course of treatment. The course at Guy's Hospital was aimed at spreading the gospel of prevention and oral health education. It defined the role of the dental hygienist in improving the dental health of the men and women of the Royal Navy.

---

* Despite the Fleet Headquarters being established at Northwood in Middlesex, this appointment remained in Plymouth until 1981, when the then incumbent, Surgeon Captain (D) G (Geoff) Sharpe, moved to Fleet HQ on the outbreak of the Falklands conflict.

Dental Hygienists were, in fact, 'invented' by the Royal Air Force, to give support to their dental officers during World War II. After the War, and in the face of some lack of enthusiasm from the dental profession, the UK Dental Board (the predecessor of the General Dental Council) decided that such ancillary support was not appropriate to general dental practice.

It was not until the mid-1960s that the Army and Navy followed the RAF in launching their own DH categories, shortly followed by the major civilian dental teaching establishments which also set up schools of dental hygiene.

Although it is seldom now acknowledged, it was, indeed, the Dental Branches of the three Armed Services, which pioneered the training and employment of dental hygienists in the UK and Philip Duly was very much in the forefront of this revolution.

Having set up the School from scratch to train to a national syllabus set by the GDC, it was his proud boast that, during his time at the school, not one DH trainee failed the national examination for the Certificate of Proficiency in Dental Hygiene. His stint at the RN Dental Training School lasted for five years and on leaving RNDTS in 1970, Duly was awarded the OBE for his services to dentistry. He was then appointed as a member of the National Board of Examiners in Dental Hygiene. By the time he was appointed as DNDS, Surgeon Rear Admiral (D) P R J Duly OBE was also Chairman of the Board of Examiners.

The creation of the integrated Ministry of Defence brought with it the "rationalisation" of the procurement and supply of medical and dental stores and in April 1968, the Army Department assumed responsibility for these functions, the Medical Equipment Depot at Ludgershall in Wiltshire becoming the Defence Medical Equipment Depot (DMed)[14]. Although this brought with it the great advantage of enhanced buying power for the Armed Forces Medical and Dental Branches, the Royal Navy continued to provide medical and dental stores through its own organisation at Greenock until January 1970.

Another feature of tri-Service rationalisation was the introduction of the "F Med" series of forms, which came into use in June 1969[15].

The Dental Envelope, F Med 271, replaced the unlamented form M.228 (Dental Treatment Form), but once again the RNDS was slow to adopt these changes and the new forms were not used by the Navy until 1973. Indeed, four months after the introduction of the F Med series, the RNDS introduced a revised version of the M.228!

With hindsight it is hard to understand the reluctance of the RNDS to adopt the new and much needed dental record forms. The origins of the

M.228 (Dental Treatment Form) have now been lost in the mists of time, but it is believed that it was in use during the Second World War. By modern dental standards the size and format of the form were inadequate for accurate record keeping and had aroused criticism by many dental officers. Even in the 1960s, it was recognised that permanent dental records were an essential ingredient for the smooth running of any dental organisation and, more importantly, for the welfare of the patient. Despite this, RNDS regulations at that time decreed that when any man or woman was drafted to another ship or establishment, their Form M.228 should be destroyed and a new one raised when joining their new ship or establishment!

During the 'Indonesian Confrontation' campaign in the Far East (1964-1966), units from all three Services sustained significant casualties. In one incident, the bodies of two Royal Marines were recovered some months after the reported loss of a number of men during a fierce action in the Borneo jungle. Their unit dental officer was asked to provide dental records to assist with identification. He had to explain that, since he had not yet been able to dentally examine all the men before they were deployed on the operation in which they met their deaths, he held no accurate dental records for the missing men. This incident resulted in the promulgation of a new order – that full dental records were to be raised for all personnel within the Far East theatre of operations and that *when the ship or unit left the theatre, these records were to be destroyed!*

Why the reluctance to adopt such a fundamental measure as keeping permanent dental records? In 1965, at *HMS Raleigh* the new entry training establishment for rating recruits, Surgeon Lieutenant Commander (D) B (Brian) Robinson and Surgeon Lieutenant (D) E J (Ted) Grant the latter of whom had recently served in the Far East in *HMS Victorious,* submitted a paper suggesting the adoption of permanent records. Their proposal was rejected with the stated reason that the RNDS did not have the manpower to be able to forward dental documents every time men or women were drafted. At that time medical documents were already transmitted from ship to ship!

January 1968 also saw the death of the 'Father of the Branch', Edward Fletcher at the age of 81[16]. His name will always be associated, not only with the founding of the RNDS, but also with the high standards of clinical excellence for which RN Dental Officers have always strived.

The same year saw the retirement of the Director, Surgeon Rear Admiral (D) Leonard Mountain, who was awarded the CB. He was superseded in February 1968, by Surgeon Rear Admiral (D) W I N (Bill) Forrest, who had joined the Service in 1937.

After the war, he pursued his interest in Oral Surgery, eventually reaching the grade of Senior Specialist in Dental Surgery. In this capacity, he served in a number of RN Hospitals, including RNH Bighi in Malta and RNH Bermuda. During the latter appointment, in 1947, he made lasting friendships with colleagues from the US Navy Dental Corps. These were to bear fruit later with the establishment of the Royal Navy/US Navy Dental Officer Exchange programme.

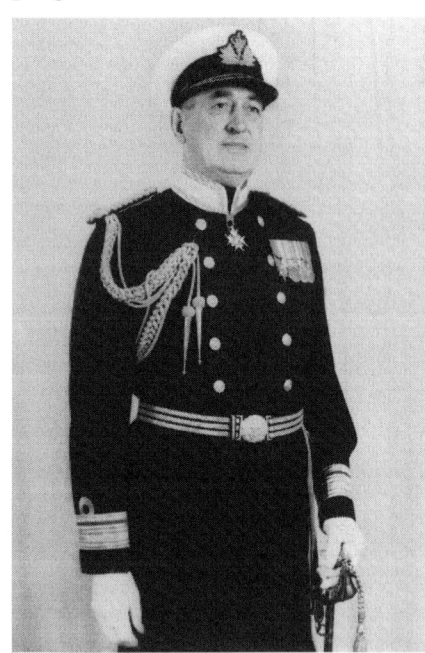

Surgeon Rear Admiral (D)
W I N Forrest CB QHDS

During the post-War years, Bill Forrest alternated between general service appointments, including a commission in the aircraft carrier *HMS Eagle* and hospital appointments where he continued his oral surgery training. Eventually, his career took yet another turn into the administrative sector, when he was appointed Assistant to the Director Naval Dental Services (Surgeon Rear Admiral (D) C J Finnegan), in 1962.

Promoted Surgeon Captain (D) in 1964, he moved from London to Portsmouth as Command Dental Surgeon on the Staff of C-in-C Portsmouth and, finally back to London as Director, in 1968.

For some years, Branch Directors had been honoured by being appointed as Honorary Dental Surgeons to the King (or Queen). In 1968, the same honours were accorded to a second senior dental officer, Surgeon Captain (D) D L Goodridge and to the senior dental officer of the Royal Naval Reserve, Surgeon Captain (D) Morris Bennett. The author believes, but has not been able to corroborate, that this was the first time that the Branch could boast three QHDSs.

Brain of the Branch?

Surgeon Commander (D) C J (Kit) Wilkinson was known throughout the RNDS, and indeed beyond the Branch, for his encyclopaedic knowledge on almost anything. In 1968, perhaps at the prompting of his colleagues, he entered the BBC Radio, "Brain of Britain" competition. He did, in fact, reach the final, but had to satisfy himself with the runner's up trophy!

It was in the late 1960s that the Labour Government of Harold Wilson announced that the Armed Forces would withdraw from all permanent bases

'East of Suez'. In practice this meant the closure of all military bases on the island of Singapore and in Malaysia as well as those in the Persian Gulf.

This drawdown of facilities and, inevitably, of personnel, had serious implications for the RNDS. At that time there were around seven permanent dental officer posts in Singapore, including the Fleet Dental Surgeon, Far East Fleet and the Singapore-based Fleet Support ships *Triumph*, *Forth* and *Hartland Point*.

The Naval Base also boasted a large clinic with a Chinese-manned laboratory at *HMS Terror* and a Families Clinic, which shared the same building as the Fleet Dental Surgeon's office and in which he would work when administrative duties permitted.

There was also a dental officer at the Naval Air Station, *HMS Simbang*. The dental strength was enhanced from time to time by visiting ships' dental officers. The Army and the Royal Air Force each had an even bigger dental establishment on the Island.

Hong Kong, being a Crown Colony, would continue to enjoy a strong military presence and the one dental officer billet at *HMS Tamar* was unaffected. Indeed, not long after the withdrawal from Singapore was complete, the Hong Kong establishment was increased to accommodate a Wren dental hygienist.

Clearly, a reduction in dental officer numbers was now inevitable and Admiral Forrest was faced with the task of reducing the strength from 105 dental officers to 93, over the next three years.

This was the beginning of a relentless decline in numbers, which was to tax successive Directors for the next two decades. Forrest firmly believed that dental officer numbers should be based on a ratio of 1:900. This was eventually accepted, but never achieved. With belts being ever tightened, the 'working' ratio remained at 1:1150.[17]

*****

Chapter 2

A Smaller World
1970 -1979

In 1970, 14 Dental Officers were serving at sea and 20 in foreign shore billets, the latter being in the Mediterranean, the Persian Gulf, Mauritius and the Far East. This, at that time represented one third of the total Branch strength. The drawdown 'East of Suez', ordered by the Wilson government was to be completed by the end of 1971.

The year 1970 saw the 50th anniversary of the founding of the Royal Naval Dental Service, a landmark noted by the Medical Director General (Naval), Surgeon Vice Admiral E B Bradbury, in his 'State of the Union' address at the Royal Navy Medical Club Dinner in September of that year. Reminding his audience of the origins of the Dental Branch, borne out of the rising awareness of the poor oral health of naval personnel at the turn of the century and of the founding of the Branch by Order in Council in January 1920, he continued: "In 50 years they have revolutionised the dental health of the Service. The Navy can be said to have pioneered and proved the undoubted value of good dental health and can take a pride in that today. Virtually no recruits are rejected, no men invalided, no illnesses are aggravated by dental diseases and no patients refuse treatment." He went on to report that Admiral Forrest had told him that: "We are now on the threshold of the preventive era of dentistry. Perhaps it has come a little late for some of us, but we all wish him well in his next 50 years."[18]

In the same year, Dr M N Naylor of Guy's Hospital, London was appointed as Civilian Consultant in Preventive Dentistry to the Royal Navy. Dr (Tony) Naylor was also, at that time, serving as Surgeon Commander (D) in the Royal Naval Reserve.

Meanwhile, despite the impending manpower cuts, it was business as usual at the operational coalface. The success of the RNDS in recruiting fully up to strength over the previous years was very much due to the exciting 'add ons' which a Service life could offer to young men and women starting out on a career in dentistry, over and above clinical expertise and experience.

As ever, news of reductions in the Armed Forces had a depressing effect on recruiting in all Branches of all Services. Dental Officers were therefore encouraged to write articles in the professional press, describing interesting experiences, outside of clinical dentistry.

In 1971, it was proposed that the British Dental Journal publish an Armed Forces issue. Sadly, this was abandoned due to lack of suitable material. However, two articles, destined for the BDJ from RNDS officers, found their way instead into the Journal of the Royal Naval Medical Service. The first was an account of 'Operation Burlap', by Surgeon Lieutenant Commander (D) E J (Ted) Grant, serving in *HMS Triumph*.[19] It is reproduced below.

Disaster!

Until the early 1970s, the area around the Ganges Delta, now known as Bangladesh, was East Pakistan. The post-war partition of India, which had created the Muslim state of Pakistan, had also resulted in the separation of the two halves of this country by several thousand miles, with the large and, to the Pakistanis, potentially hostile nation of India, between the two.

The Ganges Delta is known as the 'Rice Bowl of Asia' and much of East Pakistan consisted of thousands of square miles of low-lying rice paddy, interlaced by the multitudinous waterways which made up the delta. The inhabitants of this huge region lived mostly in primitive farm buildings on the few areas of raised ground. Communication was by boat, there being no roads. Every few years this hard existence is made worse by the cyclones to which the Bay of Bengal is prone and by flooding from the monsoon-swollen Ganges.

On 13 November 1970, a fiercer than usual cyclone, originating in the Indian Ocean, caused a twenty foot tidal wave to race northwards across the delta, destroying the rice crop, pulverising boats and dwellings and sweeping a mixed multitude of cattle and humanity to destruction. On 18 November, Pakistan requested assistance and an international relief operation was quickly organised. The affected area was so vast that it was divided into sectors, allocated to each participating nation. The British sector covered a largely devastated area in the South-West of the region, around the small township of Patuakhali. "Operation Burlap" was launched.

The nearest units of the Royal Navy, able to assist in the operation were at HM Naval Base in Singapore. A task group was quickly assembled, consisting of *HM Ships Intrepid, Triumph* and *Hydra* (a survey vessel) and *RFA Sir Galahad*. Surgeon Lieutenant Commander (D) M J (Mike) Swann, the dental officer at the Singapore Naval Air Station, *HMS Simbang*, was temporarily appointed to *Intrepid* in the absence on leave of her own dental officer. Surgeon Lieutenant Commander (D) Ted Grant was borne as the dental officer in *Triumph*. The ships of the task group spent about 48 hours, in heavy monsoon rain, loading relief stores and equipment, before sailing for the Bay of Bengal, stopping briefly to embark more stores off Penang. As well as their normal complement of RN personnel, the ships had also embarked elements of 3 Commando Brigade and 59 Field Squadron, Royal Engineers. All personnel embarked were re-vaccinated against cholera, typhoid, smallpox and polio. Grant was initially attached to the medical team and was instructed in the basic principles ➻

of public health and hygiene and the use of the 'air pressure' vaccination gun.

It had been estimated that upward of 300,000 dead, requiring burial, were in the British sector alone. In the event, the Pakistani Army had already undertaken burial of those bodies which had not been swept away by the flood waters. Although a few corpses, both human and animal were seen, survivors were probably already immune to the endemic diseases of the area. It was the men of the relief organisation who were really at risk and Ted Grant and Mike Swann were instructed in the task of supervision of the hygiene of the working parties ashore.

The waters of the Ganges Delta are shallow, hence the height of the tidal wave and the ships of the task force were obliged to anchor 27 miles offshore, apart from the smaller *Hydra*, which spent several days charting the inshore waters. A forward tactical and helicopter base was set up at Patuakhali and this was supplied by landing craft from *Intrepid* and by helicopter. The boats were manned by the Royal Marines who had a hazardous 12-hour journey each way. Supplies were distributed to the hardest hit outlying areas by inflatable boats and assault craft, as well as by helicopter. Further supplies were air-dropped daily by Hercules aircraft from RAF Changi, in Singapore.

While the Commandos were busy distributing rice, clothing and medical supplies, a detachment of 59 Field Squadron, Royal Engineers was producing potable water and repairing wells, bridges and buildings.

Swann was the first of the dental officers ashore and he set up a small dental facility at the Patuakhali 'Circuit House', within whose walls the Royal Marines had established their tactical HQ. Grant spent the first few days of the operation as a watch keeper in Operations Room, co-ordinating the dispatch of stores. On Friday 27th November, he flew ashore to join the medical team at the tactical HQ, Swann having returned to *Intrepid*. He found that the sick bay tentage had been erected on a spacious and relatively cool balcony.

Mosquitoes were numerous, as were problems of hygiene and water supplies were contaminated. A further health hazard was the copious dust whipped into clouds by helicopters and vehicles.

The sick bay staff and Royal Marines, with the help of 'press ganged' Pakistani Army personnel, also undertook the 'Augean' task of cleaning up the small local hospital, where they had found a number of sick patients lying on the floor, many in their own excrement, all beds being occupied. A few British personnel, who developed symptoms of gastro-enteritis, were immediately evacuated back to the ships for treatment and observation.

On 7 December, the Task Force Commander was advised that all possible emergency aid had been provided and that the Civil Power was now in control of the situation. All personnel were re-embarked and the Task Force returned to Singapore. ➤

> No statistics are available to show how many lives were saved by Operation Burlap, but the medical supplies, clothing, food and technical assistance brought to the stricken area prevented an horrific situation developing into one which could have been far worse.
>
> For the two dental officers, it had been an experience which truly demonstrated how the life of a clinician in the Royal Navy can demand adaptability and skills far beyond those required in the dental surgery.

It was not only those dental officers borne in the ships of the Far East Fleet who found adventure as well as clinical experience. Also in 1970, the Antarctic Survey Ship, *HMS Protector*, carried the first (and this author believes, the only) RN dental officer to accompany its annual visit to the Antarctic. The dental officer was Surgeon Lieutenant (D) J V (John) Holland.[*] An amusing account of one of his Antarctic experiences was also published in the JRNMS[20].

> ### A Cold Reception!
>
> *HMS Protector* had spent three weeks conducting a survey in an area to the south of the South Orkneys, the most northerly group of Antarctic islands. In his article, John Holland describes the tedium of quarter-hourly radar fixes, surrounded by mist and snow, with only occasional glimpses of land. Thus the chance of a 'run ashore' to visit a large penguin rookery was welcomed. The visit involved a trek across the island. Suitably attired for the climate, Holland and his colleagues were landed by boat and followed a track between high and unstable snow cliffs and across glaciers, which they had been warned to avoid, but which, if they were to achieve their destination, they had to cross, albeit with considerable care!
>
> They knew that that they were approaching the rookery, some miles before arriving there, due to the "revolting fishy smell". He describes the rookery as "enormous" and while his friends were being chased by "two ferocious fur-seals", he set off with his camera in pursuit of an Antarctic Skua, which walked in front of him, but which flew off as soon as he had fitted the appropriate lens to his camera.
>
> He continued, clambering over rocks towards the penguins and whilst focussing his camera on these, he received a sharp blow to the back of his head!
>
> Turning, to see who had assaulted him, he saw no-one but immediately received another blow to the top of his head. Turning again, he saw two skuas, which he describes as being about the size of a small goose, with a wickedly curved beak, wheeling to repeat the attack.

---

[*] Holland was not the first RN dental officer to have visited the Antarctic. Prior to joining the RNDS, Surgeon Lieutenant Commander (D) John Pidgeon had sailed with the Royal Research Ship *John Biscoe* as dental officer to the British Antarctic Survey. His experiences were covered in Volume I of this History.

> Holland took refuge, by squatting down among the penguins, but as soon as he raised his head above 'penguin level', the skuas returned to the attack, the two birds taking it in turns to make the 'bombing runs'. Eventually, he stood up and moving very slowly, managed to rejoin his party without further assault.
>
> The return trek, back to the ship passed without incident and *Protector* set course for her next landfall through Drake's Passage, bound for the Falkland Islands. En route, the next film shown in the Wardroom was Hitchcock's 'The Birds'. Holland records that he was thankful that he had not seen the film before his visit to the South Orkneys!

Surgeon Commander (D) John Holland was to return to the South Atlantic as the Oral Surgeon aboard the P&O liner *Canberra*, during the Falklands War of 1982.

While these events were taking place, closer to home the Cold War was at its height. Surgeon Commander (D) Brian Robinson was serving as Senior Dental Surgeon in the Fleet Aircraft Carrier *HMS Ark Royal*. The ship was large enough to carry two dental officers and his 'winger' was Surgeon Lieutenant (D) P S J (Peter) Gellatley. On the night of 9 November 1970, *Ark Royal* was exercising in the Mediterranean, where the two dental officers were witness to one of the more dramatic incidents of the Cold War. The following is an excerpt from Brian Robinson's personal account[21].

> ### *A Glimpse of the Cold War*
>
> The confrontation between the West and the Soviet Block lasted some forty years until the early nineteen nineties. The so called Cold War was a time of varying mistrust between the two power blocks. One of the consequences from the naval perspective was that each side would shadow the other's major assets as much as they could. When we sailed from an Atlantic port, we would invariably be picked up by a Russian intelligence gathering trawler, packed with equipment, attempting to pick up electronic and signal information from us. We would also be checked out by airborne units of the Russian Northern Fleet.
>
> In the Mediterranean, we were usually shadowed by a destroyer or frigate from the Black Sea Fleet. I have often gazed out of my surgery scuttle to see a Soviet ship steaming alongside, sometimes only 150 metres away or looked up at a helicopter taking pictures of us.
>
> [Following a ten day self maintenance period in Grand Harbour, Malta at the end of October], we sailed for an exercise in the Eastern Mediterranean and as usual, we had our Soviet shadow, this time a Kotlin class destroyer of 2,850 tonnes.

They were known in the trade as a Kotlin SAM, because they carried surface to air missiles. This particular vessel had been near us for most of the previous ten days, but had usually remained at a discreet distance. On the morning of the 9th November, our unwanted 'escort' had disappeared. At midday, another Kotlin SAM appeared over the horizon and took up station on us.

We were then about 120 miles to the south of Crete. Now the skipper of this vessel, the Kotlin SAM No. 365 named *Bravyy*, was a very different kettle of fish. As soon as he got to us, he cut close past our stern.

Eventually he got bored and settled down on our starboard side and we all got back to work. That evening we were scheduled for a night flying exercise, which got under way at about 2030. Most of the off watch officers, including me were in the Wardroom, having eaten supper. The first launch of a Phantom took place at about 2040, we felt the judder of the catapult pistons as they stopped at the end of the launch and then heard the next Phantom running up her engines on full reheat prior to launch.

Then the engines seemed to shut down and the next thing we knew was the ship seemed to be going hard astern. The whole ship was shaking as our four props strained to slow her down.

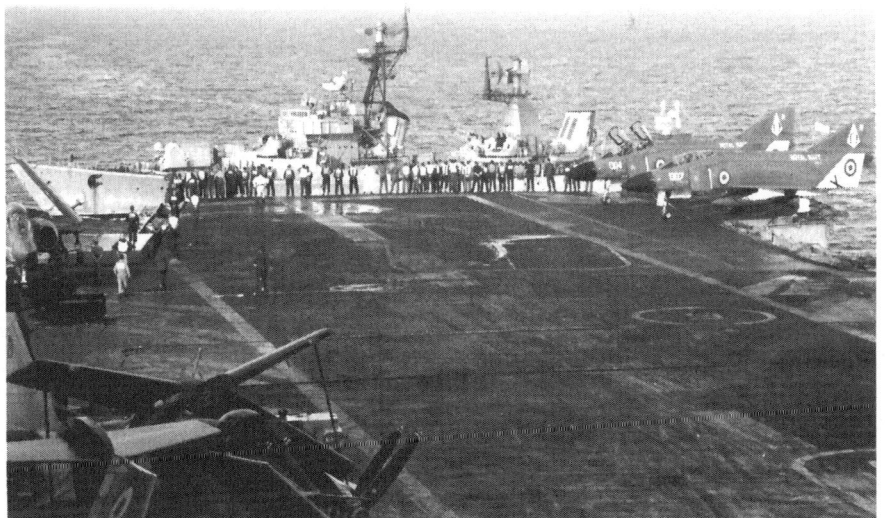

The Soviet Kotlin Class Destroyer *Bravyy* cuts close under the stern of *HMS Ark Royal*

The immediate thought was that a plane had ditched ahead of the ship, but then the alarms sounded, calling us to Emergency Stations. Everyone went scuttling to their place of duty. Finally, after what seemed like an age, the Commander came on the tannoy and said we had been in collision with a ship and we soon learned that it was our Russian friend. ➤

A ship which is flying aircraft is severely restricted in her ability to manoeuvre and shows signals or lights to that effect. Vessels in the vicinity are required to keep clear. The *Bravyy* took it upon herself to steam across our bows, coming from our starboard side.

Even if we had not been flying this would have been questionable seamanship, for although it could be said that technically she had 'right of way', it was not a clever thing to do at night and unlawful whilst we were flying aircraft. She had also been warned by voice that she was standing into danger. Despite this, she persisted. We put our engines astern, but although our speed had slowed from 25 knots down to three or four knots, we still hit her as she failed to make it across our bows. We struck her just abaft her after funnel and threw her over on to her starboard side. There had been a party of sailors working on her upper deck and seven men went over the side.

At the time of the collision, my junior dental officer, Surgeon Lieutenant (D) Peter Gellatley, having eaten a little earlier, was back aft on the quarterdeck, enjoying the night air. Apart from the port-side sentry, there was no-one else about. He recalls: "Suddenly the emergency klaxon sounded and the ship started to shudder. I immediately thought that it was the 'Man Overboard' signal. I rushed to the starboard side and, on looking over, to my horror I saw a face in the water, which I assumed was an *Ark Royal* sailor. I grabbed a lifebelt and threw it over and then watched the face disappear in the wake turbulence. I later learned that one of the Russian sailors was picked up, clinging to an *Ark* lifebelt!"

Both ships stopped and we lowered sea boats to look for survivors. We had our helicopters up and our escorting frigate *HMS Yarmouth* joined in the rescue and her sea boat found three men.

Within a couple of hours, half the Black Sea Fleet seemed to be in the area, by dawn we had about twenty Soviet ships nearby. The two missing sailors were never found. The *Bravyy* was lucky to be afloat and we were lucky that she did not drive her bows into our side, for there would have been a much greater loss of life on both ships. As it was, the Russian sustained a lot of damage on her port side and it appeared that the hull had been twisted lengthways. We sustained a 4x3 foot hole in our stem, about five feet above the water line, to which we made emergency repairs to stop the water entering.

I went along to the sickbay to see the Russian sailor. He was physically unharmed, but a bit shocked. What stood out was the very poor clothing that he wore. We gave him a hot shower and kitted him out with a brand new set of clothing. He spoke no English and, the only person we had on board with linguistic skills was a midshipman who spoke rudimentary Russian. It was clear that he could not give us any useful information so, as soon as the doctors deemed him fit to travel, we took him back to his ship in our sea boat. ⇒

> The poor sailor climbed the gangway and at the top of the steps, he was stripped of his new clothes which were thrown to the 'Mid' in charge of the boat.
>
> We returned to Malta to make more permanent repairs to our bow and to hold a Board of Enquiry into the collision.

Into 1971 and as that year progressed, so did the drawdown of UK Forces in the Far East. All families and dependants had left Singapore and Malaysia by October and the last ship to leave the Naval Base, *HMS Triumph*, sailed for the UK in November, in company with *HMS Glamorgan* and *RFA Tidespring*, leaving behind the 'rump' ANZUK (Australia, New Zealand, UK) force. ANZUK was to last barely three years and by 1974, the largest RN presence outside the UK had been replaced by one Royal Navy Liaison Officer and a small staff.

A particularly sad but touching event which marked the end of the large RNDS presence in Singapore, was the superb Chinese banquet given in a restaurant, by the Chinese dental technicians and chairside staff in *HMS Terror* to the remaining RN dental officers.

As the withdrawal from South-East Asia continued, so also, did the withdrawal from Bahrain and the Persian Gulf. By the end of 1971, with the exception of Hong Kong, there was no remaining permanent British Armed Forces presence East of Suez.

> ### *Fun in the Sun*
>
> Although the withdrawals were accompanied by sadness and nostalgia in all who had served in these far-flung and exotic bases, there were still some enjoyable times to be had. En route for the UK, *Triumph* and her escorts spent six weeks in Kilindini Harbour, Mombasa, whilst her Fleet Maintenance Group gave technical support to the Persian Gulf withdrawal operation. This period covered Christmas 1971 and the New Year and her ship's company, including the dental officer, Surgeon Lieutenant Commander (D) Ted Grant, took due advantage. Although, it was 'business as usual' in the dental clinic, time outside normal working hours was spent on the beaches, at the delightful Silver Sands RN Leave Centre or on Safari.
>
> Because Christmas would be spent away from home and loved ones, the MoD in its wisdom, engaged a number of entertainers, including the dancers, Pan's People, to perform for the ships' companies, in the period leading up to Christmas. Leave warrants were also issued to enable personnel to travel on the night sleeper train to Nairobi, an attractive city, with its own small game park.

> During these several weeks, numerous RAF flights shuttled stores, service personnel and entertainers between UK and Mombasa. Advantage was taken of these to fly out wives and sweethearts on 'indulgence flights' to spend a week or so in the tropical paradise which was then Kenya. This idyll ended when three consecutive RAF flights became unserviceable in Mombasa due to "contaminated fuel". Some wives and Pan's People had to return by commercial flights from Nairobi.

During his time as DNDS, Bill Forrest was to introduce or initiate several innovative measures. Among these were the Royal Navy/US Navy Dental Officer Exchange Programme and the Harvey-Fletcher Prize and Medal.

The US Navy Exchange was, as has been previously noted, borne of Forrest's contacts made during his service in Bermuda, shortly after the end of World War II. One of these, Rear Admiral Ed Raffetto, was now Admiral Forrest's opposite number in the US Navy Dental Corps. The seed which had resulted from their earlier acquaintance, now germinated and the exchange programme commenced in 1972. The first participants were Surgeon Commander (D) D A (David) Coppock and Commander Steve Mach DC USN. David Coppock, an extrovert and well known raconteur within the RNDS, destroyed all of his USN colleagues' preconceptions about 'typical British reserve'. His time was spent at the US Navy Hospital, Bethesda, Maryland, close to Washington DC and included a postgraduate course in the Navy Graduate Dental School. He was an inspired choice and he is well remembered in the USN Dental Corps to this day. He was, however, as this author can testify, a hard act to follow!

Another item high on Bill Forrest's 'wish list' had been to inaugurate a prestigious prize within the RNDS, to recognize outstanding scientific or administrative achievement by Royal Navy dental officers.

It was his thought that such a prize should also honour the founding fathers of the RNDS, Staff Surgeon Christopher Harvey, who was the first to recognize the need for a Naval Dental Service and Surgeon Rear Admiral (D) Edward Fletcher who set up the RNDS and who nurtured it to maturity during his long years of service. Thus was the Harvey-Fletcher Prize conceived.

Its gestation period was protracted and required the setting up of a trust fund and the approval of the Admiralty Board. The prize was to comprise a medal and a sum of money. The medal was to bear the image of St Apollonia, the patron saint of dentistry, as originally designed for and used on the London-Haslar Gold Medal. * The latter had been awarded to dental officers who excelled in the Branch entry examination, before the Second World War.

---

* The face of the Harvey-Fletcher Medal is depicted on the back cover of this History.

The obverse would bear the title of the prize, the date and the name of the recipient. Early medals were struck in silver and were made in the Command Dental Laboratory, Portsmouth. Later the work was to be carried out by the Royal Mint.

Although Bill Forrest initiated the work leading up to the establishment of the Harvey-Fletcher Prize, it was carried forward by his successor as DNDS, Surgeon Rear Admiral (D) John Hunter. Following an appeal both within and outside the Branch, the Trust Fund was set up in 1973 under the auspices of the United Services Trustee. It is not generally known, but the fund was initially primed by generous donations from both Bill Forrest and John Hunter. It was decided that an Award Committee would meet every three years, but the first award was not made until 1980.

Bill Forrest is remembered with affection as an innovative Director who was always approachable and who strove to raise the profile of the RNDS with its 'customers' in the Fleet. His dictum to his officers was "Treat sailors like admirals and admirals like sailors." He was awarded the CB upon retirement.

Surgeon Rear Admiral (D) John Hunter, a distinguished looking man with a neatly trimmed white beard and moustache, had joined the RNVR in 1940 and his war service took him to sea in *HMS Kenya* with the 2nd Cruiser Squadron, Combined Operations and the Pacific Fleet.

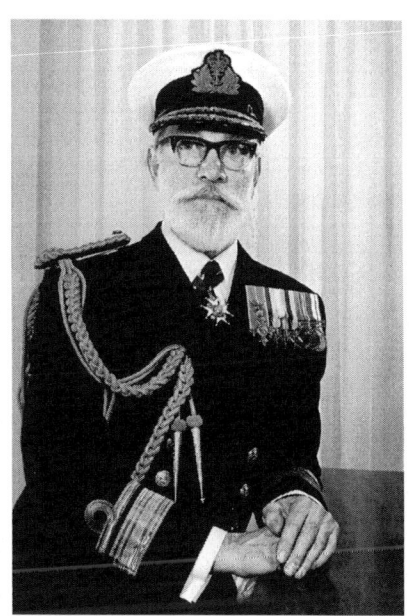

Surgeon Rear Admiral (D) John Hunter
CB QHDS

Whilst in *Kenya*, he had experienced both the North Atlantic convoys and the Malta convoys. During one of the latter, in June 1941, *Kenya* was damaged, but not sunk, by a torpedo.

In 1991, he was one of only two surviving RN dental officers to be awarded the Malta George Cross Fiftieth Anniversary Medal*. Hunter ended the war in the battleship, *HMS Howe*, in the Far East. In 1946, John Hunter transferred to the regular Navy. After various clinical appointments and, by then in the rank of Surgeon Commander (D), his career took him to Queen Anne's Mansions as Assistant to DNDS (Surgeon Rear Admiral (D) P S 'Titch' Turner).

---

* The other recipient of the Malta George Cross Fiftieth Anniversary Medal was Surgeon Commander (D) Bill King-Turner, who, at the time of writing the above [2004], was approaching his 100th birthday. At age 101, he became the oldest ever emigrant from the UK, joining his family in New Zealand, where he died in late 2009.

Promoted Surgeon Captain (D) in 1963 he filled a number of senior Fleet, Command and Staff appointments before his promotion to Surgeon Rear Admiral (D) in August 1971.

In his address at the 1971 Dinner of the Royal Navy Medical Club, the Medical Director General, Surgeon Vice Admiral Sir Eric Bradbury suggested that 1971 would be remembered as "the year of the committee"[22].

Among the committees set up during that year were the Armed Forces Committee on Postgraduate Medical and Dental Education and, perhaps the most significant, the Committee of Enquiry into the Medical Services of the of the Armed Forces, chaired by Sir Edmund Compton.

The terms of reference of the Compton Committee were "to review the arrangements for providing Medical, Dental and Nursing Services for the Armed Forces at home and abroad, for peace and war, in the light of developments in defence policy and to make recommendations."

This was not the first and would certainly not be the last such investigation of the structure of the Defence Medical Services. Indeed, Admiral Bradbury, in his address referred back to the Waverly Committee of 1956, which had had almost identical terms of reference. The chairman of the 1971 committee (Compton) was superseded by Sir Clifford Jarrett in January 1972, who issued his report the following year. For Service Dentistry, the Jarrett Report held no 'nasty surprises'.

Indeed, in many respects, it was more than helpful, recognizing the need for increases in establishment of both dental officers and support staff, in order to meet the fitness standards of the modern Armed Forces and the support manpower needed to practice 'four-handed' dentistry. Jarrett also suggested that the Armed Forces Dental Services should recognize the increasing complexity of dental postgraduate training and should match the rising standards of training in civilian dentistry[23].

This undoubtedly led to John Hunter's decision to initiate 'specialist' training for Naval dental officers and in October 1971, Surgeon Commander (D) D L (David) May joined the Institute of Dental Surgery (the Eastman) as the first of many RNDS officers to undertake a course leading to a Master of Science degree in the different disciplines within dentistry – in his case in Restorative Dentistry.

On a different note, Jarrett also recommended that Dental Hygienist training for all three Services, should be concentrated in one training establishment and that the RNDS should recruit and employ uniformed dental technicians, to overcome the problem of recruiting civilian technician of suitable ability and in sufficient number[24].

It is also of note that one of the members of the Compton/Jarrett Committee was one Dr Henry Yellowlees. He was to become a significant player in the story of the Defence Dental Services some years later and we will meet him again.

In 1972, *HMS Intrepid*, with 40 Commando embarked, took part in an amphibious exercise with the US Navy in the Philippines – Exercise SUBOK. This gave yet another dental officer the opportunity to discover how different is Service dentistry to that practiced in 'High Street, UK'.

The ship's dental officer, Surgeon Lieutenant (D) G L (Graham) Wickens later wrote an account of his Filipino adventure[25].

Caries & Coconut Milk

Travelling along the coast by Land Rover, accompanied by the doctor of 40 Commando, *Intrepid*'s Chief Medical Assistant and two Leading Medical Assistants, one of whom was dentally trained, Wickens landed on a beach on the Island of Luzon, the largest in the Philippines archipelago, with the last wave of assault troops. With 40 Commando HQ Company, they set up base in a dry river bed outside the town of Caba. The medical/dental team were not directly involved in Exercise SUBOK and their aim was to provide medical and dental assistance to the local population, where and when possible.

Having established their base camp, under canvas, they made themselves known to local medical staff, who showed them the government-sponsored health centre, which had been set up to provide care for children and pregnant women. Dental treatment, such as it was, was provided on a private basis.

After a visit to the nearby *barrio* (village) of Wencslao and a meeting with local officials, it was decided to set up a temporary clinic in the village school. That evening the team was invited to supper by the school's head teacher and very much enjoyed sampling the local food as well as listening to their host's views on the Filipino way of life and politics.

On the second morning, the dental staff set up clinic at 0800. Working only with the contents of a dental valise, enhanced with local anaesthetic and some silico-phosphate cement, they saw about 100 patients, including most of the children in the school. Sadly, and despite the local diet consisting mainly of fish, rice and vegetables, they found rampant caries to be rife. The only treatment possible, in most cases was extraction of painful teeth, although some teeth were dressed with silico-phosphate, in the hope that they might be properly restored later.

Most of the school teachers could speak English and gave help when language problems were encountered. The children were somewhat overawed by Wickens' chairside assistant, who stood 6ft 4in and weighed 19½ stone! Few Filipinos achieve such dimensions.

During the morning, the dental team was sustained with welcome glasses of fresh coconut milk. After lunch and a refreshing swim in the sea, the team ▶

> moved five miles inland to the village of San Gregario, where they set up shop in yet another school. Here they saw another 40 patients, mostly adults.
>
> In his article, Wickens comments that among the patients seen, signs of betel nut chewing were common. An even more alarming health problem was the habit among local village women of 'reverse cigar smoking', done apparently to avoid smoke getting into their eyes whilst working. As a probable direct result of this habit, he saw a number of cases of leukoplakia and one in which there were probable carcinomatous changes, in a 27 year-old woman.
>
> After another night under canvas, the team returned to the ship, finding time *en route,* for another refreshing swim. ❧

The early 1970s were the time when, within UK dentistry, the transition was being made from the 'bad old' method of treating the patient with the chair upright, to four-handed dentistry with the dentist and his assistant seated and the patient supine. Previously to this, the dentist was obliged to stand on one leg (in order to operate the Rathbone foot control, which required the lever to be pushed sideways with the toe), and with his head and neck at an awkward and potentially debilitating angle.

A good ten years before, the Medical Services Coordinating Committee had recommended that dental equipment in the Armed Forces should be brought into line with the then existing civilian standards. This had led to a gradual replacement, as funding permitted, of the old Rathbone units, with the modern 'Air Hostess' unit manufactured by DMCo. In August 1973, DNDS directed that the replacement programme should be complete by 1975.[26] Between 1971 and 1973, a number of Murray Ranger stools had been procured, with the intention that all chairside staff should work seated. The programme to provide suitable chairside stools was complete by 1977.

The third component required to practice four-handed dentistry was the provision of 'Flowline' chairs, designed to fit on the existing Rathbone hydraulic bases. These allowed the patient to adopt a supine position during treatment.

The task of providing dental services to ships lying alongside, in order to reduce the time naval personnel spent away from their places of duty, had long been recognized and caravans and trailers, converted to dental use, had been deployed on a number of stations during World War II. Their use was revived in the 1960s, when two converted Bedford buses were used in Malta and the Far East and the Mark I Dental Caravan was designed and produced for use in home dockyards. In the 1970s, the design was twice updated (Marks II and III) and these were fitted with DMCo 'Bel Air units, a 'cut down' version of the 'Air Hostess'.

Although the presence of a Dental Caravan alongside delighted first lieutenants, who were loathe to accept the time loss engendered by letting their men go to the Naval Base Clinic (often via the NAFFI!), dependence upon the Principal Stores and Transport Officer (Navy) for the movement of caravans around the dockyards was a constant source of frustration. Thus it was that thoughts began to turn towards designing a self-propelled 'Prime Mover', not only with its own automotive power, but with an integral water supply, drainage and with a generator to provide power to the dental equipment when not available from a mains source. Surgeon Captain (D) A A (Alan) Davies was tasked with the development of this idea, which came to fruition in 1978 with the production of the prototype Prime Mover[27].

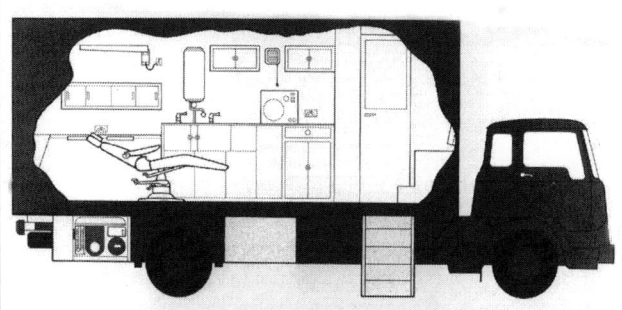

Plan view of Alan Davies' Prime Mover

Another 'revolution' in modern dental practice, which was quickly adopted by the Armed Forces Dental Branches, was engendered by the appearance at that time of a new and potentially very dangerous viral liver infection, originally known as Australia Antigen, but now identified as Hepatitis B.

This blood-borne virus was found to be resistant to even prolonged boiling in the then available boiling water sterilisers.

The Chief Scientific Adviser to the Government of that time was the much respected scientist Sir Solly Zuckerman. After deliberating for some time on the potential dangers of Australia Antigen, he issued a report which recommended that any health care worker, who, consequent to treating an infected patient, contracted Hepatitis B, should cease, <u>permanently</u>, to practice their profession! This recommendation caused great disquiet among the health professions and in 1973, the British Dental Association set up a committee to look into the implications for dentistry, of the CSA's pronouncement. In the meantime, the Dental Branches were quick to replace the old boiling water sterilisers with 'Little Sister' steam-pressure autoclaves.

Fun and adventure were not only the prerogative of the young. In 1971, Surgeon Captain (D) E B (Mac) Mackenzie, then serving at RNH Gibraltar, took the opportunity to take part in a boar hunt in Morocco. His particularly well written account of this adventure was published in the Journal of the Royal Naval Medical Service the following year[28]. It is reproduced here in its entirety.

Moroccan Boar Hunt

Pepe said it would be cold, but who could believe this of Morocco? I pulled on another woolen sweater and Charles and I stepped out into the Tangier night. It was 5 a.m. and all lights were on. Arabs, shrouded in their hooded djellabahs, squatted on guard at the entrances to private premises, while merrymakers in European dress, on their way from some mysterious and obviously exciting activity, shouted at each other.

We took a short cut through narrow, gloomy streets, passing huddled forms sleeping in corners, hearing strange music drifting from dimly lit passages and 'pop' blasting from an open window above a flashing neon sign. Most people were indoors, but life obviously went on apace through the night in this one-time international city. Doorways exhaled heady incense, a whiff of spices, the smell of mint and sometimes exotic perfumes.

We met our friends and there seemed much to do. Guns, food and wine were piled into the Land Rover, followed eventually by men and dogs. Soon we were off through the early morning traffic: overburdened peasant women arriving in the city, backs bent and laden with massive piles of vegetables; donkeys and carts stacked high with boxes of fruit; taxis, bicycles, all hustled along with business in mind.

We pulled up by a café. The pavement was crowded and the tables and chairs spilled into the street, all in the fierce glare from the restaurant within. So many people so early. The sound of the jumbled babble of a dozen languages. Men were wrapped up in sweeping garments and a cluster of Arab women, fully veiled and robed, flashed bright eyes from their covered faces and enamelled toenails in high heeled sandals showed below to belie the ancient coverings. Groups of young Arab girls in minis giggled with their oddly-clothed hippy boyfriends, just like anywhere in the modern world.

All were drinking coffee out of glass tumblers, hot and sweet, and with fresh buttered toast to start the day. It was the last weekend of the hunting season and many of the crowd sported bandoliers of cartridges around their shoulders. Altogether the throng on the pavement, illuminated in a dark street, looked highly dangerous and, to an untutored eye, might well have forecast revolution. Soon we were off into the Moroccan countryside. Long straight roads made the journey smooth and now and then, all but the driver were lulled to half awake dreaming of the day ahead.

An hour and a half later we turned off the main road and were bounced into full awareness. We climbed up a sand track leading through scrub to cork woods, ➤

winding in and out, up and down, splashing through streams and eventually through trees, to halt in a clearing. There was a huge fire blazing in the middle and we gathered round. The flickering flames lit up the faces of a ferocious looking crowd of Arabs and their even hungrier looking dogs, dozens of them. The men were our beaters.

It was getting light now and before we set off, there was to be the ritual jumping through the fire which, we were told, ensured that we would find boars and shoot well. No one got burnt, but there was a strange smell about and the whole process amused, and I think softened, our fierce audience.

Soon we were off, with the sun getting higher and the temperature rising rapidly. We pushed through scrub covering a very rough, wooded hillside till, sweating, we were quietly shown where to stand and wait.

Three or four overgrown paths led from the small clearing, looking like the entrances to tunnels through the thick green. We were told that to miss would mean jumping fast, as the beast knew where he was going and meant to get there. There was not much room for two.

After a while the silence was shattered by a shot, the breaking out of a wild voice of hounds and the crashing of undergrowth. Excitement grew and the noise got very near, coming our way. There was a terrific feeling of expectation, tension and hope. Another shot cracked nearby and the crashing pursuit ended. The hounds stopped calling and men shouted. The boar was dead, shot by the gun at the next stand.

By midday we had shot our quota of four pigs, plus a dog which was suddenly produced by one of the beaters. It looked a long dead dog and no one would admit to the crime. It did not even look like a boar. It turned out to be the best hunter in the pack and could find a pig if it was the only one in the country. It was also a dear friend of the family. Much haggling and a good many dirhams eventually converted this distraught and heart-broken man into an exceedingly happy and proud Arab. Perhaps it was good that the season was ended. The deceased could not have lasted much longer!

When the excitement was over, we had our bread and wine and noticed the beaters squatting in groups, not eating or drinking, but passing the Kif pipe round the circle.

In the afternoon we came to different territory, a vast reed-covered swamp, through which our beaters advanced, chanting and shouting strange noises. Snipe came forward, offering very high shots and sometimes as tricky as snipe can be. This was a more familiar kind of shooting, but a good ending to an unusual day's sport.

The early 1970s were also a time that saw the retirement of a number of the senior RNDS officers who had seen service through or during the Second

World War and who had then chosen to continue their careers in the RNDS. Surgeon Captain (D) B F S (Ben) Popham, who retired from the Service in 1973, was one of these.

Qualifying from the Turner Dental School in Manchester in 1940, at the same time and from the same dental school as John Hunter, he joined the RNVR shortly after Hunter, after a short time in civilian dental practice. Ben Popham joined the Service in *HMS Pembroke* at Chatham and shortly afterwards was appointed to *HMS Europa,* the headquarters of the Royal Naval Patrol Service at Lowestoft. Here, he was able to observe at close hand, the valiant work of a flotilla of North Sea trawlers, equipped as minesweepers, in their efforts to keep clear the coastal shipping lanes, following the nightly forays of German E-Boats and fast minelayers.

From *Europa*, Ben Popham was appointed to *HMS Argus*. *Argus* had been one of the first RN aircraft carriers. Converted from an Italian cruise liner, by laying a flush flight deck above the hull, she had seen service during WW1. At the time Popham joined her, she was in use as a training carrier, but following the loss of three front line carriers, early in the war, she was pressed into operational service. The end of World War II found Ben Popham in *HMS Saker,* the RN establishment on the East Coast of the United States, which accommodated Royal Navy personnel waiting to join the 'Lend-lease' and 'Liberty' ships being built or converted in the USA.

A series of shore appointments followed and in mid-1946 he joined the light fleet carrier *HMS Ocean,* serving on board her for the next three years. *Ocean* was at that time part of the Mediterranean Fleet and took part in operations in the Eastern Mediterranean during the Palestine Crisis. Ashore again at the end of 1949, he married his wife, Jane in early 1950 and another series of UK appointments followed, including two years in *HMS Seahawk,* the RN Air Station at Culdrose in Cornwall. In 1955 he joined *HMS Terror,* the Naval Base shore establishment in Singapore as the Senior Dental Surgeon, in the rank of Surgeon Commander (D). Two and a half years later, he returned to the UK. Promoted Surgeon Captain (D) in January 1966, the following year found him in *HMS Daedalus* the Naval Air Station at Lee-on-the-Solent as the Command Dental Surgeon to the Flag Officer Naval Air Command. In 1970 he moved across Portsmouth Harbour to the Naval Base as Command Dental Surgeon to the C-in-C Naval Home Command, from which appointment Ben Popham took his retirement.

In 1974 another provision of equipment brought the RNDS into line with modern practice. It was recognized that dental staff must be both prepared and properly trained to resuscitate patients who suffer serious medical emergency in the dental surgery. As well as providing the necessary training, all clinics were provided with a Vickers Portagen/ Modulaire resuscitation apparatus.

In August 1974 and after three eventful years during which he had firmly led the RNDS through a period of significant change, Surgeon Rear Admiral (D) John Hunter retired and was succeeded by Surgeon Rear Admiral (D) A E (Ted) Cadman. Hunter was awarded the CB on retirement.

Educated at Dover Grammar School, Ted Cadman qualified at Guy's Hospital Dental School in 1941. During his time at Guy's, which was close to London Bridge, he experienced the night raids on London docks during the Blitz. On many such nights, he acted as a 'firewatcher' including one when a stick of 250lb bombs hit the hospital, causing extensive damage.

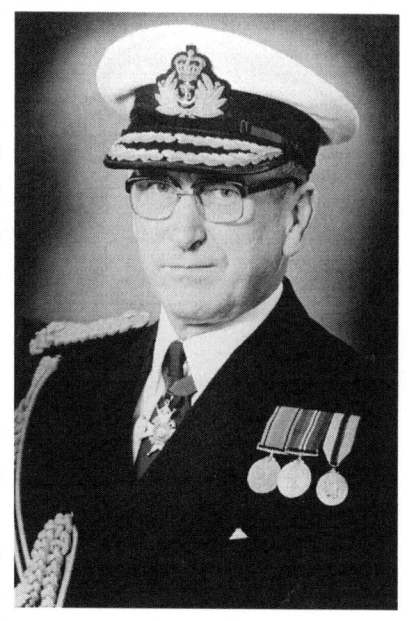

Surgeon Rear Admiral (D)
A E Cadman CB QHDS

In May 1942, he joined the RNVR as a Temporary Surgeon Lieutenant (D). During his New Entry courses at RN Barracks Portsmouth, he yet again experienced the German air raids – this time on Portsmouth Dockyard. Transferred to *HMS Collingwood* at Fareham, he was once again on the receiving end, when during one raid a bomb hit one of the mess huts, causing many casualties. It was probably with some relief when, later that year and after an arduous rail journey to Scotland, he found himself embarked on *SS Aquitania* bound for the United States.

Arriving in New York, he was assigned to the dental clinic in a newly established RN training facility at Asbury Park, a small city in New Jersey, a short distance south of New York City. Amongst his colleagues in the busy dental clinic, (they treated upward of 600 patients a month), he met Surgeon Lieutenant (D) K E J (Ken) Fletcher, son of the Branch Director, Surgeon Rear Admiral (D) E E Fletcher, the 'father' of the Branch.

Returning to the UK at the end of the European phase of the WWII, (hostilities against Japan were still ongoing), in 1946, he was appointed to the heavy cruiser *HMS Cumberland*, which was deployed to the Far East, to take part in the repatriation of British and Australian troops. In early 1947, Cadman was offered a transfer from the RNVR to the Royal Navy on an 'Extended Service Commission' for four years. This he accepted.

He was promoted Surgeon Lieutenant Commander (D) in August 1950, at the end of his four-year regular commission. This had coincided with a moratorium on releases from the Armed Forces, following the commencement of hostilities in the Korean War. Thus, in August 1952, he made the decision to transfer to the Permanent List of the Royal Navy. Then followed a series of appointments at *HMS Ceres* (the Supply and Secretariat School near Leeds), *HMS Heron* (the Naval Air Station at Yeovilton) and the RN Barracks at Chatham and Portsmouth.

In June 1956, Cadman was promoted Surgeon Commander (D) and in 1963, he joined the fleet carrier *HMS Victorious,* as the Senior Dental Surgeon (of two dental officers). The ship immediately deployed to the Far East to relieve the *Ark Royal,* which had become unserviceable. Returning to the UK in mid-1964, he was appointed again to the RN Barracks in Portsmouth and thence, in 1965 to the Royal Marines Depot at Deal, as Senior Dental Surgeon and in 1967, he was appointed to the Ministry of Defence as Assistant to the Director of Naval Dental Services – at that time Surgeon Rear Admiral (D) W L (Leonard) Mountain, and as Staff Dental Surgeon to the Admiral Commanding reserves.

In December 1967, whilst still in this appointment, he was promoted Surgeon Captain (D).

His next appointment was as Command Dental Surgeon to the Flag Officer Naval Air Command at *HMS Daedalus* in Lee-on-the-Solent and on 16 August 1974, he was promoted Surgeon Rear Admiral (D), succeeding Surgeon Rear Admiral (D) John Hunter as DNDS. In addition to his service as a general dental practitioner and senior staff officer in the RNDS, Ted Cadman had given much time and support to Navy sport, serving at various times as President of the RN Hockey Association and as Vice-President of the United Services Rugby Club.

As with many of his predecessors and, indeed, those who were to follow him, Cadman found himself living in difficult times. At the annual dinner of the Royal Navy Medical Club, held in the Painted Hall of the RN College, Greenwich on 12 September 1975, the Medical Director General, Surgeon Vice Admiral Sir James Watt stated that "for the Medical and Dental Services the past year has often brought anxiety, turbulence and frustration as the Defence Review following hard on the heels of the Defence Medical Services Inquiry, has overtaken the first fruits of much painstaking and constructive planning, to challenge each new initiative and every aspect of our medical and dental organisation."[29]

The senior managers of both Branches were having to learn to live with something which was to become a way of life for those in the Directorates; namely, that no sooner had they commenced planning to implement the last set of political directives, events would be overtaken by the next 'bright idea'!

In 1977, a new version of the Frigate Portable Dental Unit was built at *HMS Sultan* and was trialled in *HMS Arrow* in April and May of the same year. The Mark I FPDU had been modified many times since its debut in 1964 and the new model was designed to fit standard Service, air-transportable "Lacon" boxes. Experience with the Mark II was to lead to further updated versions in the 80s and 90s.

It was also in 1977 that the Branch found itself facing crisis. As had happened many times in the past, HM Government was looking for economies, many of which fell upon the Ministry of Defence. A decision was made at high level to downgrade the post of DNDS from Surgeon Rear Admiral (D) to Surgeon Commodore (D). This decision caused outrage amongst the career officers of the RNDS and their cause was taken up by the President of the General Dental Council, Sir Rodney Swiss.

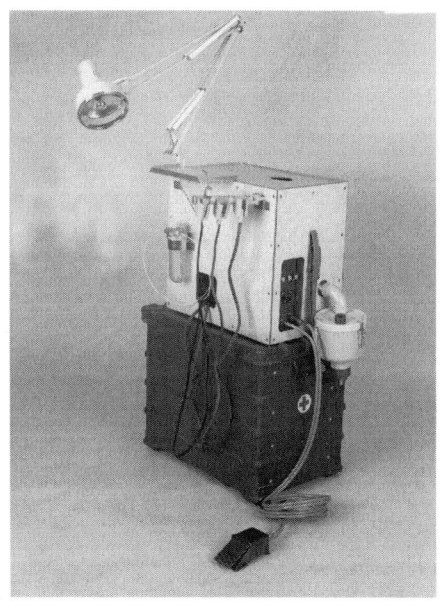

Mark II Frigate Portable Dental Unit with Lacon Box – Circa 1977

He wrote to the Under-Secretary of State for the Royal Navy, requesting "…earnestly (that) their Lordships … reconsider their verdict."[30] The letter went on: "This would appear to be a demotion in the rank of the Director, Royal Naval Dental Services, which can only adversely affect the morale of the whole dental profession."

The Minister, Patrick Duffy, replied on 4 May 1977:[31]

"I can assure you that this decision in no way reflects the esteem which the Dental Service has rightly enjoyed throughout the Royal Navy for so many years. … I would not, however, wish to hold out any prospect of a change in the decision, as I believe, albeit reluctantly, that the appointment of a Surgeon Commodore (D) as Director is necessary and will not unduly prejudice the existing effectiveness of the central direction of this Department".

Needless to say, these exchanges did little to improve the morale of the Branch and since this crisis coincided with the retirement of Surgeon Rear Admiral (D) Ted Cadman, the succession 'automatically' fell to the next most senior RNDS officer, Surgeon Captain (D) B F (Brian) Rogers who was thus set to succeed Ted Cadman in the rank of Surgeon Commodore (D). However, the matter had not yet been put to rest.

Further negotiations (in which, RNDS officers had no part) continued 'behind the scenes'. On 5 September 1977, the Minister, Patrick Duffy, wrote yet again to Sir Rodney Swiss:[32]

"You will be pleased to learn that the Secretary of State and I have reconsidered the matter and in the light of our continuing studies, have decided that it is premature to reduce the rank of the Director at this time. Surgeon Captain (D) B F Rogers will therefore succeed Admiral Cadman on 16 September in the rank of Acting Rear Admiral."

The significant phrase in this letter was, however, "… at this time …" And although parity with the Directors of the Army and Royal Air Force Dental Branches, was now restored, this problem would return before too long, to haunt all three dental services.

Surgeon Rear Admiral (D) Ted Cadman was awarded the CB upon his retirement.

Surgeon Rear Admiral (D) Brian Rogers had qualified in December 1945 and immediately joined the RNVR, serving for two and a half years with the Fleet Air Arm. He then left to go into general dental practice, but rejoined later, when he perceived that the conditions of service had improved. During two spells of sea service in *HM Ships Ocean* and *Eagle*, he spent 256 days at sea in one year! Service ashore had taken him to Scotland, Malta, Dartmouth and Deal.

In 1978 a new 'Clinical Rig' was introduced for Wren Dental Surgery Assistants and Dental Hygienists. This had followed some 'unofficial trials' some four years earlier in the RN Dental Training School, when the trainee hygienists were allowed to wear a standardised white tunic top and black trousers. So keen were the Wrens to wear this new rig, that they bought the necessary material and made their own garments – back to the real 'Make and Mend' days! The new rig, finally approved by the Director of the Women's Royal Naval Service was almost identical to the RNDTS 'trial' version. Category badges were worn on the white top, but not rank badges.[33]

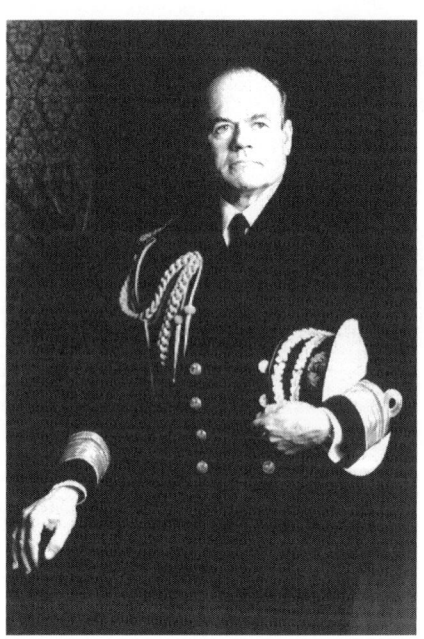

Surgeon Rear Admiral (D)
B F Rogers CB QHDS

The advent of 'four handed', seated dentistry having rendered the old, white, wrap-around overall inappropriate, in January 1979, a gentleman

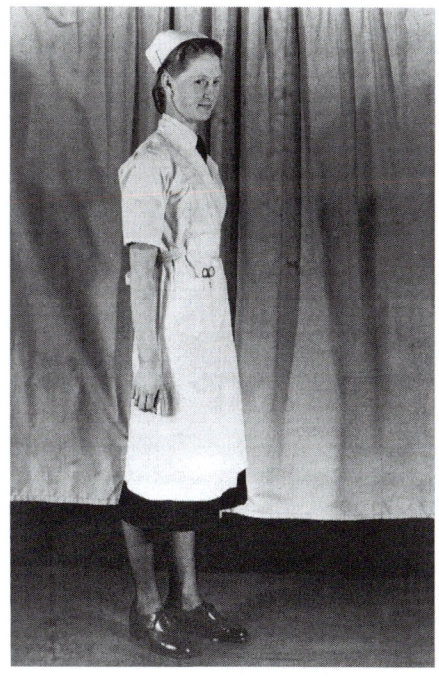
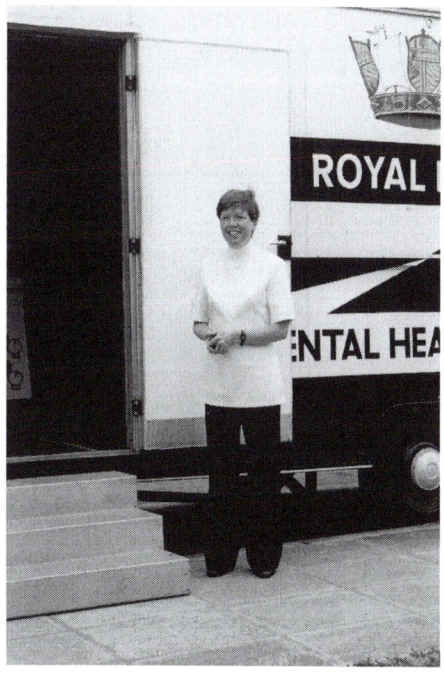

Wren DSA Rig 1950s • Wren DSA/DH Rig 1980s

named Bernard Campion, who dubbed himself 'The Bard of Plymouth' and who was a regular contributor to *Navy News*, wrote a poem, in that publication, regretting the passing of the old rig.

The poem expressed the now very 'non-PC' view that 'Jack' would no longer be able to enjoy the sight of the Wrens' legs, while in the dental chair, being "detoothed". A letter dated 12 January 1979, was sent to and published in *Navy News* from the RN Dental Training School. It is reproduced below:

Rigs & Rhymes

Dear Sir,
We are your neighbours
Next door to Barham Block
The Naval Dental Training School
Where all the sailors flock!

We must Sir, lodge a protest
At Bernard Campion's slur
Upon our image and our job
He does our wrath incur!

It must be hard for Plymouth's bard
To view the changing scene
With Wrens in tights and other sights
On which he isn't keen

And now Sir, Wrens in trousers!
What's going to happen next?
We hope Sir, that you'll give us space
To tell you why we're vexed!

We're DSAs, Hygienists too
Why does your poet fuss?
If there's "detoothing" to be done
It won't be done by us!

In days of yore
Now gone before
Toothache was all the rage
That other bard, his life was marred
"Sans teeth" in his old age

Now Jack's a charming fellow
And it makes us sad and blue
To see his bright and shiny smile
Discarded like a shoe

And now Sir, here's our message
This is the crucial bit
There is no need for gums that bleed
And dentures that don't fit

We'll teach Jack how
And this we vow,
To KEEP his teeth – No jest!
And he'll be back,
(We know our Jack)
'Cos we fill trousers best!

During the late 1970s there had been a general move within the Royal Navy to standardise the structure of training. In 1979, this trend caught up with the Medical and Dental Branches and, in line with all other branches, Provisional Professional Examinations were introduced.

These exams were to be taken in the rating's own establishment, but were marked and graded at the RN Dental Training School and had to be passed before the candidate was permitted to attend the Professional Qualifying Course and Exam at the school. Success in the latter examination led to eventual advancement to Leading or Petty Officer Wren[34].

The Commander-in-Chief Naval Home Command, at that time Admiral Sir Richard Clayton, bore responsibility for all naval training and the commanding officers of all RN training establishments were directly accountable to him, through his Chief Staff Officer (Training), for the efficiency and effectiveness of their schools.

In June 1979, again as part of the process of standardisation in naval training, the C-in-C directed that the RN Dental Training School would become a 'Direct Command School'. Before this change, RNDTS had been a department within *HMS Nelson*, the Navy's Portsmouth support establishment and barracks.

Now, the Officer-in-Charge, Surgeon Commander (D) E J (Ted) Grant, found himself to be elevated from 'Head of Department' to Commanding Officer, with defined but limited powers of executive command. These included the responsibility of dealing with Requestmen and Defaulters at his own 'Captain's Table'.

It was traditional, when signals of a congratulatory or observational nature were exchanged between senior officers or ships and establishments, to use 'coded' biblical references. A Concordance Bible was an essential possession for any Commanding Officer.

On 29 June 1979, the OIC RN Dental Training School received the following signal:

"From: CINCNAVHOME to RNDTS. Welcome on becoming the twenty-seventh Direct Command Establishment of Naval Home Command. Psalm 32. Verse 8".

The Bible revealed the reference to be: "I will instruct thee and teach thee in the way thou shalt go: I will guide thee with mine eye."

After some research in the Concordance Bible, the OIC sent back:

"Very many thanks. I am delighted at last to be made legitimate. Amos 4. Verse 6."

This reads: "And I have also given you cleanness of teeth in all your cities, and want of bread in all your places: yet have ye not returned unto me saith the Lord."

This verse was felt to be doubly appropriate, since the Chief of Staff had recently failed to keep an appointment in the Dental Hygiene Clinic!

One new duty imposed upon the recently elevated CO, was attendance at C-in-C's three-monthly Commanding Officers' meetings. These were interesting affairs, where Grant was able to get a good feel for the administration and accompanying problems within the RN training world.

The meetings were held in different training establishments around the Command. On these occasions, the majority of participants would arrive in smart, black staff cars with ship's badges, pennants and flags much in evidence. Although the Officer-in-Charge RNDTS could on occasion, call upon a 'pool' car, at one such meeting held in *HMS Vernon*, he chose to arrive on his bicycle, so that he could continue his usual journey home at the end of the afternoon. On stating the purpose of his visit, he was met with some incredulity by the *Vernon* gate staff, who were lined up to salute the arriving VIPs! After consultation with the C-in-C's Bridge Card, he was allowed to proceed.

Despite the acclaim with which the RN Dental Training School became part of the 'Big Navy', its History was to be short-lived.

*****

Chapter 3

Threats and Opportunities
1980 – 1982

No decade during the existence of the Royal Naval Dental Services could have been described as 'uninteresting', but the 80s were to prove at least as challenging, for dental officers and ratings, as the years of conflict during the two World Wars.

Not all of these challenges were encountered 'in the face of the enemy'. Many were administrative, brought about both by politicians seeking political survival or a Navy seeking to squeeze itself into the fiscal strait jacket thrust upon it by its political masters. Some of the latter were to threaten the very existence of the Branch. Dentistry and the cost of running the RNDS, did not always take on great importance, in the eyes of the Sea Lords and Chiefs of Staff, when weighed against the need for more manpower, more modern weapon systems and the ships and aircraft to carry them.

In the last chapter, we left the RN Dental Training School trying its wings in its new environment as a Direct Command School in the Naval Home Command Training organisation. Very early in the new decade the School was to learn that it now had to 'fly' by itself.

As part of the Naval Training organisation, the RNDTS found itself very much under the microscope and the Officer-in-Charge and staff got very used to three-monthly visits from either the Chief of Staff or the C-in-C himself, both of whom clearly enjoyed their visits to this 'mini-establishment'. However, some initial panic ensued, when the Officer-in-Charge received a signal in early 1980, announcing that the School would undergo C-in-C's biennial inspection in the middle of that year. Such inspections had previously been carried out as a department of *HMS Nelson*, but now the school was on its own and the OIC was, as part of the inspection process, required to give a 'Pre-Inspection Presentation' in the Naval Headquarters, to the Chief of Staff and assembled staff officers. For this daunting task, much preparation was required. A script and appropriate visual aids were prepared and these were rehearsed and amended with valuable support from staff in the neighbouring RN School of Education and Training Technology.

The day of the Presentation arrived very quickly and the OIC attended at the Headquarters, supported by his Deputies, Surgeon Lieutenant Commanders (D) A J (Alan) Woodman and M J (Martin) Lovell, who were in the process of a handover of the appointment. Also present was the Senior Instructor, Chief Wren DSA Lynne Allitt, who acted as projectionist. Despite awful rumours of other COs being 'eaten for breakfast' at Pre-Inspection Presentations, the presentation seemed to be well received by the staff and was followed by nearly 40 minutes of questions, fielded, as appropriate, by the different members of the team.

A few days later, came the 'on site' inspection by the Admiral himself and despite the considerable age of the premises, this too seemed to go smoothly. The OIC, Surgeon Commander (D) Ted Grant, would have been very content if the result of the inspection had been a "Satisfactory", so it was with huge delight on the part of both training staff and students that on 29 July 1980, the OIC received a signal from the C-in-C, Admiral Sir Richard Clayton

The signal read: *"I much enjoyed my inspection this morning and congratulate you on the effort that had clearly gone into preparation for it. Within the limits of your works position the school looked immaculate and, as always, I was impressed by the enthusiasm and dedication of students and staff. Overall a very good inspection. Well done."*

A good start for both the School and the Branch in a new decade.

In March 1980, Surgeon Rear Admiral (D) Brian Rogers was succeeded as Director Naval Dental Services by Surgeon Rear Admiral (D) P R J (Philip) Duly OBE. Admiral Rogers was awarded the CB upon his retirement.

A Londoner by birth, Philip Duly had trained at the London Hospital, qualifying in 1947. Joining the Royal Navy in 1948, he transferred to the Permanent List in 1956. His early appointments were with the Fleet Air Arm at Lee-on-the-Solent and in Malta, whilst later serving in the carrier *HMS Hermes* and at the Gosport submarine base, *HMS Dolphin*, as Staff Dental Officer to the Flag Officer Submarines.

As recounted in Chapter I of this volume, in 1965, Philip Duly was appointed as the first Officer-in-Charge of the RN Dental Training School, where he set up the first training courses for Wren Dental Hygienists. This was undoubtedly a turning point in his career and, by his

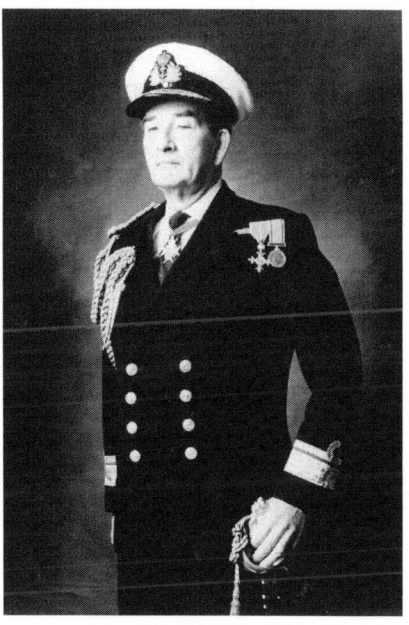

Surgeon Rear Admiral (D)
P R J Duly CB QHDS

own reckoning, certainly one of his highest achievements. After five years in the post, his success in setting up the courses and in seeing several courses of students all pass the National Examinations for Proficiency in Dental Hygiene, were recognised by the award of the OBE. Also in recognition of these successes, in 1969, the General Dental Council appointed him as a member of the Central Examining Board for Dental Hygienists, a body of which he was to become Vice Chairman of External Examiners in 1976 and Chairman in 1977.

After leaving the Dental Training School in 1970, Philip Duly was appointed as Assistant to the Director, in which job he was promoted to Surgeon Captain (D).

A number of senior staff and administrative appointments were to follow, including Director of Dental Training and Research and Command Dental Surgeon to the Flag Officers Naval Air Command and Naval Home Command. Thus he took the helm of the RNDS with a wealth of staff experience under his belt; well qualified to steer the Branch through ever increasingly, stormy waters.

On taking up his appointment, Admiral Duly wrote in the newly launched RNDS Newsletter (see below):

"All dental officers and uniformed dental staff are fully part of the Navy, with the dental technicians being very closely allied to the Service. I am totally convinced that being a full part of the RN is correct in every respect and hope that this policy is now firmly accepted in all quarters."

Since their inception, the uniformed medical and dental branches of the Royal Navy had been seen by their colleagues in other branches of the Navy as being apart, and sometimes aloof, from the rest of the Service. Sadly, this dichotomy of purpose was sometimes encouraged by a minority of medical and dental officers. It was Philip Duly's view that rational integration within the larger Service was essential to the long-term survival of the Branch.

Although there had dwelt a lengthy pause between the launch of the Harvey-Fletcher Prize in 1973 and its first award in March 1980, the news of the award of the Medal and Prize to Surgeon Lieutenant Commander (D) G W (Geoff) Myers, was warmly received by the Branch. * The award was made in recognition of Geoff Myers' achievements in enhancing the reputation of the RNDS, particularly through his service in Hong Kong and Naples[35].

In the Spring of 1980, Surgeon Captain (D) B (Brian) Robinson, at that time Director of Dental Training and Research at the Institute of

---

* A list of recipients of the Harvey-Fletcher Medal and Prize is shown at Appendix 2.

Naval Medicine in Alverstoke, introduced the Royal Naval Dental Services Newsletter. The idea of such a publication had been suggested to him in 1979 by Surgeon Captain (D) D A (David) Coppock, the then Deputy Director of Naval Dental Services. This 'demi-official' publication was widely welcomed by all members of the Branch. Intended as a vehicle of communication for all ranks, it carried news and views, policy statements, clinical update articles, accounts of adventurous training and of visits in Her Majesty's Ships to many exotic parts of the world, news from the clinics and the training world and appointments and drafts. It also carried from time to time, personal accounts by RNDS personnel who took part in a number of military operations. It was to appear approximately three times a year until the late 1990s, when its 'hard-copy' format was overtaken by the Electronic Age. Its first Editor, Brian Robinson, set a high standard from the start and this eminently readable publication was to continue under several different editors, whose job it was to 'bully' Branch members into producing suitable copy and then to render all contributions suitable for publication – a demanding, but always enjoyable task for those concerned. In its heyday, the Newsletter achieved a number of issues of over 100 pages! From the point of view of this author, the Newsletter has also provided an invaluable archive.

The RNDS had, for some years, under the talented guidance of Surgeon Captain (D) D A (David) Coppock, been involved in the making of a series of Dental First Aid and Oral Health Education films. At the time of his Harvey-Fletcher Award, Geoff Myers was the project officer for the making of the RNDS' first recruiting film: "Toothie RN", which had just been released. This brought to the screen the aspirations and opportunities encountered in the lives of RN dental officers. The film, in video cassette form, was distributed to dental schools and libraries and was shown whenever circumstances permitted, by RNDS personnel.

It was premiered in February 1980 in front of the Second Sea Lord, the Medical Director General (Naval) and the Director Naval Dental Services[36]. In an early issue of the Newsletter, Geoff Myers wrote an amusing account of the making of the film, giving an insight into a world apart from routine naval dentistry[37]. An abridged version of his article is reproduced below.

The Making of Toothie RN

I should perhaps have realised more, when I was told that I had been selected for the job – the normal terminology for "We haven't got anyone else". Anyway, my first introduction to the work was a hurried read of the script and the shooting programme, followed by a frenzied dash down to the Sandbanks Hotel in Poole for a brief with the (film's) director and production manager. Slowly it started to ⟫

dawn that the next few weeks were going to be pressurised and that film crews have an enormous penchant for whisky.

Umpteen phone calls and letters later saw a gathering of the crew and equipment in the Wardroom, *HMS Nelson,* one Sunday evening. Problems over 'dress in the mess' reared their ugly heads instantly, but fast talking seemed to work. Much discussion over future days' filming took place in the bar, following which, I found myself the next day with illegible notes and a need to swallow large doses of Vitamin C in order to prolong the useful life of my liver.

The logistics of moving six people plus hundredweights of equipment into Her Majesty's Ships, standing off in Portsmouth Harbour, are not easy, but eventually all was achieved and we were ready to start shooting.

This was when I learned that even a very brief and simple shot can take hours to achieve and that my role involved asking captains of ships in fleet formation, taking part in an exercise, if they could "steam the other way, as the sun is in the wrong place". (In retrospect I think I would have had more joy in speaking to the padre about moving the sun!). Even when things are going well, snags can crop up, such as; having got a Sea King helicopter to hover beautifully over the stern of *HMS Blake*, with sundry ships delightfully in the background, it can be frustrating to be confronted by a breathless lieutenant, informing you that the filming has to stop, as the downdraft from the helicopter is drenching the official guest's at the Captain's cocktail party on the quarterdeck!

There can be, however, immense satisfaction in watching others perform tasks for the film whilst you can stand back. Such as having a dentist going up and down a Sea King winch like a yo-yo, or nearly drowning two dentists, one with sub-aqua gear in the swimming pool and the other in combat kit on Woodbury Common.

One of the recurrent problems in making '*Toothie*' was having to explain just why establishments' routines should be disturbed by men leaping about the place making a film on dentists. It's not easy to be discrete when filming, like trying to hide four people plus camera behind a figure-head during Dartmouth Lord Mayor's Divisions, or explaining to young children why they have to keep singing 'Happy Birthday' many times without having a nibble of the cake, and No! It's not Blue Peter!

It is difficult to describe the exact feeling of seeing the first products of one's labour in the screening of the rushes. Still at least you know that there will finally be an end product. But then, back to the coal face and dealing with such problems as losing equipment on Woodbury Common, providing sandwiches, beer, whisky, glasses in the middle of nowhere – bad enough in itself, but trying to get ice there as well, is not easy! "He does moan a lot", you are probably thinking, "But what about the Gibraltar shots? Can't be bad – a few days over there!" Um – touchy subject! You see it was decided that it was preferable for the filming of those particular sequences, that the tricky dealings out there would be ⇒

> best dealt with by someone more senior than a Lieutenant Commander. (Passes on quickly before more points are lost!)
>
> So – can we have a Sea Harrier on Monday and a nuclear submarine on Tuesday, and could you please arrange for a Wasp helicopter to take a cameraman plus Production Manager to film a Type 21 Frigate off Portland, and then fly around Dartmouth, where we can get some Wooly-Pullies and khaki shirts, and aren't those white bath towels excellent value, and do they only have Teacher's here, no Bells or Grouse? – Yes they're back!
>
> Downhill leg now. Smoke flares setting light to the superstructure of *HMS Intrepid*, getting Tony Shepherd to virtually do the Green Beret Course all over again and still trying to find a ruddy nuclear submarine.
>
> And then it's all over; with memories of the prima donna actor of the Branch: "Can't do those shots", "Don't you think I should show my other profile?", "Just how long will I be seen in the actual film?" Thank you Steve T…..! But then, there you are again in the studios, advising on which bits to use and seeing the whole thing take shape, with commentaries to be recorded, titles to be made, the sound track tidied up, until finally the Preview, acceptance and it really is all finished.
>
> By the time you read this, you will have seen this epic of the Silver Screen. I have seen it many times and still find it pleasurable – but then I can see all the behind the scenes activities as well and, despite my moans, I would do it all again. The film crew are an amusing bunch, the technicalities of film-making are interesting, the insight into the workings of the Navy, are beneficial and I did enjoy the work – but next time, please can't I go to Gib?

Almost since the birth of the RNDS there had been debate as to what should be the defined role of dental officers in combat, emergency and disaster situations. It was generally accepted that their primary role in war was to provide dental care as close as possible to the 'front line', in order to maintain the fighting effectiveness of all service personnel. Clearly, in a 'hot' combat or disaster situation, the provision of primary dental care was not an option and, in such circumstances, dental officers in all three Services had been variously employed as triage officers, anaesthetists, and as surgeons and even, on one occasion, in a public health role.

For some years, in addition to dental officers in Specialist (Oral Surgery) grades, some dental officers had received training in resuscitation techniques, in order to be able to give support to medical officers in war or emergency. It was now felt that the time had come to identify a formal war role for RN dental officers and that appropriate training should be given to all.

In May 1979, Surgeon Captain (D) Brian Robinson attended the US Navy's Combat Casualty Care Course. Combat Casualty Care training had existed in the USN Dental Corps since the early sixties and had evolved over a number of years, but in 1979 the course had been completely redesigned and was now a very comprehensive programme. He was joined on the course by Surgeon Commander (D) R S (Dick) Hambly, the officer then serving in the RNDS/USNDC Exchange appointment[38].

The arrival of Robinson and Hambly on the course, run by the Regional Dental Center in Norfolk Virginia saw, for the first time, an exercise using the USN's ship damage control facility for a mass casualty exercise. The simulator (known 'affectionately' as *USS Buttercup)*, and similar to the one now used by the Royal Navy, was capable of being flooded and tilted – difficult conditions in which to practise the skills required to triage, resuscitate and maintain casualties and to evacuate them to second line medical care.

The five-day course, which included both classroom and exercise elements, covered such subjects as Cardiopulmonary Resuscitation (CPR), physical examination and life-support procedures (using a very technologically advanced manikin), triage, rescue and movement of casualties, the management of obstructed airways, intubation, intravenous infusion and bandaging and splints.

With this experience under his belt, Brian Robinson returned to the UK and wrote a report on the USN 'C4' course, which eventually reached the desk of the Medical Director General (Naval), Surgeon Vice Admiral John Harrison.

In 1980, having recently taken up the appointment of Director of Dental Training and Research at the Institute of Naval Medicine, Robinson was directed by MDG(N) to design and introduce an RN version of the C4 course. To assist him in this demanding project, Robinson requested that Surgeon Commander (D) T J C (Timothy) Hall be seconded to his team. The course, both in the design phase and once up and running, received invaluable assistance from a number of medical consultants and from the Aircrew Survival School at Seafield Park near Lee-on-the-Solent.

The new course would last for two weeks and would be run during the winter months, (February and October), twice a year. It was based at the Institute of Naval Medicine, where Brian Robinson, in addition to being DDTR had now been appointed as Head of the Training Division, giving him easy access to the excellent complex of classrooms and lecture theatres as well as to INM's own team of training officers and senior rate instructors.

The course syllabus covered not only most of that included in the USN course, but also such subjects as the Geneva Conventions and the management of casualties under nuclear, biological and chemical attack. The latter included a night exercise at Browndown Army Camp, near Alverstoke, when the students were introduced to the difficulties of carrying and treating 'gas contaminated' casualties, whilst wearing full NBCD suits and respirators in conditions of low visibility!

Other exercises included the evacuation of casualties from the engine room of the harbour training ship *HMS Devonshire* and the DRIU (Damage Repair Instructional Unit), a 'disaster' exercise at Fort Grange, Gosport and, the centre piece of the course, the New Forest Weekend!

The latter, viewed with some trepidation by each new course of students, was designed to demonstrate to them how their medical skills could be degraded, when they, the students, were debilitated by lack of sleep, lack of food and strenuous effort. Many of the exercises undertaken during the 'Weekend' were devised and supervised by staff of the RN Air Survival School from Seafield Park, near Lee-on-the Solent.

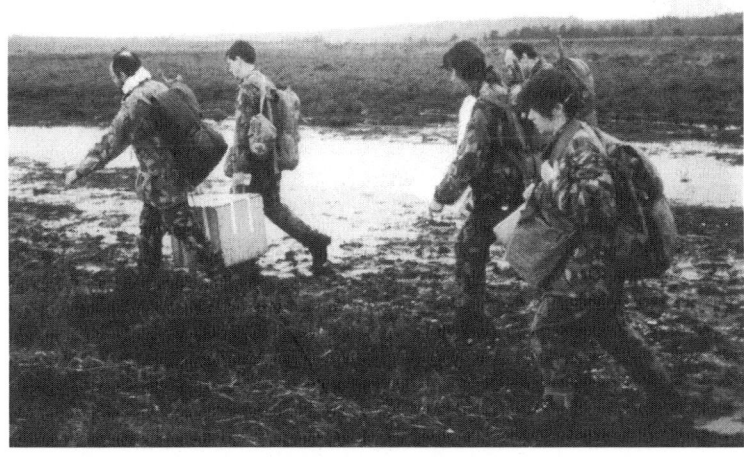

Combat Casualty Care Course – Dental Officers on New Forest Exercise in arduous conditions (Photo. E J Grant)

A typical New Forest Weekend is described below:

A Weekend in the Forest!

Immediately after the completion of the Browndown casualty handling module on a Friday evening, the students were piled into a bus at around 2200, and driven to a lake at a 'secret location' on the edge of the New Forest. Here they were searched for 'contraband' food, their cash and other personal effects having been 'taken into care' earlier, and they were then required to don ➤

> 'Once Only' sea-survival suits, which had often been used more than 'once only' and which were, consequently, prone to leaks! Once suited up, the students had to swim to moored, eight-man survival rafts and, often with twelve to fifteen to a raft, to spend an uncomfortable and cold night, trying to catnap, albeit with one man awake and on watch at any given time.
>
> The following morning, Saturday, the cold and somewhat damp students were disembarked from their rafts and set off, without breakfast, on a trek of about 10 kilometres, during which they would encounter and have to deal with, a number of simulated 'medical' incidents. At least one of these would result in each team, of about eight men and women, having to stretcher, either a team member or a suitably weighted dummy, for a considerable distance. As they were to discover, this was an exercise in both strength and endurance. The goal, for that night, was an old road bridge at Long Slade Bottom, in the heart of the Forest. Underneath the bridge, it was dry and much used as a shelter by New Forest ponies in inclement weather. Despite copious amounts of pony dung, with the addition of dry bracken, this was to be 'home' for that night. In the eyes of most students this was a huge improvement on their previous night's accommodation! Before the exhausted dental officers were allowed to turn in, the Seafield Park staff demonstrated how to build a shelter and how to catch, kill and cook a rabbit. Since it was very unlikely, in the time available, that the course members would successfully snare a rabbit, live rabbits were provided for this exercise. The resulting stew, to students who had spent the previous 36 hours with no food and from whom had been demanded considerable physical exertion, would remain in their memories as one of the best meals ever!
>
> Turning in at last, but leaving again, one man on watch, the students were roused in the middle of the night to deal with a 'crashed helicopter' incident. Once this exercise was completed, they were then left in peace until dawn, when they were again roused and given ten minutes vigorous PT, to get cold limbs moving once again. During a final, but shorter leg of their trek, the teams would again encounter various incidents and initiative tests before arriving, at about Sunday midday, at a most welcome pub, where they were reunited with their money and personal effects and would quickly embark upon eating virtually everything the pub had to offer, as well as downing a much anticipated pint or two of beer!

The Combat Casualty Care Course was to exist in this form, under a succession of Directors of Dental Training and Research, with some modifications until 1991, when the post of DDTR was abolished.

At the outbreak of the Falklands Conflict in April 1982, 14 RN dental officers were deployed operationally with both Naval and Royal Marines' units. Seven of these were graduates of the C4 course, which undoubtedly stood them in good stead. Four others had attended Resuscitation Courses in RN Hospitals[39].

After the conflict, the Branch's achievement in this area did not go unnoticed by the Medical Director General (Naval), who directed that all New Entry Medical Officers, would, henceforth, do the course. The course had already been expanded to include RNDS reservists and some dental officers from the Royal Netherlands Navy. Subsequently it was expanded further to include RN Medical Services and QARNNS (Nursing) Officers.

At the time of the abolition of the DDTR post, the RNDS lost control of the course. The New Forest Weekend was rapidly dropped and all practical exercises confined to Browndown ranges. A retrograde step in the eyes of not only the ex-directing staff, but also many C4 'graduates'.

The Spring of 1980 brought with it the announcement of the death of Surgeon Rear Admiral (D) Leonard Mountain CB OBE. After a distinguished career, he had been Branch Director from 1964 to 1968 and died on 19 February 1980.

On a happier note, it also brought the commissioning of the first of the 'through deck cruisers' * – *HMS Invincible*. The first dental officer to serve in *Invincible* was Surgeon Commander (D) Keith Pendrill. He has written an amusing account of the first few months of the commission in the RNDS Newsletter[40].

On 20 March 1981, the second ever Wood Lecture and Clinical Day was held at *HMS Nelson*. The Wood Lecture was inaugurated in 1973 to celebrate the memory of Surgeon Captain (D) James Thomson Wood, the second Director of the RNDS, and his dedication both to high clinical standards in the RNDS and to a viable and attractive career structure for RN dental officers. His inestimable contribution to the development of the Branch is well chronicled in the first volume of this History.

There had been a seven-year gap since the first event, but the Wood Lecture Day would now become a triennial event and would be held once during the tenure of each Director. The 1981 Wood Lecture was delivered by Mr Norman Rowe CBE, Civilian Consultant in Oral Surgery to the Royal Navy. The lecture day was enhanced by a dental trade exhibition and table demonstrations by dental officers, technicians and hygienists. The main event was preceded by lectures from dental officers who had obtained MSc degrees in various dental disciplines and was followed by the Director's Dinner, held in the Wardroom at *HMS Nelson*[41].

---

* The Invincible class aircraft carriers were designated "through deck cruisers" at an early stage of design, because the then HM Government had decreed that the future RN had no further need for fixed wing carriers!

With the continued shrinking of the Fleet and an ever smaller number of overseas commitments, opportunities to send dental officers to sea were becoming few and far between. Thus it became policy to deploy dental officers with Frigate Portable dental equipment, whenever an opportunity presented. Additionally a number of exchange appointments were arranged with the Federal German Navy, the Royal Air Force in Germany, the Royal Air Force in Cyprus and the Army in Aldershot as well as the continuing exchange with the US Navy. There were also two RNDS officers seconded to the British Army-led dental service which provided treatment to the Armed Forces of the Sultan of Brunei. The Branch could still provide travel and adventure to all ranks and it was calculated that during one month in 1983, no less than 42 foreign ports were visited by RN Dental Officers.

It was in September 1980 that Surgeon Lieutenant (D) R J (Richard) Leworthy, borne in the frigate *HMS Naiad* in the Far East, managed to transfer his equipment to another ship in company, *HMS Alacrity*, becoming the first RN dental officer to visit China since 1949. At that time, China was still very much a 'closed' country and was seldom visited by Europeans, apart from the occasional politician or diplomat. Richard Leworthy has written an amusing account of his visit in the RNDS Newsletter[42], an abridged version of which appears below.

Shanghaied!

HMS Alacrity led *Antrim* and *Coventry* as we headed up the Yangtze estuary and then turned left into the Whangpo River on which Shanghai stands. At the berths there was an impressive welcome with flags, banners, sailors, bands and dignitaries waiting for us.

The Chinese had arranged a full programme of events, which started with a welcoming banquet on the first evening. On the next day there was a tour of their East China Fleet, a lunchtime banquet and a show afterwards. The following day saw a tour by train to Hangzhou, their main seaside resort. About 400 men were required for each of these visits and the organisation was impeccable. The transport of about 50 cars and coaches always left on time and every detail went like clockwork.

My only trip was to the East China Fleet. We were raced across the city with all traffic stopped for us and crowds lining the streets. On our arrival we walked through an avenue of clapping sailors and flower waving sailor girls. We clapped back, since this was the polite thing to do. Their ships [although old in design] were immaculately clean and the paintwork sparkled. The banquet of twelve courses included stewed sea slugs on fried rice crusts (the other eleven were delicious!). In between dishes, we were required to drink toasts to various ➤

> people, friendship and whatever we could think of next. We were toasting with an evil brew called Moutai and we were expected to drink the whole glass and then hold it upside down! In the afternoon (yes, I do remember the afternoon!), we had a show of singing and dancing by sailors of the Fleet.
>
> The [British] ships were open to visitors for three days. On the first day the Chinese flooded the ship with their experts, who sketched everything they could and paced out all dimensions possible. They can now probably produce a copy of the Types 21 and 42.
>
> The city, when I went around it, seemed drab and dirty. There were no neon lights, few private cars and much atmospheric pollution. There were hundreds of bicycles. The people, although dressed in dull-coloured clothing were extremely friendly and impeccably honest. Quite often we were stopped in the street by people who wanted to practice their English and express their friendliness.
>
> The Chinese went out of their way to make the visit a success. They even had a special franking made for all postcards and letters posted while the ships were there. After four days of a very hectic programme, I was glad to get back to sea for a rest! It was a remarkable experience and one I shall never forget.

It is interesting to compare Leworthy's descriptions of the drabness of Shanghai with the spectacular city which exists today.

In January 1981, the Prime Minister, Margaret Thatcher, appointed Mr John Nott Secretary of State for Defence, with the remit to cut the spiralling cost of the Armed Forces. Nott, a banker and accountant, understood this brief much better than the actual business of running operationally efficient forces and on 25 June of that year, he published the Defence White Paper "The Way Forward". From the Navy's point of view, never was a Government Paper less aptly named. It quickly became apparent that the Secretary of State's vision was that Britain no longer required a Navy with global capability and that her defence interests would best be served by the Royal Air Force, with the Royal Navy being reduced to a coastal defence force and the Submarine Flotilla, providing the nuclear deterrent. The three Invincible Class aircraft carriers, one of which, *HMS Ark Royal*, had yet to be commissioned, were offered to be sold, with Australia showing considerable interest and the amphibious warfare support ships *HMS Intrepid* and *HMS Fearless* were also to be sold or scrapped. Many frigates and destroyers were also to be disposed of and manpower would be cut accordingly.

In the RNDS, this would mean a reduction in the number of dental officers from 102 in 1981 to around 80 in the following year. Redundancies would be available if necessary, although it was hoped that the numbers would be achieved mainly through a moratorium on recruiting.

Little was it realised that reprieve from these draconian cuts would come in the form of a particularly unpleasant South American dictator – but with a cost to pay. The events which were to cause a rapid and significant U-turn in the Government's policies for the Armed Forces were still over a year ahead. In the meantime, life in the RNDS went on and despite the implications of the White Paper, dental officers still found time to do intrepid things, whilst continuing also to develop their clinical and other professional skills.

Over Easter Leave 1981, Surgeon Commander (D) M D (Malcolm) Hocking, an enthusiastic and experienced skier, embarked upon a challenging ski-trek across the Alps via the 'Haute Route'. A graphic account of his adventure appeared in the Summer 1981 issue of the Newsletter.[43]

Also in 1981, Surgeon Lieutenant (D) Catherine White, a new entry dental officer and an experienced climber, was selected to lead a climbing expedition in the Russian Caucasus Mountains. With the Cold War still rumbling on, this was something of a first for a British Naval Officer. Her account of this, also in the Newsletter, tells the story of an expedition which turned out to be no picnic! An abridged version of her article appears below[44]. The expedition was planned to celebrate the 25th anniversary of the Duke of Edinburgh's Award Scheme and the idea of a climb in the Caucasus came from Lord Hunt of Everest fame.

Caucasian Climb

In January of this year, I received a letter asking me if I would like to be the leader of [the Caucasus] expedition. I was delighted and felt most honoured at being asked, but thought that, now I was a member of the Services, the letter was destined for the round file on the floor.

After finishing at Dartmouth and taking up my first appointment at *HMS Raleigh*, I mentioned the matter to Surgeon Captain Lindsay. He was most keen that I should go and initiated the wheels of security clearance. Very soon, I was clear to go.

[Flying from Gatwick with a mountain of equipment, White and her party arrived in Kiev and then transferred to a train for the 16-hour journey to Simferopol in the Crimea.]

From Simferopol we caught an internal flight to Mineralnie Vody (mineral waters in English), which is the nearest town to the mountains. There followed an eight-hour coach ride up into the mountains. The scenery was exceptional, which is more than could be said about the state of the roads and the ability of the driver.

Eventually we arrived at a rather luxurious mountain hut in the heart of the Caucasus. ⟫

The Caucasus is a range of high mountains situated between the Black Sea and the Caspian Sea. We were in the central area, where most peaks are over 16,000 feet. The weather [there] is best described as variable. Poor weather is a constant hazard, with heavy rain and snow possible at any time of the year.

After settling into the hut, I had to meet the Director of the USSR Sports Council, the Director of Mountain Training and the Chief of Mountain Rescue for the area. After this, I was introduced to the three Soviet climbers who were going to climb with us. Speaking mainly French or German and using our interpreter, we had a long and fruitful discussion.

My first shock came when I went to investigate the rations we were to take with us into the mountains. The food for a group of three for four days was as follows: 2 x 30 cm salamis, 2 x blocks of salt meat, 1 x packet of tea, sugar, and semolina. In the words of one of the group: "Not a lot!" The second shock was the Soviet tents. These were made of a simple layer of silverised cotton, with no pegs, only ropes for putting around rocks. Fortunately we had taken a couple of British tents with us.

At 1700, with all our gear packed, we were taken a few miles down a track. The walk up a beautiful tree-lined valley continued until dusk, when we set up camp and prepared a meal – well, peeled the salami! During 'supper', one of the group came to me complaining of lower abdominal pain. Something clicked in my mind and I realised these were classic symptoms of appendicitis. I examined him and, to my mind there was no doubt. I … explained the situation to the Soviets, who were at the time, talking to a party going down to the valley. These people said that they would ask Boris [the Russian doctor] to come up the next day. [At 0330], early breakfast consisted of yet more salami and a cup of tea. Chris, our suspected appendicitis case was no better, but started walking at about 0600. Boris caught us up and confirmed my diagnosis. He took Chris back down to the valley.

The early start paid off, as we had done most of the snow work before the sun became a nuisance. Cheget, at 16,500 feet was the relatively easy peak ascended that day. During that day, I really got to know Slava, Igor and Victor, the Soviet climbers. When climbers meet and start discussing gear, routes climbed, etc., all else fades into insignificance.

I ended up doing a fast descent into the valley with Slava and Victor to recce a campsite. The mineral spring, found by Slava, tasted just like Champagne – it was [even] aerated! Three hours later, we [were] back up the mountain again, helping to bring down other members of the group with the following injuries: John: broken bone in left foot, Howard: cartilage problems in right knee and a case of heat exhaustion. Slava and I spent the evening and most of the next day arranging a helicopter to casevac these people back to base. [Having dispatched the casualties], Slava, who came from the nearest village, arranged a 'run ashore' for the remaining members. »+

The local hooch was very potent and the hot food, provided by the kindly villagers "went down a treat".

The following day, we set off up another valley in a cabbage truck. The driver stopped many times along the route to sell his wares. We became very hot and drank our way through a crate of warm beer to stave off dehydration. Again we were dropped and walked up the valley until nightfall. On the way up I lanced and dressed an abscess on a foot, did some temporary fillings on some local people in a small settlement and extracted some periodontally involved teeth for an old man. They had heard we were coming!

An early start the next day and a mind blowing ascent up some fantastic rock to Kavkaz peak, 17,900 feet. Severe headaches and dyspnoea were suffered by two members of the group. However, as this was the day of the Royal Wedding, we flew our Union Flag and drank our Champagne – I was glad not to have to carry a full bottle anymore!

The descent, again caused problems, as Mick, when glissading on a snow slope, did not brake at the bottom and hit a boulder field with force … He was unconscious after the fall [and], from the way he fell, I thought that he must either be dead or … very seriously injured.

However, when I actually got over to him and started to examine him, during which he regained consciousness, he did not seem to have any serious injuries, apart from a possible dislocation of his right shoulder. …. As he was generally very sore, I gave him an ampoule of morphine and Victor and I helped him slowly down. We had to get him off quickly as we were still at 12,000 feet and the sun was really beginning to melt the snow. Avalanches were thundering down everywhere. It took five hours to reach the nearest point for evacuation – a cable car station – a very long and tense time.

[From the bottom, Mick and the other casualties were evacuated by truck, an uncomfortable, three-hour drive, to a local hospital]. The hospital was small, old fashioned, but functional. They dressed wounds and took radiographs. The surgeons seemed to be highly esteemed, as I learned that one had to stand every time a surgeon entered the room. They also wore 'Chef' type hats made of lace! I [was told that Mick had] only strained his shoulder and that the other injuries were no more serious than the original diagnoses. Chris' appendicitis had settled with antibiotic treatment. [Back at the hut, in a happier frame of mind] as it was our last night, a dinner had been arranged for us – Champagne and caviar – a good time was had by all.

The following morning, [we were] presented with various climbing medals and I was greatly honoured in being made an honorary member of their rock climbing association.

[After some problems with tickets, they flew back from Moscow to Gatwick] Looking back, it was an amazing trip and one I will never forget!

Despite the gloom engendered by the Nott defence cuts, the Branch leaders did not lose sight of the *raison d'être* of dental staff being trained and deployed in support of the Fleet. The continual push to attain higher professional standards continued and, in September 1981, the Conservative Dentistry Refresher Course was introduced. This course, held at the RN Dental Training School, was designed to pass on to other RN general dental practitioners, the information and expertise gained by those dental officers who had gained their MSc degrees.

Also, for the first time, Dental Branch wrens, both Dental Hygienists and Dental Surgery Assistants, studied for and sat the examination for the Diploma in Dental Health Education awarded by the Royal Society of Arts.

All four of the first batch of wrens to sit the exam, were successful [45].

The range of exchange appointments with other uniformed dental organisations has already been mentioned. It may therefore be pertinent to see such an exchange from the opposite point of view. Like any institution or corporation, uniformed or otherwise, we grow comfortably into the traditions and jargon of our own organisation and it is sometimes interesting to hear how others see us. Major John Aitken RADC, the then current Army exchange officer, wrote a brief, but amusing and complimentary article on his temporary transition from 'Fang Farrier' to 'Toothie' [46]. Part of which is reproduced below:

A Khaki View

Arriving at the Wardroom at the end of a fairly long car journey, my first words were, "Where's the gents?" "The heads are down the corridor to the right sir", was the reply. Oh well, you can't win them all. Once I had sorted out that my cabin was two decks up on the starboard side, everything was, as you might say, 'plain sailing'! …. My next rather traumatic experience was when it was announced that there was going to be a departmental 'run ashore'. Surely, I had not left the Army and its fitness tests, only to be caught up in something even more horrendous? You can imagine my relief and pleasure when I discovered the real meaning of the words.

A few weeks later I 'went over the brow' of a warship [*HMS Cardiff*] for the first time. It was my first taste of the sea and I found it quite an experience, not only from the dental point of view, but as an insight into the working of a ship.

'Going ashore' then, really meant what it said. Somehow, it didn't have quite the same ring to it when I was at *HMS Mercury*. Mentioning *Mercury*, reminds me of the first time I went there. On asking the hall porter at *Nelson*, what I should do before going away on temporary duty, I was told that I must "moor myself out". An interesting expression really! ⟫

While I was away, this last summer, on the Gulf [Armilla] Patrol, people kept apologising for it being so boring. I must admit I enjoyed every minute of it. For me it was fascinating and was literally the experience of a lifetime. … I am very grateful for having been given the opportunity.

So …. What will I remember? I think that the attitude in the Navy to dental treatment is different to that found in the Army, partly because it is more easily available and partly because of various other factors.

I think that the dental condition of the average person in the Royal Navy is better than that of his equivalent in the Army – a pleasure in itself. What a splendid arrangement it is to have a dental branch in the Wrens. Fellows are fine, but perhaps they do lack a little something. The availability of stores was another pleasure. All these little things and the general atmosphere led to a most enjoyable two years. For me, being on an exchange to the Royal Navy, was far from a hardship and, had I woken up one morning to find myself wearing blue instead of khaki, it would have given me little pain.

*****

Chapter 4

"Down South"
The RNDS Contribution during the Falklands Conflict
April to July 1982

It was now 1982, a fateful year for the United Kingdom, its Armed Forces and for the RNDS. In order to distract his own people from a rapidly deteriorating economic and political situation at home, the leader of the military junta which governed Argentina, General Leopoldo Galtieri, had decided to divert the attention of his increasingly disaffected citizens to a 'popular' cause, by invading and annexing 'Las Malvinas', as the Falkland Islands were there known.

It seems reasonable to suppose that he had been encouraged in this by the 'signals' sent by the Nott defence cuts, which were to include the Antarctic survey vessel *HMS Endurance*. The *Endurance*, as part of its routine task, had made recent courtesy calls at several Argentine naval ports, following which, its captain, Captain Nick Barker, acting on information gleaned during social contact with senior Argentine naval officers, had signalled to the Ministry of Defence, warning of pending crisis.[47] Sadly, these signals were largely ignored and following an initial foray on to the island of South Georgia by an Argentinian 'scientific group', in April 1982, Galtieri launched a full scale invasion of the Falkland Islands.

Now the Prime Minister, Margaret Thatcher, and her government, sprang to life. Against a background of frenzied diplomacy, led by President Ronald Reagan of the United States and 'shuttle diplomacy' exercised by his spokesman, General Alexander Haig, the Falklands Task Force was born.

The Armed Forces and particularly the Royal Navy were plunged into a period of huge activity as the spending 'brakes' were taken off and warships, ships of the Royal Fleet Auxiliary and merchant 'ships taken up from trade' (STUFT), were prepared for their various roles in the coming conflict.

In the Dental Branch, the number of dental officers, already serving with ships and Royal Marines units, was enhanced by the addition of others to RN and STUFT ships, which would not normally carry dental officers. These included three oral surgeons, Surgeon Commanders (D) J V (John) Holland in the P&O cruise liner *Canberra*, G H (George) Rudge, assigned to a Surgical Support Team and destined to work ashore in the makeshift, second line surgical facility at Ajax Bay and G B (Geoff) Keeble in the *SS Uganda*. The latter ship was to be designated a hospital ship and carried appropriate Red Cross markings, but the Canberra, despite having hospital facilities, was designated a troop carrier and had no such protection.

Many other officers and ratings of the RNDS were employed in support of Operation Corporate, as the Falklands conflict was designated[*].

Personal accounts of the experiences of both those deployed and those working in support are chronicled in the RNDS Newsletter and the Journal of the Royal Naval Medical Service [48] [49] ¶.

The invasion started on 2 April, with an overwhelming attack on the Falklands capital, Port Stanley, and after a fierce three-hour battle, the small Royal Marines detachment, the only British military presence on the islands, was obliged to surrender. The following day, a smaller force invaded and took South Georgia after brief resistance from the Royal Marines detachment from *HMS Endurance*, which had been landed prior to the Argentinian action. Against a background of frantic diplomatic activity at the United Nations and elsewhere, HM Government announced that it was assembling a task force in order to force the withdrawal of enemy forces from these British territories.

At the time of the invasion, a group of about 20 RN warships and their seagoing support (the Royal Fleet Auxiliaries) were exercising in the Atlantic, a short distance to the west of Gibraltar. They were under the command of Rear Admiral John (Sandy) Woodward. The exercise was rapidly abandoned as the Ministry of Defence announced the formation of the Task Force, which would sail for the Falklands areas as soon as the necessary preparations were complete. At Gibraltar, Admiral Woodward, who was named as Task Force Commander divided his ships into two groups, those which would sail, within a day or two for the South Atlantic and those which would return to the UK. The latter were stripped of all 'detachable' stores and ammunition to the benefit of the Task Force ships.

For the Armed Forces in general and the Navy in particular, taking into account recent Government plans to run down the Armed Forces, the speed with which the Task Force was prepared and dispatched was astonishing. The vanguard of the force sailed from Gibraltar and the UK on 5 April, with Admiral Woodward flying his flag in *HMS Glamorgan*. In the meantime,

---

* For a full list of RN dental officers deployed on 'Operation Corporate' see Appendix 3.

¶ The story of the Falklands Conflict, as seen through the eyes of all those dental officers involved has been distilled from the above accounts and other sources. The author is aware that there are those who played significant roles in these memorable events, whose contributions are not acknowledged in these pages. Attempts have been made to contact some of those whose stories have not been thus recorded, where possible, but 25 years on and more, there remain some gaps in the story.

civilian (STUFT) ships were being modified and stored in the home port naval bases, including Gibraltar. Among these were the cruise liners *SS Canberra* and *SS Uganda* and later, the Cunarder *QE2*. All had to undergo significant modification, enabling them not only to provide full 'third line' hospital facilities, but also to receive helicopters on deck.

To give an idea of what was involved and achieved in such a short time, at the time of the invasion, *SS Uganda*, an elderly cruise ship, then employed in taking large parties of school children on 'History cruises' around the Mediterranean, was in the port of Alexandria. Her students having been disembarked and repatriated, she sailed for Gibraltar. At the same time, all stores required to equip her as a tri-Service field hospital were embarked on the RN Auxiliary Service ship *Throsk*, which sailed from Portsmouth for Gibraltar on 12 April. On Friday 16 April, *Uganda* entered dry dock in Gibraltar. Although a good deal of preparatory work had been completed on passage, by RN medical and dockyard staff who had joined her in Naples, a huge amount of work remained to be done, including the construction and welding of a sturdy helicopter flight deck above her stern sports deck.

Three days later, on 19 April, *Uganda* sailed from Gibraltar fully equipped as a 200 bedded hospital with intensive therapy unit, reception, resuscitation and x-ray facilities as well as a laboratory and operating theatre – and of course the landing deck!

In the meantime, Her Majesty's Government had already announced a 200-mile Total Exclusion Zone (TEZ) around the Falkland Islands effective on 12 April, the Advanced Group had reached and passed the Ascension Islands and the Carrier battle Group had reached Ascension, where Admiral Woodward transferred his flag to *HMS Hermes*.

In order to make the political point that the Task Force 'meant business', the Advanced Group (those ships which had sailed from Gibraltar with Admiral Woodward and from the UK on 5 April), were ordered to continue to the Falklands area and enter the TEZ

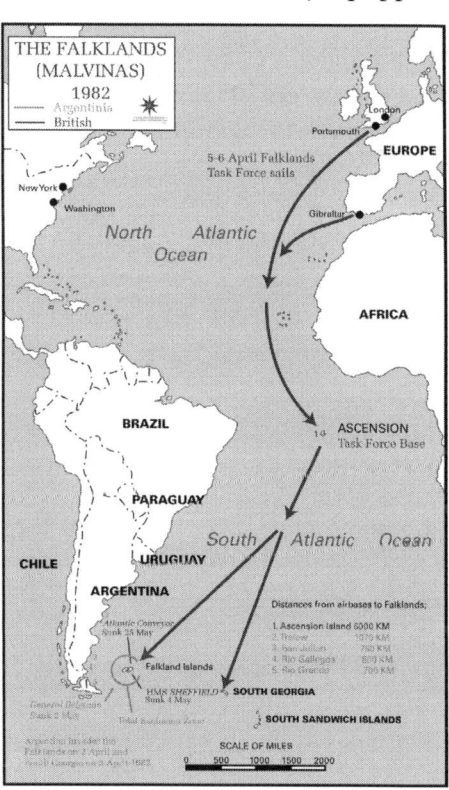

Map Showing April 1982 Route of the Task Force to the Falkland Islands & South Georgia

55

"with all dispatch", a Government decision which did not entirely please the Task Force Commander, who would have preferred to have kept the Force together.

In the event the Task force finally formed up on Sunday 25 April, by which time the 'hot war' had already started with a detached flotilla, led by *HMS Antrim* re-taking South Georgia.

Since this is the story of the Falklands conflict as experienced by RNDS personnel, let Surgeon Lieutenant Commander (D) G H (Godfrey) Rhimes, who was embarked in *HMS Antrim*, tell the South Georgia story.

Rhimes, who, like many others, had been recalled from Easter leave, found himself rapidly transported to Ascension, in company with RN medical staff and a large pile of stores, in the back of a Royal Air Force Hercules. After a few days, he joined *HMS Antrim* which headed south to rendezvous with *HMS Endurance*, which, as already stated, had been involved in the initial resistance to the invasion of South Georgia and which was now 'keeping her head down' somewhere to the north of those islands. The following is Rhimes' personal and very graphic account of the taking of South Georgia[50].

Action in South Georgia

Antrim eventually left Ascension on Easter Sunday and, four days later, we had a very emotional reunion with *Endurance*, who turned to join us for the passage to South Georgia. By 21st April we were near enough to fly the SAS onto Fortuna Glacier, but that night we had a blizzard with force 11 winds. Due to the atrocious weather, the SAS had to be evacuated the next day. During this operation we lost two helicopters in the total white-out conditions.

The flight commander eventually brought all 17 people to safety, for which he was awarded the DSO. Miraculously, there were only a few cases of frost nip and a couple of facial lacerations amongst the survivors.

A number of those who had already survived two crashes were later to die, when a Sea King ditched in the sea, a few weeks later. On the 23rd, the SBS were landed, but two of their boats went adrift.

One was picked up a few hours later, floating out to sea; the other managed to get ashore and only radioed for help when they knew that the island had fallen. Later that day we made our approach to re-take the island. At midnight, we suddenly went to action stations and I was thrown out of my pit [bunk] as the ship violently altered course and increased speed. We had a radar contact at only four thousand yards, thought to be an enemy submarine.

As we sped away to the north, it became known that the contact was the *Plymouth*, but it gave us a nasty fright. After this series of potential disasters, morale had reached its low point. ➤

> Just after 0900 on the 25th the [Argentinian] submarine *Santa Fe* was spotted on the surface by our helicopter, which dropped depth charges. As we raced in towards the boat, which was now heading for Grytviken, trailing oil, morale went sky high and a feeling of intense excitement rapidly spread.
>
> When Northwood came on to 'the growler', asking to speak to the Captain, the young radio operator replied "I'm sorry sir, but he's sinking a submarine at the moment, could you phone back later?"
>
> That afternoon we bombarded the area around Grytviken with our 4.5 inch guns and at 1705, their white flag went up. We only had one casualty, an Argentine whose right leg had been blown off by an AS12 [missile], when he was on the fin of the *Santa Fe*. I managed to get ashore for a look round the old whaling station, before we left South Georgia on 2nd May.

Within and around the TEZ, the war was hotting up. It was also on 2 May that the Argentine cruiser *General Belgrano*, perceived to be a serious threat to the ships of the Task Force, was sunk by the submarine *HMS Conqueror*. On 4 May, *HMS Sheffield* was hit by an Exocet missile, launched by an Argentinian Super Etendard aircraft. On 9 May, the Argentinian trawler *Narwhal*, which had been shadowing the Task Force, was sunk by two Sea-Harriers and on 12 May, *HMS Glasgow* was damaged by bombs. On the same day, *SS Uganda* entered the TEZ and admitted her first casualties *.

During the following days, leading to the establishment of a beachhead at San Carlos Bay, the war began to intensify. The Amphibious Group entered Falkland Sound en route for the designated anchorage in San Carlos Water. The ships were held up from approaching the intended landing areas, whilst awaiting the outcome of some initial 'clearing' operations by the SBS and SAS to remove a small detachment of Argentinian troops from Fanning Head, overlooking the Bay and to halt an advance by part of the Darwin garrison towards the intended beachhead.

These operations were supported by gunfire from *HM Ships Antrim* and *Ardent*.

The Amphibious Group comprised *HM Ships Fearless* (Surgeon Lieutenant Commander (D) R C (Chris) Sanderson) with 40 Commando (Surgeon

---

* During her rapid 'refit' *Uganda* had been painted white with red crosses on her topsides, funnel and decks. She had been registered as a hospital ship under the Geneva Conventions. Whilst, this afforded her appropriate protection from enemy attack, it also restricted her movements. SS *Canberra*, although similarly equipped, was also used as a troop transport and could therefore not be designated as a hospital ship. Thus, whilst anchored in San Carlos Water, she was subjected to numerous Argentinian air attacks, miraculously, sustaining no hits.

Lieutenant (D) A M (Andy) Prosser; *Intrepid* (Surgeon Lieutenant Commander (D) P L (Peter) Titchen) with 3 Para; *SS Canberra* (Surgeon Commander (D) J V (John) Holland) with Surgical Support Team 2 (SST2) (Surgeon Commander (D) G H (George) Rudge) and 42 Commando (Surgeon Lieutenant (D) P (Peter) Hodgson; *RFA Stromness* with 45 Commando (Surgeon Lieutenant (D) N R (Nigel) Sturgeon and *MV Norland* with 2 Para. These ships were accompanied by a further seven supply transports.

By 21 May, the beachheads were established, with 40 Commando and 2 Para the first ashore, the Royal Marines to defend the landing area and the Paras to move south to prevent the Argentines from Darwin occupying the high ground of the Sussex Mountains.

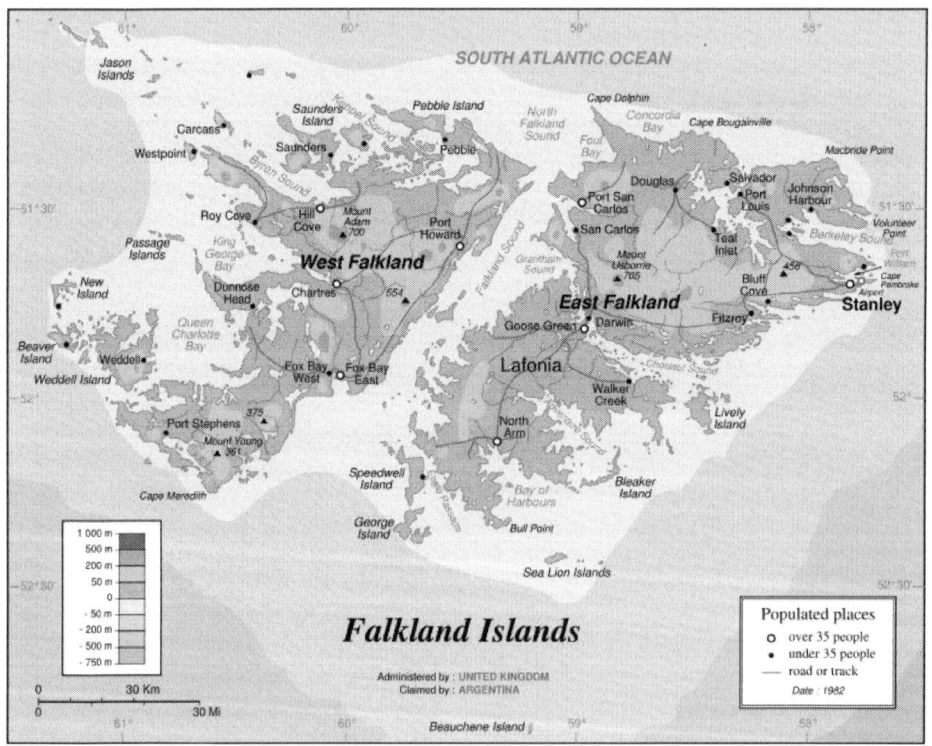

Map of the Falkland Islands

These landings were followed by 45 Commando at Ajax Bay and 3 Para at Port San Carlos thus encircling the beachheads, which were further protected by the Rapier [missile] batteries of 29 Commando Regiment, Royal Artillery. 42 Commando in Canberra was held in reserve but was landed the following night. The landings had taken place unopposed, but this early stage was not to be without its casualties.

The beachheads established, the twelve ships of the Amphibious Group now moved into the close confines of San Carlos Water in order to offload support teams, ammunition and supplies and there began a sustained aerial attack by aircraft of the Argentinian Air Force and Navy.

It was one of the miracles of the Falklands conflict that with so many ships at anchor in such confined waters, few telling hits were sustained, although there were many 'near misses'. A number of ships did, however, take hits from bombs which failed to explode. Sadly, *HMS Ardent* was hit and had to be abandoned due to a bomb which did explode and the subsequent, uncontrollable fire. The only other fatalities sustained during that eventful day were the loss of two Royal Marines Gazelle helicopters with three aircrew, to Argentine gunfire. A significant number of Argentine aircraft were destroyed on 21 May and during the days which followed, shot down by gun and missile fire from both the ships at anchor and the Harriers of the Carrier Group.

Close behind the commandos and the paras came one of the two Surgical Support Teams (SST2), which set up a Field Dressing Station in a disused slaughterhouse and meat refrigeration plant at Ajax Bay. This team, which was to become known as the 'Red and Green Life Machine', after the colours of the berets of those who manned the facility. It was under the command of Surgeon Commander R T (Rick) Jolly. As previously stated, Surgeon Commander (D) G H (George) Rudge was oral surgeon to the team.

Having set the scene and recounted the early, eventful days of Operation Corporate, it would not be appropriate in this History to follow every action of the Falklands Conflict. Thus, the rest of this account will confine itself mostly to the experiences of those members of the Royal Naval Dental Services who took part.

Surgeon Lieutenant (D) R E (Rupert) Brown had joined *RFA Resource* on 1 April. The ship, which had been stored for an April deployment on the Armilla Patrol, in the Gulf, was now in readiness to deploy for the South Atlantic, for which she sailed on 5 April.

In addition to stores and ammunition, *Resource* was carrying a detachment of some 200 Royal Marines, including members of the SBS, and some SAS personnel. Sailing via Ascension Island, she arrived in the TEZ on 1 May, just in time for the most intense period of the air/sea phase of the conflict. Here, let Rupert Brown take up the story[52]:

> ### *The War in Close Up!*
> Saturday 1st May brought the first 'Air-raid Warning Red' and hands went to emergency stations. The atmosphere was very tense, but everybody stayed very calm. ➤

The 4th May brought the terrible news of *Sheffield* being hit by an Exocet and of the crew abandoning ship. The following day, half of the survivors were transferred to *Resource*. This event made everybody realise how serious the situation was. All of the survivors were offered treatment, but only about forty were seen before they left the ship on 12th May. I spoke at length to the medical officer of the *Sheffield* about what he had come up against during what must have been a terrifying experience.

The situation seemed to have calmed down to some extent, from the day *Sheffield* had been hit, so I decided to try and move the PDU [portable dental unit] to another ship. *Yarmouth* advised me that they had a large number of patients wanting treatment. I arranged to move to *Yarmouth* on 13th May, however, it took nearly four days at a few hours notice, before I was finally transferred.

Four full days' work was all that was possible and even this was continually interrupted by air-raid warnings. I found that by working early mornings and evenings this could be avoided.

All equipment was stowed away on 20th May, in preparation for the landings on the following day. We went to emergency stations at midnight, but were relaxed at about 0200.

The ship was attacked on numerous occasions throughout the day, which I spent, mostly in the sick-bay, listening to what was going on.

At about 1800 we went alongside *Ardent* to take off survivors. The sight of *Ardent* burning was something that shocked everybody, but within a very short while, we were working with the casualties brought onboard. Two hours were spent treating them before they were transferred to *Canberra* in San Carlos Water.

That evening *Yarmouth* moved into San Carlos, which gave everybody a feeling of security, being surrounded by hills with Rapier batteries. The Saturday was surprisingly quiet, but the Sunday was very different.

I was on the bridge at lunchtime, when there was a surprise attack, which was the most incredible sight, with an aircraft falling out of the sky in flames and *Antelope* being hit – all most unreal!

On Monday 24th May, *Resource* came into San Carlos to offload stores and, that afternoon, was narrowly missed by two bombs. I felt that I would probably be of more use in *Resource*, where there were few trained first-aiders, so I transferred later that evening.

Tuesday 25th May was another day full of air-raids. The morale of everybody on board noticeably improved from the previous day as the 'novelty' of the air-raids wore off.

Resource finished her work in San Carlos and, at midnight, moved out to join the main task group. The ship was then to rendezvous with *MV Saxonia* at South Georgia.

HMS Yarmouth had, in fact, changed stations with *HMS Ardent* shortly before the latter was attacked. The ship had been attacked from astern and as Yarmouth closed Ardent to take off the injured, those on deck could see that the quarterdeck was an inferno. There were two men in the water. One had dragged the other, who was injured, through a hatch on the quarterdeck, helped him into his life jacket and had pushed him over the side, before, himself, jumping in. They were rescued by Surgeon Commander Rick Jolly, who was winched into the water from a Sea King helicopter, which had arrived to give assistance.

A number of other ships had suffered (unexploded) bomb damage including *HMS Antrim* (Surgeon Lieutenant Commander (D) Godfrey Rhimes) which had received a 1,000 pound bomb in the tiller flat. Since seeing action in South Georgia, *HMS Antrim* had transported the rescued British Antarctic Survey Team "together with their ducks and penguins", almost halfway to Ascension, handing them over to *HMS Antelope*. [*Antelope* was later to suffer the same fate as her sister ship *Ardent*, during an attempt to defuse an unexploded bomb]. *Antrim* then returned to the Total Exclusion Zone (TEZ). Let Rhimes, once again take up his story [53]:

On the Receiving End!

[Thursday 20th May] The weather was wet and foggy as we sped across the TEZ at 29 knots, to land our SBS team around Fanning Head and to open the D-day bombardment. Again, there was an atmosphere of intense excitement and relief that we were at last going in. By the time we arrived in Falkland Sound it was a clear starry night with no moon.

I was on the bridge when the first two ranging shells were fired. The SBS spotters reported direct hits and so the order was given, "Four point five inch, engage, 20 rounds, rapid fire". From the reports coming back, it was apparent that we were causing a lot of damage and occasional flashes could be seen ashore as enemy ammunition dumps were hit. It struck me as odd at times, how I could stand there, quite unmoved, as if watching a 'Space Invaders' game in progress, whilst the several hundred rounds that we fired that night were causing untold deaths and mutilation to the enemy troops.

A few hours later, things were so very different. I was again on the bridge when we went to 'Air Raid Warning Red' and, had hardly hit the deck when the first raid came in. A dozen bombs were dropped and landed within yards of the ship, but we took no direct hits. The deck was shuddering as the engines went to full speed and the ship started weaving to avoid the incoming aircraft. When this raid had passed, I picked myself up and scurried down the ladders to reach the sick bay. As I reached the bottom of the ladder, the second wave of planes came ➤

in. A 1,000 pound bomb entered the ship aft, but did not explode.

It came to rest in the junior rates' heads, just a few feet from the magazine. "Lucky" *Antrim* was living up to her reputation. During this attack we were peppered with 30mm canon shell, which gave us a dozen or so casualties, all from shrapnel wounds. As I lay on the deck I could hear the shrapnel ricocheting off the bulkhead next to me. Rather than fear, I had a feeling almost of exhilaration, tinged with the unreality of it all. In my wildest dreams I had never thought that I would see active service, before this incident occurred.

The bomb was safely ditched 12 hours later and we put to sea to repair our damage. The following Sunday afternoon [23rd May], I was on my pit 'doing a deckhead survey', when there were three enormous roars, which sounded just like jets overflying us. I was off my pit and halfway to the sickbay before the action stations alarm went off. As I lay on the deck in the sickbay, it was announced that the three roars were our chaff [a missile defence decoy] being fired, as an Exocet radar was being picked up. To say that I was frightened would be an understatement. With the sickbay being midships and above the waterline, we were, to say the least, poorly placed, should we receive an Exocet hit. We lay there for what seemed like an eternity, in utter silence, until the threat had passed. It's amazing the thoughts which race through one's head at times like these!

Once we were seaworthy again, we went off to meet the *QE2*, off South Georgia and picked up the Army Command Unit for transfer to two days later. During the passage, I shared my cabin with an RAMC major, who was later killed at Bluff Cove.

After this, we went back to our old haunt at South Georgia to act as 'Queen's Harbourmaster'. Whilst here, I was asked to take an alginate impression of the inside of the gun breeches, to see how badly they had been scratched and pitted. As a result of this, the gun barrels were changed. So I was, at least, of some use to somebody on this deployment!

In fact Rhimes' last comment, above, was overly modest. During the events of 21 May, as a Combat Casualty Care Course 'graduate', he was involved in giving first aid to several casualties, some with serious shrapnel wounds. Once afforded primary treatment, the casualties were then transferred to the Hospital Ship.

Following the Argentinian surrender in mid-June, Rhimes, as did many of his colleagues in the Task Force, reverted to his normal professional role – providing primary dental care.

The experiences of these two dental officers in *HM Ships Yarmouth* and *Antrim*, were not untypical of those encountered in the front line, by the dental officers afloat throughout the Task Force.

The oral and maxillo-facial surgeons, deployed in *Canberra, Uganda* and with the Surgical Support Team ashore at Ajax Bay, were kept equally busy, providing both the skills and experience of their own specialties and, not infrequently, also acting in general surgical roles.

Meanwhile, the dental officers in the ships of the Carrier Battle Group were afforded a grandstand view of the war in the air; a view which, at times proved to be less than comfortable! Surgeon Commander (D) Neil Harkness, the Senior Dental Surgeon in *HMS Invincible,* gives his account in a well written report.[54]

> ## *A View from the Flight Deck*
> On 21st April we had our first contact with the Argentine Air Force when a Boeing 707 reconnaissance aircraft approached the force. It was successfully intercepted by a Harrier but the pattern continued for a few days.
> As the ship approached the Total Exclusion Zone, the majority of the ship's company made wills, joined the RN Dependents Fund and checked life insurance policies. Everyone received a 'dog tag' identity disc, and the officers and senior ratings were issued with two monojects of morphine.
> First Aid lectures were also given. The prospect of war loomed large at this stage, particularly following the recapture of South Georgia when the submarine *Santa Fe* was disabled and the island retaken without loss of life.
> We entered the Total Exclusion Zone on Saturday 1st May for the first time. There was an air of relief about the ship that at long last all the uncertainty had gone and the procedures which we had practised so many times were to be put to the test. An atmosphere of quiet confidence pervaded, but action soon followed with the Vulcan strike on Port Stanley airport. A high level of air activity continued throughout the day but it was early evening before either side inflicted damage on the other. Our success came when a Mirage and a Canberra were shot down by *Invincible's* 801 Harrier Squadron with reports of another of each type of aircraft as possible hits. Another Mirage was hit by Argentine shore batteries as it crossed the coast but with the onset of darkness the Argentine air activity ceased. We had been closed up at action stations over 9 hours during which time 24 Sea Harriers and 24 Sea King sorties were flown. By then we were under no illusions that the war had begun!
> The next few days were relatively quiet as both sides took stock of the confrontation. Meanwhile, on 2nd May we heard news of the sinking of the *General Belgrano* to the South West of the Total Exclusion Zone. Our sympathy went out to the sailors pitched into a freezing sea in darkness, but events moved quickly and 4th May was to see the first Exocet attack on the Task Group. The ships had literally minutes warning of the raid which resulted in *Sheffield* being hit amidships at about 1415. Power was lost and the fire spread uncontrollably ➤

until the order was given to abandon ship at 1730. A second missile dropped harmlessly into the sea ten minutes later between *Alacrity* and *Invincible*. This was too close for comfort and the Group withdrew to the south-east section of the Total Exclusion Zone to reappraise the situation. The events of the last 24 hours had shocked us and there was a tense disbelief at the frightening speed with which fortunes could change.

It was on Thursday 6th May that *Invincible* suffered her first and only casualties of the war period. Two Harriers sent into low cloud to investigate a suspected enemy contact, appear to have collided and their pilots killed. The double tragedy of *Sheffield* and this loss brought the realities of war home to us. Much of the early bravado had evaporated and this was replaced by a quiet determination to see the conflict through to a successful conclusion.

During the middle of May, *Fearless*, *Intrepid* and the Amphibious Group arrived in the area and this started the chain of events leading to the recapture of the islands. The events of the landing on 21st May have been well described in the media. The repeated air attacks on our ships and the loss of *Ardent*, *Antelope* and *Coventry*, and damage to *Antrim*, *Argonaut*, *Brilliant* and *Broadsword*, were a high price to pay but their presence proved an essential element in achieving our goal.

The fact that these and other escorts bore the brunt of the Argentine Air Force attacks and, together with Sea Harriers from *Hermes* and *Invincible*, were to destroy approximately 50% of the aircraft sent against them, were major factors in achieving a successful landing. Had the Mirage and A4 pilots concentrated solely on the amphibious forces, the outcome might have been different.

Another interesting feature was the number of Argentine aircraft which, on seeing the Harriers, jettisoned their bombs and turned for home. This proved to be the height of the air battle, and it transpired that the Argentine nickname for our grey painted Harriers was "The Black Death".

25th May saw the attack on *HMS Coventry* and its subsequent loss. It was whilst we were wondering about casualty figures that the Carrier Group again came under Super Etendard attack. Radar contacts were picked up several miles from the ship as the enemy aircraft climbed to release their missiles. Our own anti-Exocet manoeuvres were instituted but within minutes *Atlantic Conveyor* had been hit on her port quarter about eight miles north east of us. Its range was rapidly closing and at 14 nautical miles we fired three salvos of Sea Dart missiles. Whether or not we hit anything remains a mystery, for the approaching darkness combined with the need to recover survivors precluded a search for wreckage.

Despite the losses of *Coventry* and *Atlantic Conveyor*, the day had not gone entirely the Argentines' way. They had again lost aircraft over the Amphibious Operations Area, and they had failed to hit their primary Task Force targets which were *Hermes* and *Invincible*.

The day after the capture of Goose Green and the taking of over 1,000 Argentine

> prisoners, came the third and final attack on the Carrier Group. This time the two Super Etendards closed the force from the south and, but for a displacement of ten miles to the west, might have found *Invincible* as their first contact.
>
> In the event, it was *Avenger*, detaching herself to go inshore, who found herself at the centre of their attention. Once again, the same attack pattern emerged, of radar contacts as the Etendards climbed, released their weapons and dived away to the south. As everyone watched, waited and listened for the Exocet missiles, several A4s suddenly appeared from the same direction and carried out a low level bombing attack on *Avenger*.
>
> Both *Exeter* to the north and *Avenger* herself engaged these aircraft with Sea Dart and guns respectively. One, possibly two, was destroyed. Whether the Exocet missiles were also destroyed, or merely failed to find a target, is not known. However, this was the first unsuccessful attack on the Carrier Group. Our Exocet experience had been hard won and the learning curve was steep, but refinement and practice of Exocet countermeasures had proved successful.
>
> The final days of the land battle are now a matter of History. The impressive advance of the Commandos, Guards and Paratroopers over appalling terrain, the bombing of *Sir Galahad* and *Sir Tristram* and the surrender of Port Stanley are events which we, like the rest of the Task Force, learned of with a mixture of admiration, concern and elation.
>
> Our own support of the operations continued with 594 Sea Harrier sorties and 1172 rotary wing launches during the 45 days of war. We spent 270 hours at action stations and steamed a total of 51,462.5 nautical miles from Portsmouth to Portsmouth – half her total distance since *HMS Invincible* was built.

It is worth here recording the exact role of the dental officer borne in front-line units in time of conflict. Until the unit is actually engaged with the enemy, the general duties dental officer will provide a primary dental care facility, within that unit.

Oral and maxillo-facial surgeons are and, were during the Falklands conflict, borne to provide second and third line levels of treatment to personnel suffering both soft tissue and bony injuries to the head and neck.

All general dental practitioner dental officers, deployed to the Falklands, were involved in ships' or Royal Marines' first aid and casualty handling organisations. Normally, they were involved in leading a first aid team which covered one area of the ship. Some dental officers were employed in the primary reception of casualties and in triage, whilst others assisted with the running of emergency operating theatres.

All the ships' dental officers deployed took part in the treatment of casualties. This ranged from simple first aid (e.g. the application of bandages and shell dressings) to the setting up of intravenous infusion sets, suturing lacerations and the administration of drugs, both intravenously and intramuscularly. Some were also involved in the organisation of CASEVAC (Casualty Evacuation) procedures.

The oral and maxillo-facial surgeons, deployed in the Hospital Ship *SS Uganda*, in *SS Canberra* and with the Second Surgical Support Team (SST2), were able to take a larger part in the treatment of the injured, due to their surgical training and experience.

SS Canberra had sailed from the UK, believing that she was to be designated a hospital ship, whilst temporarily carrying troops. Under the Geneva Conventions, this status was not allowed. Having spent several days in San Carlos Water disembarking her troops, she was withdrawn to a safer distance. It was a miracle that, despite having been attacked a number of times, she did not sustain any direct bomb hits. Painted white (and known affectionately as the Great White Whale) she must have made a tempting target for the Argentine aircraft. The oral surgeon on board, Surgeon Commander (D) J V (John) Holland records the disappointment of the medical team when they were pulled back from the front line. Despite this, over 70 casualties were treated on board.

Surgeon Commander (D) G H A (George) Rudge (another oral surgeon) was also borne in *Canberra*, where he took on the role of executive officer to the medical team, but was then deployed ashore with Surgical Support Team 2 (SST2) to set up the Ajax Bay Field Hospital. Here, he was called upon to act as both maxillo-facial and general surgeon, treating injuries to most areas of the body. *

SST2, at Ajax Bay lived and worked in difficult and squalid surroundings. These were not improved when, on 27 May, the old refrigeration plant and slaughterhouse, in which they were accommodated was hit by a stick of bombs.

Fortunately, only one of these exploded, but this killed five men and injured 27. After some reappraisal of their situation, the Surgical Support Team continued their essential and difficult work, with two unexploded bombs as near neighbours![55]

The landings at the San Carlos beachhead marked the beginnings of the land battle for the Falkland Islands. Three Commando-trained RN dental officers were deployed ashore with the Royal Marines of 3 Commando Brigade. They too had their stories to tell. Needless to say, these dental officers also had another part to play aside from clinical dentistry and all three formed

---

* The details of dental officer participation on this page were gleaned from a demi-official report by Surgeon Commander (D) J V Holland – "Operation Corporate – Dental Report".

up with the Regimental Aid Posts (RAP) of their respective Commandos. As ever, it is best to let the dental officers involved tell their own stories. First, Surgeon Lieutenant (D) N R (Nigel) Sturgeon of 45 Commando, whose diary of the campaign does much to bring alive the tedium, discomfort and horrors of the land battle. The author makes no apologies for reproducing his account in full [56]:

> ## *Teach Yourself Yomping!*
>
> Having landed at Ajax Bay, on 'D'-Day, 21st May, 45 Commando stayed in defensive positions around the disused refrigeration plant for nearly a week. This account of the now-famous walk across East Falkland is mainly unaltered from my diary.
>
> Thursday 27 May
>
> Up early. Kitted out ready for 33 kilometre march to Douglas Settlement. Landing craft at first light to Port San Carlos – Nearly saw Peter Hodgson [Surgeon Lieutenant (D) P Hodgson of 42 Commando] as we assembled. Apparently he was treating some of the local kids. Set off on 'yomp' with rucksack, webbing, medical bag and weapon. Very slow going, whole Commando in a 'snake' about 2kms long. Slogged all day. Quick cup of tea, just before dusk – no time to cook a meal. Then spent six hours to travel another six kms to bivouac area. Routine: shuffle 25 metres, stop, wait, shuffle, stop, find yourself standing in a bog with boots topping up, shuffle, etc. Weight of kit very unpleasant, although I was carrying far less than some of the rifle company boys – grenades, mortar bombs, rocket launchers etc. Going got worse – very boggy and wet. Eventually arrived bivvy area about 0230. Got into bag inside 'waterproof' outer and slept like the dead until 0600, when it started to belt down. Lay in bag for another hour, feeling water drip through the outer. Eventually gave up trying to get back to sleep. Got rigged and sat shrouded in waterproofs for three hours, until daybreak.
>
> Friday 28 May
>
> A couple of exposure cases seen; five marines CASEVACed [evacuated as casualties] by helo, due to ankle and knee injuries. First meal for 24 hours – 'Arctic breakfast' of instant porridge and hot chocolate – made a big difference to the way I felt! Stopped raining at 1200 and we set off again, this time without rucksacks, which were dumped to move by helo. Walked about six kms until Douglas came into view – then got lucky and hitched a lift in a tracked vehicle for the last three kilometres – bliss! Arrived Douglas Settlement about 1900, set up Regimental Aid Post (RAP) in half built house. Dug trench in back garden, then had some food – Arctic curry again, but nevertheless, very welcome.
>
> At this point heard some bad news. Ajax Bay was bombed on the previous evening. A 400kg bomb went off in the unit's main galley, part of the refrigeration »

plant. Five dead, approximately 20 wounded. Unfortunately two of the dead were stretcher bearers who were the other half of the RAP at the time. The MO (he stayed behind and was there during the attack), spent five hours in his trench, while all the ammo piled around 'cooked off' with huge bangs.

Despite being inside, not much sleep on Friday night – the previously dumped rucksacks did not arrive – therefore, no sleeping bag! Very cold lying on concrete floor, shivered the night away. No rucksacks due to the Paras having a go at Darwin/Goose Green, therefore all helos used for ammo to re-supply them.

Saturday 29 May

Good Day. Rucksacks arrived, rations arrived. Dug trench, completed RAP. Nice weather, so everyone dried their kit out. Saw lots of marines with blistered feet, pulled ligaments, early trench foot. Troops we saw all cheerful, so if we stop here for a day or two to 'shake down', should be no problems.

Wash, shave, meal of sausages and mash. Only thing missing was a run ashore! Buzzes [rumours] flying around about what next. – Possible move tomorrow p.m. Talked to locals.

Apparently about thirty enemy here (one of whom had his sixteenth birthday), until two or three days ago. Treated villagers pretty badly – locked them in the hall, stole their valuables etc.

Apparently the Argentinians got wind of 45's imminent arrival and sent in a helo to lift their troops a couple of days before we arrived – when the enemy here saw it arrive, they assumed it was us and showed the white flag!

Sunday 30 May

Left Douglas at 1430. Yomped about two km, then returned via civilian Landrover to see eight-year-old with toothache – quick extraction of deciduous tooth. Caught up with RAP. Good day for walking, mainly sunny, very cold, so ground frozen. Hard walk of 20 km to Teal Inlet. Arrived 2200. Pretty tired and hungry. RAP moved into large house already in use by Paras.

Large kitchen with peat-fired 'Rayburn' ensured a hot meal of baconburgers and beans, probably the most enjoyable meal of my life. Also had wash and share in hot running water. Amazing stuff! Turned in about 0100, but despite being exhausted, full and warm, could not sleep. Ached all over and kept thinking about the possibility of another day's march in a few hours' time.

One amusing incident today. During march, message was passed down the column, starting from the front. Originally started out as: "Air raid warning red", by the time it got to the back, two kilometres later, it was: "Galtieri is dead and they've surrendered". No wonder those at the front could not understand why those at the rear of the column seemed to be overjoyed and throwing their berets in the air at the prospect of coming under attack by Pucaras. ➳

Tuesday 1 June

Yesterday and today static at Teal Inlet. Lots of blistered feet dressed – about 120 cases in all – even the Padre was at it! The result of spending six weeks at sea, feet have 'gone soft', through not walking and running in boots. The soft 'squelchy' terrain probably does not help.

Thursday 3 June

Have been ready to move east for the last two days. Poor weather has stopped flying. Unit has set off on yomp of 32 kilometres, so as to be in position as soon as possible. Main RAP has stayed at Teal Inlet, until us and stores can be moved forward by air. Ironically the weather is now clearing, a couple of hours after the unit has left.

We have been loaned another MO from Medical Squadron. The strength of the RAP is now two doctors, myself, POMA, LMA, plus about a dozen stretcher bearers. The forward medical support consists of an MA per rifle company, four in all.

Saw Peter Hodgson, who has moved up with 42 [Commando]. His moustache is better than mine!

Monday 7 June

Bluff Cove Peak. Moved to this location by helo, with stores, on Friday. Unit legged it here. They took all day. We took 10 minutes in a Wessex. Never having flown tactically before, I think I would rather walk in future. It was hard to tell if the helo was actually airborne, or just taxiing at 120 knots! RAP now set up in tents for the first time – a 12' x 12' and a 9'x9', joined together, to form a triage/reception area and a separate major treatment area.

Ground very wet, especially after yesterday, when it poured all day. Surrounded by two batteries of guns, so there are lots of 'bang-whizzes', although we are starting to hear a few 'whiz-bangs' as well, which keeps people on their toes.

Tuesday 8 June

Still here! Quiet day for us, everyone is wondering how much longer we are going to sit around. The marines continue to 'harry' the Argentinians, with night patrols attacking specific targets, such as machine gun posts. Heard sound of jet aircraft on the other side of Bluff Cove Peak. Later came the news of *Galahad* and *Tristram* being hit.

Saturday 12 June

Finally move east yesterday, to Mount Kent's northern slopes. Five minute helo ride, took RAP initially to old Argentinian position – two burned out enemy helicopters, plus thousands of rounds, rockets, grenades, etc.

None of us liked the look of setting up near here, so we moved three hundred metres, behind the slope, out of sight from the east – just in time to enjoy the spectacle of 155 mm artillery rounds landing near the first position. »→

During the early evening, 45 Commando moved up into position for a full scale attack on Two Sisters, a twin-peaked mountain about six kilometres to the east. Part of a five-unit attack that night. Mortars and artillery gunfire all night, with unit's attack starting at 2359. First casualties reported at 0300. Due to landing site coming under fire, helicopter could not ferry wounded back to us for another three hours. Sounds of battle coming from over the hill, made us think that casualties would be heavy. First casualty arrived about 0700 – a serious head injury, who was very quickly moved back to operating facilities, but unfortunately died. During the course of the night, about another ten, not so serious casualties passed through the RAP, mainly shrapnel wounds. Four marines and a sapper were killed outright on the slopes.

After first night, we saw several Argentinian casualties, two serious, a head injury and a sucking chest wound; plus another three, lightly wounded. Attack successful, position secured by first light. Did especially well considering it was a very cold night – approximately -5°C.

Footnote

On the same night as the attack on Two Sisters, Mount Longdon and Mount Harriet were taken. Two days later, Mount Tumbledown and Mount William to the south and Wireless Ridge to the north-west of the capital were taken. By midnight on June 14, the Argentinians had surrendered.

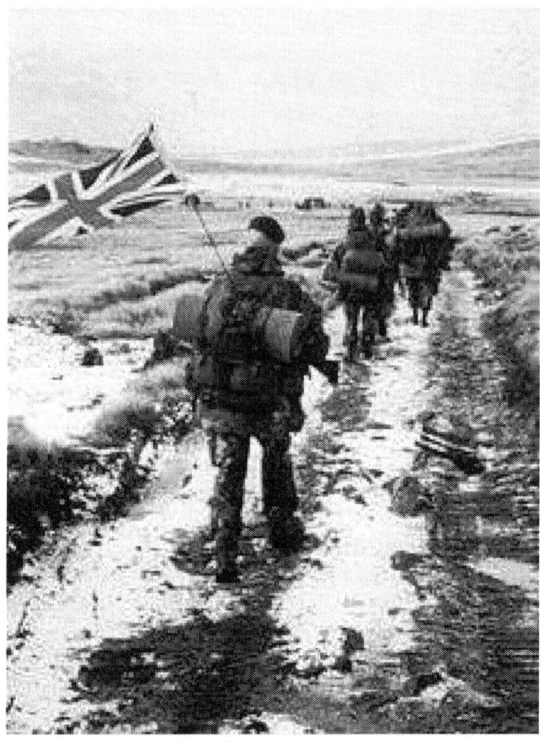

Iconic photograph of the Royal Marines 'yomping' into Port Stanley following the surrender of the Argentinian Forces. Published by permission of the Imperial War Museum. Negative no. FKD 95

Surgeon Lieutenant (D) A M (Andy) Prosser was deployed with 40 Commando. His campaign was somewhat different from that experienced by Nigel Sturgeon. Unlike his colleague, Prosser did not experience the 'yomp' across the island. Like Sturgeon he was disembarked from *SS Canberra* on 21 May.

The following extracts from his written report[57], paint a graphic picture of the intense activity which followed 40 Commando's disembarkation, whilst also coping with frequent attacks from the air and treating incoming casualties.

Taking the Heat

At 0630 [21 May] at San Carlos (Blue 1 Beach) 40 Commando went ashore, the three rifle companies separating to clear the small airfield, the settlement and the low ground to the South. The Union Flag was raised by 9 Troop, 'C' Company. The medical staff were deployed – two MAs [Medical Assistants] per company (normally only one); MO with the Tactical HQ and the dental officer and petty officer MA to initially run the RAP [Regimental Aid Post].

After clearing the immediate area, the companies began digging in on the reverse slope to the East of the settlement, and the low ground to the South. At first light there was a massive effort to get as much of HQ Main and the artillery and air defence ashore, before the first of the predicted air strikes. This in fact, was not possible and HQ Main came ashore by LCU [landing craft] during an air attack.

At 1900, in a large air attack, *Coventry* was severely damaged and *Atlantic Conveyor* hit and abandoned, by Exocet missiles, fired by Super Etendard aircraft. *Broadsword* was again, slightly damaged, when a bomb passed through the flight deck.

The rifle companies were put at short notice to move the next day; 'C' Company to Ajax Bay to protect the Medical Squadron Field Hospital and 'A' and 'B' Companies to, as yet, undisclosed destinations.

On 27th May, an Argentinian soldier was captured on the ridge overlooking our trenches. He was found to be a Lieutenant Commander of Marines and possibly part of a larger patrol, which had come under fire from 'A' Company on the previous night. He was lightly equipped and could have been a forward aircraft controller, a fact borne out some 30 minutes later, when an air strike came in on our position.

Skyhawks, flying very low, dropped parachute bombs (presumably to give the bombs time to arm, following the failure of some dropped on the Fleet). It was suspected that they were aiming for a large wool shed, which had been filled with troops earlier in the day. The bombs landed around the shed, amongst our trenches, several not exploding, despite the parachutes. All five medical personnel were required during this and a subsequent raid, to treat casualties. ➤

One sapper died in his trench, despite my efforts to resuscitate him, from the almost direct effects of the blast. Several serious shrapnel wounds were flown direct to *Intrepid* or Ajax Bay, while the remainder were treated in the RAP, before being bedded down, or flown to *Uganda*.

I flew to Goose Green on 30th May to treat a civilian patient, one of the 130 civilians who had previously been held for 29 days in a church hall. Conditions were disgusting, with only one toilet and no washing facilities, resulting in many cases of diarrhoea, particularly amongst the children.

There were over 1,400 prisoners to be processed and the grim task of dealing with some 250 Argentinian bodies, many unrecognisably mutilated. Casualties were flown to Ajax Bay, *Canberra* and *Uganda*.

Major General J J Moore, Commander Land Forces, arrived in the Falklands on 31st May, as 'B' Company prepared to move to Port San Carlos.

Another bombing raid that night damaged a helicopter and left a string of 11 foot craters towards 'A' Company position.

The move to Port San Carlos did not, in fact, occur until 2nd June, when 5 Infantry Brigade arrived and began to move through our position. The defences at San Carlos were, by now, stretched pretty thinly and it became increasingly difficult to man all the trenches and send out the regular clearing and fighting patrols.

Air raids at San Carlos had now ceased [and] the general mood became more relaxed. The weather also deteriorated during this period and, [on] the high ground, near arctic conditions caused many problems of trench foot in the wet trenches. The only successful treatment appeared to be rest with the legs elevated in a warm environment. This was achieved as best we could, by taking the men out of the trenches and [placing them] under cover (in the bunkhouse at San Carlos and in a schoolhouse at Port San Carlos).

The medical officer and I moved between San Carlos, Port San Carlos and Ajax Bay as necessary, to treat patients. The regular Gazelle and Wessex flights made this comparatively easy and we were seldom unable to see patients within a short time of being called on the radio net. Treatment was also provided for civilians and several dental extractions were performed, in particular for local children, who were normally only able to see a dentist annually.

On the afternoon of 8th June, at Bluff Cove, three waves of Argentinian planes attacked the *Sir Galahad, Sir Tristram* and *HMS Plymouth*, who were taking the Welsh Guards to their new location. That evening, many of the survivors, shocked cases and minor casualties, were brought back to San Carlos, before moving to *HMS Fearless* and other ships in the fleet for rest and re-equipping, having lost most of their equipment in the fire.

Fifty men from the Welsh Guards and Field Ambulance were killed and 160 injured, of whom 75 to 80 were walking wounded; mainly shock or minor burns.

On 12th June 'B' Company captured 11 prisoners and three casualties at New House, North-East of Port San Carlos. Meanwhile, 'A' and 'C' Companies had joined the Welsh Guards in their advance. On 13th and 14th June, the Argentinian troops came under heavy attack on the high ground they were defending around Stanley – Mounts Longdon and Harriet and later, Tumbledown, Mount William, Wireless Ridge and Sapper Hill. Despite early stiff resistance with artillery and mortar, each successive objective fell and the Argentinians retreated into Stanley before very heavy fire power from our gun batteries, mortars, armoured vehicles and company weapons. Casualties in 40 Commando, were suffered from mines and small arms, with, fortunately, no loss of life. The white flag was raised over Stanley on the afternoon of 14th June.

At dawn the next morning, [with] one company of 40 Commando, plus elements of HQ, I flew to Port Howard in the West Island, to raise the Union Flag and to accept the surrender from the local Argentinian commander. Not convinced of the reception we could expect, the Wessex flew straight into the middle of the settlement and the marines deplaned, as if for an opposed landing. However, we were soon greeted by the pitiful sight of hundreds of young Argentinian soldiers, coming down the hill dragging their kit bags behind them. Unlike most of the prisoners at Stanley, they were, in many cases, genuinely undernourished and under clothed. The civilians told us of instances of indiscipline, resulting from the struggles to obtain food, and of a number of occasions on which they had broken into civilian homes to steal food. The majority had no webbing and were often without sleeping bags or waterproof clothing.

My first task was to deal with the 39 casualties, housed in their field hospital. They ranged from malnutrition and trench foot to casualties of the Harrier cluster bomb attack, in which they had lost four men. These were quickly CASEVACed via the MO of *Intrepid* and the doctors and medical staff of the hospital were searched and processed with the other officers.

Disarming and searching the 800 odd prisoners, took the whole day and it was dark by the time they had all been despatched to ships for homeward transmission.

The mountains of weapons and ammunition had then to be sorted by nature and type. The hospital which was sited in the local community centre had to be cleared out. It was by any standards in a disgusting state, by then the all too familiar hallmark of Argentinian occupation, but nonetheless, surprising in a medical facility.

The majority of medicines and drugs appeared to be very old and, in many cases, well out of date; probably coming from a reserve stock. The surgical equipment was very rusty and barely serviceable. I used a working party, for two days, to clean and pack the kit into the 80 wooden boxes, it had been brought in. Most of the useful items (drips, dressings, bandages and some instruments), were offered to Stanley hospital.

One of the problems confronting the British Armed Forces as they planned Operation Corporate, (the military code for the Falklands operation) was to be able to keep the front line ships, aircraft and men supplied with ammunition, general stores and food, at the end of a much extended supply line.

Both the Argentinians and some of our allies underestimated our ability to overcome such problems. During the short period of preparation, before the Task Force sailed, all units involved, having been living through the rigours of the Nott defence cuts, found suddenly that the purse strings had been loosened and the store cupboards unlocked! To keep doctors and dentists at sea and in the field supplied with essential stores, was just as much a problem as with any other section of the fighting force.

Despite the tri-service medical stores system, located at the Defence Medical Equipment Depot (DMED) at Ludgershall in Wiltshire, the RNDS had for some years used an 'intermediary' Command Dental Storekeeper, on the staff of the Command Dental Surgeon to C-in-C Naval Home Command.

He was Mr Ron Coote, an ex dental-trained Petty Officer Sick Berth Attendant.

The success of Ron Coote's operation during the period of conflict is well summed up by Surgeon Commander (D) John Holland in his demi-official report on Operation Corporate, to DNDS.[58] In this, he records: "Before ships left Portsmouth, their stores were checked and re-stocked by the Command Dental Storekeeper. He also checked and re-stocked all the FPDUs [Frigate Portable Dental Units] put on Portsmouth based ships [as well as] *Canberra* and *Uganda*.

Most dental officers took increased supplies of dental stores, particularly those items they favoured. *HMS Fearless* took sufficient stocks to be able to supply other ships in the TEZ [Total Exclusion Zone], when necessary.

A system of re-supply boxes was devised by the Fleet Dental Surgeon, at the request of C-in-C Fleet, to be distributed by DMED, alongside the medical system. In fact, these re-supply boxes were used only by the large ships and then, infrequently. For one item required, a whole box of stores would arrive, most of which was unwanted.

The re-supply system, favoured by dental officers, was that of a letter [or signal] to the Command Dental Storekeeper. His personal knowledge of individual dental officers, allied to his experience in dental stores, overcame communication difficulties which could have arisen with dental officers 8000 miles away. The system worked rapidly and most satisfactorily."

Despite the unremitting trend towards centralisation within the Armed Forces, once involved in such a challenging scenario, it had been shown that the single-Service, more personalised system, worked well and enabled all deployed dental officers to perform their duties effectively, within the constraints of local operational conditions.

John Holland, was, as previously mentioned, one of the three Oral and Maxillofacial Surgeons, deployed with the Task Force. The experiences of Surgeon Commander (D) George Rudge, with the Surgical Support Team, in the makeshift hospital at Ajax Bay, have already been briefly described.

Holland, deployed in the *Canberra*, elaborates on the tasks performed by the oral surgeons in the same report, a further extract from which is shown below[59]:

> ### *Specialist Support*
>
> When *Canberra* sailed from Southampton on 9 April 1982, the belief amongst the medical teams on board was that she was to become a hospital ship. However, the requisitioning of *Uganda* as a hospital ship, freed *Canberra* to undertake her role as an 'assault ship' with a large medical capability. Due to operational and political restraints, the medical facilities were under used.
>
> On the outward passage, she acted as the local hospital for the accompanying, invasion force ships. Several cases were treated under general anaesthesia, using the ship's hospital and wards. Cases included appendicectomies, a hernia, a fractured nose, a branchial cyst and a soldier who had exploded a grenade detonator in his hands.
>
> A casualty reception route was organised on the games deck, where, it was expected, the majority of casualties would be landed. The maxillo-facial surgeons [Holland and Rudge] were involved in the primary reception of patients and the treatment of minor injuries. SST2 [Surgical Support Team 2] was incorporated into this organisation, until they were put ashore on 21 May 1982.
>
> *Canberra* took two loads of patients, whilst in San Carlos. On 21 May all the casualties received that day, were transferred from accompanying ships and the forces ashore. Of the 50 received, 20 were minor casualties. The rest required more major surgical treatment, under general anaesthesia. Later these cases were transferred to *Uganda* or *QE2* in South Georgia. On 2/3 June a further 30 cases were received. These were mostly Argentinians, who had received primary treatment at Ajax Bay. They were eventually disembarked at Puerto Madryn, Argentina, having received prolonged treatment in the intervening three weeks.
>
> Facial injuries were minimal, five requiring lacerations suturing. After hostilities ceased, a further casualty was received from the field hospital in Port Stanley. A soldier had been shot in the left cheek by a negligently discharged pistol, at close range. However, the cartridge was faulty and the bullet did little damage, being removed through an incision in the side of his neck. On the homeward ⇢

> passage, a P&O steward was treated for a bilateral fractured mandible, under general anaesthesia.
>
> SST2 was put ashore with all its stores on 21 May, to set up a field hospital with the RAMC units attached to the Parachute Regiment, in a disused refrigeration plant in Ajax Bay. The field hospital acted as a second line facility, but also received patients direct from the fighting zone, transported by helicopter. Although the proportion of head and neck wounds was as expected (16%), the number of those with bone injuries was remarkably low (1.2%). This meant the maxillo-facial surgeon [Rudge] was free to treat other types of wounds and acted as a general surgeon. Primary surgery of war wounds is quite simple and a maxillo-facial surgeon has more than enough surgical skill to treat wounds of the limbs and trunk.
>
> The limited size and facilities of the field hospital necessitated the early CASEVAC of casualties, after initial resuscitation, surgery and stabilisation, to the hospital ship *Uganda* or *Canberra*. The building gave a warm, dry environment, although dusty and dirty. Part became unusable when hit by bombs – two remained unexploded. However, wound infection was almost non-existent, underlining the advantages of early debridement [wound cleansing] and delayed primary suture.
>
> After the Argentine forces surrendered, the RAMC set up a small facility at Port Stanley and SST2 was able to pack and move to Port Stanley to be embarked on *Canberra* for the homeward passage.
>
> *Uganda* was converted to a hospital ship. The hospital staff included a Consultant Maxillo-Facial Surgeon [Surgeon Commander (D) G B (Geoff) Keeble], but little equipment with which to work. A FPDU [Frigate Portable Dental Unit] was flown in from Portsmouth and a second was borrowed from Gibraltar and the surgical instruments combined to give an operation set. The remaining equipment, with a dental chair from Gibraltar, was used to set up a dental surgery. The maxillo-facial surgeon was incorporated into the Casualty Reception Team, giving primary care to those wounded, arriving on board and arranging their accommodation in the ship. Initially, he was also part of the team assisting the Plastic and General Surgeons, but arrival of more doctors, made this no longer necessary.
>
> The small number of maxillo-facial casualties treated on board – all had been primarily treated at Ajax Bay – occupied only a small proportion of the time. The rest of the time was used to treat the dental pain cases amongst the civilian crew and the embarked forces and patients.

Thus it was that a significant number of RN dental officers experienced the thrills, horrors and privations of war. Of those who experienced the conflict at first hand, many were to carry with them vivid memories, both good and disturbing, of their three months 'Down South'. Nor should those who did not sail with the Task Force, be forgotten. As well as continuing with their 'day jobs', a significant number of RNDS staff gave invaluable and dedicated support to their colleagues in the front line.

Many lessons had been learned for the conduct of the Branch in future conflicts and current thinking on the war role of RNDS personnel had been well and truly tried and tested! The Royal Navy Dental Services had acquitted themselves supremely well.

*****

Chapter 5

After the Storm
1982 – 1985

As the dust began to settle following the challenges and turmoil of the Falklands Conflict, the Royal Navy and the RNDS had to reappraise, once again, its position and purpose in the greater scheme of that enterprise known as the Defence of the Realm.

The lessons of war were analysed and learned and, although Secretary of State John Nott had 'moved on' – back to the world of banking which he better understood – both the Navy and the Dental Branch had to face yet again that war of attrition symbolised by a continuing series of Defence Reviews and Defence Medical Services Reviews.

Amongst the honours awarded in the 'Post Falklands' list was a British Empire Medal to Leading Wren Dental Hygienist Kim Toms. The war had not only touched and affected those men and women in the Task Force, it had also changed to a huge extent the lives and working routines of those personnel who were not deployed. Kim Toms had been seconded to the Casualty Care Cell in *HMS Nelson*, which worked long hours, keeping in touch with and disseminating (often distressing) information to the dependants of deployed personnel. Kim Toms' BEM was awarded for the sensitivity and dedication with which she handled this difficult task. A Flag Officer's Commendation was also awarded to Surgeon Commander (D) Geoff Myers, for his work in the same organisation.

We have read, in the previous chapter, of Surgeon Lieutenant (D) Andy Prosser's exploits when deployed with 40 Commando Royal Marines. Shortly before the outbreak of the Falklands Conflict, he and Surgeon Lieutenant (D) Catherine White (whom we last met leading a mountaineering expedition in the Russian Caucasus Mountains), had been selected as members of the British Joint Services Hovercraft Expedition to Peru – Exercise Andes Rover. The expedition had been due to take place in early 1982, but, for obvious reasons, had been deferred. It had now been re-launched and, both gluttons for punishment, the two RN dental officers joined the expedition in September of the same year. Their account of their experiences, once again made good reading in the RNDS Newsletter.[60] It is copied below in abridged form.

Up the Creek ...

Standing in 105 degree heat on a remote jungle airstrip in the Amazon headwaters, clutching nothing but a toothbrush, is surely no way to take up a new appointment and is surely an extravagant way to give oral hygiene instruction. However it was in exactly this way that we began Exercise Andes Rover.

[After a nail-biting flight across the Andes in an overloaded light aircraft, they arrived at their designated base camp.]

From the air, San Francisco, the site of our base camp, appeared almost civilised and a number of quite substantial buildings could be seen adjacent to the girder bridge, which spans the river at this point. How wrong could we be? On the ground the 'substantial buildings' turned out to be hundreds of shanties built on the hillsides either side of the river, many with no roof, all without electricity and water – the only common denominator being the filth and stench of rotting vegetables. Unmade streets were littered with the debris of a daily market, washed by daily downpours, which turned them into quagmires.

Our first introduction to the local people, however, left us in no doubt that appearances can be deceptive. A banner-waving and cheering crowd escorted us proudly to the 'Operations Centre' of the "Servicio Medico Fluvial". No roofless hovel this. Rather a newly completed garage/hangar complex, capable of housing four hovercraft with ease, together with a medical store, workshop, tool room and office, equipped with typewriter and duplicating machine. We were still more amazed when they showed us the concrete ramp which had been built, to allow the hovercraft to run straight up to the doors. It was almost embarrassing to tell the locals, at this point, that our hovercraft were still detained in customs.

After a sleepless night in sweltering heat, without mosquito nets, the team set to, the following morning, to unpack the stores and erect the base camp. To avoid any potential clash with the [drug cartel] terrorists, our camp was sited on the opposite river bank, overlooking the shanties but adjacent to the airstrip. Nine 150lb. tents were erected for accommodation, with a separate marquee for eating and additional tents for stores. The whole area was fenced with chain-link on three sides, the remaining side being open to the river.

The engineers were preparing the first hovercraft, which had [now] arrived, whilst we started to unpack a mountain of medical equipment. As we undid box after box, it became apparent that not all of what we had could be put to good use. Endoscopes and contrast medium for cholecystography, in particular, had us scratching our heads. There is no better way of learning pharmacology than to stand, MIMS [an official periodical pharmaceutical guide] in hand, in front of 15 hundredweight of assorted drugs, with the task of sorting them out on to shelves.

In the absence of the hovercraft, the medical team, complete with doctor, nurse and two dentists, decided to set off up river by local transport and make our first ⟫→

visits to some of the clinics.

[After a full day's journey in a 21 metre dugout canoe, powered by two outboards and taking in some fearsome rapids, they arrived at their first destination.]

On arrival at Lechemayo, we were taken to the new village clinic, a blue concrete building standing in a fenced enclosure at the edge of the village and far more substantial than we had imagined.

It had both roof and mosquito nets on most of the windows, quite a luxury by local standards. By now a large crowd had gathered and stood silent but curious, as we walked in. The locked front door posed no problem to the village elder, who had herded the donkeys out of the grounds when we arrived. His son was told to climb over the top and open it from the inside. The purpose of the first visit was to complete a survey of the villages and to complete a questionnaire on birth-rate, longevity, most acute medical problems and condition of the water supply, in order that we could correctly plan our future visits.

Needless to say, when presented with scores of beseeching faces, our intention weakened and we ended up providing treatment, gaining our first insight into the scale of need. A small child with rickets, so obvious that we dentists could recognise it, presented, not as a patient, but pushing a wheelbarrow, containing a far more seriously ill baby, who was later diagnosed as having typhoid. It was dark by the time we prepared our compo meal and settled down to sleep on the clinic floor.

[The following day they visited two more villages, ending for the night at San Martin].

As we sat around our camp fire that night, two local boys arrived and tried to persuade us to walk with them to a settlement some 10 kms. away, where, they said, some 20 to 30 people were in advanced stages of TB. At this point we were unable to do anything without depriving another clinic of our time, but promised to do what we could on a subsequent visit. As we stared into the fire, I'm sure that each of us wondered how empty those words really were. The problem of treating tuberculosis is twofold; firstly the combination of drugs is very expensive and we had all too few at our disposable and secondly, third world peoples do not understand the necessity for continuing the treatment after the presenting complaint has cleared up. In the case of TB, this is for several months.

[After visiting yet another village, the medical team returned to base camp to refresh themselves, before commencing a second journey downstream].

Our first visit to a Campa village was made at Otari. These stone-age people hide themselves away in open, thatched huts, well into the jungle and we experienced considerable difficulty in locating them. When we did, we found that most of the villagers had fled and that those who were left had very hostile expressions on their painted faces. We sat in silence for some time, as a few more Indians gathered around, none of us daring to show a camera, which, we had been told, was a passport to a King Harold impersonation. Eventually, the chief appeared, with his feathered headdress quivering and delivered a lengthy tirade directed at the government, Lima, white people in general and anyone else he could think of. We were unmoved by his speech, he, being unaware that we could not understand it and [thus] he seemed surprised when we shook him by the hand. Whilst the doctors and we worked in the clinic, he took our engineer to one side and directed his attention to an enormous and ancient Mercury outboard. His mood visibly softened when he learned that it might be possible to repair it. The following week, he presented himself for dental treatment.

By now the engineers had two hovercraft on the water, but were struggling to overcome an overheating problem.... therefore, we took to the canoes again for the next few trips. The routine was the same with the doctors starting to implement height and weight recordings of small children, whilst we worked steadily through long queues of dental patients. The general standard of mouths seen was very poor, many children developing caries in teeth, still only partially erupted. This was attributable to the lack of oral hygiene and to the high carbohydrate diet.

Sadly, the ubiquitous Coca-Cola turned up in all but the most remote villages and was drunk in preference to the contaminated water. It also found its way into infant feeding bottles and was highly implicated in the rampant caries seen in many infants. We worked using a portable scale of kit based on the field valise, with the addition of some equipment for cold sterilisation and boiling. Most patients complained of actual pain or gave a History of pain and examination invariably demonstrated a number of grossly carious teeth.

In order to see the maximum number of patients, we confined ourselves to the extraction of the tooth causing the presenting pain (except in the lower jaw, where grossly carious teeth in the same quadrant were removed). In all some 600 patients were seen and over 500 teeth extracted. The majority of patients showed no fear and a very high pain threshold.

The incidence of pathology was less than we had expected and only two cases of neoplasm were seen; both in men. One had spread from the antral floor to involve the tuberosity and the other involved the soft palate and throat, with several enlarged nodes. Biopsy material was sent to the University Hospital in Lima for [pathologist's] report. Many farm workers chew coca leaves to stave off hunger and fatigue, consequently having very flat occlusal tables, correspondingly caries free, although the periodontal condition deteriorated markedly. For each patient seen, a full charting and gingival examination was made and recorded on a WHO form. During the two months that we visited the clinics, we were able to teach five of the 'Sanitarios' (health workers), the principles of extraction and [local] anaesthetic technique. By the time we left, each was able to infiltrate, give blocks and extract teeth with some confidence.

[During their three months in Peru, the medical/dental team continued to visit »→

> the villages around the area on a weekly basis and even managed to run a healthcare symposium for 50 local teachers and health care workers, to train them in basic primary care techniques].
>
> [Meanwhile the engineers struggled to maintain the hovercraft and also were able to train two local men in the basics of hovercraft handling].
>
> Once running at normal temperature, the hovercraft performed well and even attracted the interest of the President [of Peru], who requested a trip whilst visiting a convent 200kms. down-river. The craft, accordingly, went down in one day and met him. He was suitably impressed and, subsequently, invited a group of us to lunch at the Presidential Palace in Lima, on our return.
>
> We sadly took our leave of San Francisco on 9th November and commenced an epic 1,000 kms journey to Pucallpa, the first major port on the Amazon, with one hovercraft, two Geminis and a canoe loaded with fuel, acting as a 'tanker'. Taking five days, we experienced several mechanical failures, extreme sunburn, arrest by the police and eventually, a night spent fighting the craft through a log jam in a mosquito-infested backwater. The hovercraft was then delivered to the workshops of a Wycliffe Bible Translators' camp, where they were already running six float planes in the area.
>
> After a welcome shower and a chance to wash some extremely smelly kit, the party went its separate ways for the last week prior to departure. Some to Cuzco to see the Inca remains, some to Lima to demonstrate a hovercraft at a trade fair and the two dentists and two engineers, back to the mountains. We hired a four-wheel drive vehicle and, with a borrowed wind-surfer tied on the top, drove to Lake Chocla Cocha, the highest in Peru (approximately 15,000 feet), where Sergeant Jim Mundie set the World Altitude Wind-Surfing Record – a suitably triumphant note on which to end what, for us, had been a memorable three months, during which, hopefully, we were able to impart just a little of our knowledge to people desperate for help.

November 1982 saw the retirement of Surgeon Captain (D) R L (Roy) Travis, the Branch's Consultant Adviser in Dental [Oral] Surgery, after 33 years in the Royal Navy. Roy Travis' distinguished career had taken him to sea in *HMS Centaur*, to Malta, Gibraltar and Singapore as well as long periods of service in the RN Hospitals, at home and abroad. Passing his fellowship in Dental Surgery in the late 1950s, he was appointed Consultant in 1968. Following his retirement, Roy Travis took up an appointment as a Consultant Oral Surgeon in Saudi Arabia.

1983 started on a sad note, when the RNDS learned of the untimely death of one of its younger members, Surgeon Lieutenant (D) Peter Hodgson. Awarded a Dental Cadetship in 1977, Hodgson had graduated at Kings College Hospital Dental School in 1979 and was promoted Surgeon

Lieutenant (D). After initial appointments, he joined the Commando Training Centre, Royal Marines at Lympstone, where he gained his much prized green beret in 1980. Hodgson had served ashore during the Falklands conflict with 42 Commando, when like his Commando colleagues, whose accounts of the conflict we have already read, he endured that hard fought campaign across East Falkland. On return to the UK, he married his fiancée, a professional opera singer, in August 1982. The beginning of 1983, found him in Norway, undergoing Arctic Warfare Training with his Commando. During a routine exercise, he and the squad of men, for whom he had responsibility, were caught in un-forecast, rapidly deteriorating weather. In full blizzard conditions, he spent time supervising his men in the digging of snow holes for shelter. Sadly, during this procedure, Hodgson himself and one other marine became wet and very cold. Both died of hypothermia before rescue could be effected. Peter Hodgson's death shocked and saddened all who knew this quiet, but determined and self-contained, young officer. It undoubtedly cut short what would have been a distinguished career.[61]

At a clinical meeting at the Royal Naval Hospital Haslar, on 22 March 1983, the Director, Surgeon Rear Admiral (D) Philip Duly presented the Harvey-Fletcher Prize and Medal to its second recipient – Surgeon Captain (D) Brian Robinson.

Amongst his many achievements, Robinson could boast two which had had particularly significant impact on the RNDS. Indeed, one of these, the design, setting up and running of the Combat Casualty Care Course (C4), had had notable effects well beyond the Branch. These have been documented in the previous chapters of this History and need no further explanation.

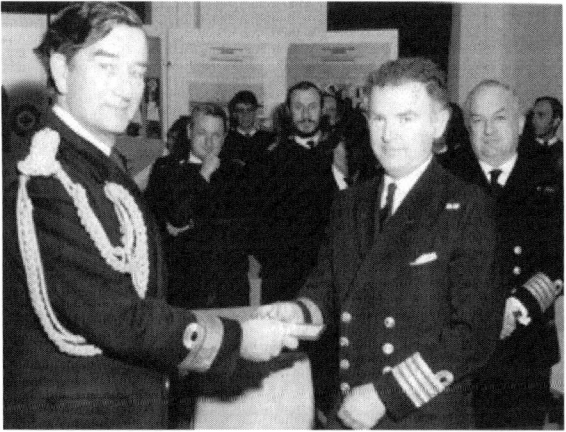

Surgeon Captain (D) Brian Robinson receives the Harvey-Fletcher Medal from Surgeon Rear Admiral (D) Philip Duly

Robinson's other major achievement was the launch of the RNDS Newsletter, which had become an invaluable organ of intra-Branch communication. As its first editor, he set a high standard, which was to be continued for many years. Brian Robinson's selection for the major Branch award was a very popular choice.

Also early in 1983, Surgeon Captain (D) C T (Clem) Stacey, the Fleet Dental Surgeon, serving in the Fleet Headquarters at Northwood, Middlesex, became the first RN Dental officer to hold a NATO appointment. He was given the additional appointments of Dental Adviser to C-in-C Eastlant and C-in-C Channel.

In May 1983, a new Dentists' Act was passed by Parliament. Amongst other innovations, it produced a new 'generic title' for dental hygienists and dental therapists, who became known collectively, as Dental Auxiliaries. The act also introduced the possibility of suspension from the right to practise on medical grounds.

By now, the day to day routine of dental officers and ratings 'at the coalface' had returned to normal and the RNDS Newsletter of Summer 1983 records, among other things an Armilla Patrol deployment to the Gulf by Surgeon Lieutenant (D) S J (Steve) Robey, during which he sailed in *RFA Pearleaf* and *HMS Avenger*, visiting Rhodes, Djibouti, Cochin, Bahrain, Doha, Abu Dhabi, Singapore, Bangkok and eastern Thailand and Colombo in Sri Lanka.[62] Quite a travelogue! The same issue of the Newsletter includes a description of his successful attempt at the London Marathon by Surgeon Lieutenant Commander (D) C (Chris) Howell RNR[63] and an account of yet another deployment in *HMS Invincible* by Surgeon Commander (D) N (Neil) Harkness, whom we last met in the same ship during the Falklands Conflict and who seems to have spent most of the latter half of his career in that ship![64]

An abridged version of his account is reproduced below:

Caribtrain 83

During a conversation with the Appointer, early in 1982, I was enthusiastically reciting the Far Eastern ports which *Invincible* was scheduled to visit, following my appointment to her. "You should be crossing my palm with silver for sending you to such a marvellous ship", he observed, sounding green with envy. [However], General Galtieri's untimely invasion effectively cancelled our well laid plans and a 5½ month period followed, during which we were embroiled in the rigours of the South Atlantic. This proved a testing interlude for the ship, but she acquitted herself well and there was a real feeling of pride and achievement on board, when she returned to Portsmouth on that memorable September day.

We had been told that normal business was to resume in February 1983, with a leisurely deployment to the West Indies.... Officially the aim of the deployment, known as Caribtrain 83, was to exercise with other NATO navies and undertake »→

a series of port visits. Privately however, those who had been to the Falklands and had experienced three successive winters, were intent on seeking as much sunshine as possible.

[After a period in the dockyard repairing the ravages of the recent campaign, including updating some of the weapons fit, *Invincible* sailed for Mayport, Florida, undertaking a series of exercises *en route*. During the passage....] there was an unscheduled serial, when one of our Sea Harriers located a Russian submarine, on the surface some 70 miles from the ship!

Mayport is an artificial basin, dredged out of reclaimed marshland and is a sort of US Navy version of Portsmouth with sun and Budweiser beer. The Naval Base, in true American style, is very big and those who took their bicycles were able to avoid the three-mile walk to the main gate! The facilities available were tremendous and all the sporting fiends were able to indulge in tennis, golf, swimming, squash etc. However, the Americans were intrigued with our cricket team … as they practised for their West Indian tour.

From the USA, the ship proceeded to Nassau [Bahamas], prior to carrying out anti-submarine warfare exercises on a special US Navy underwater range. *En route*, it was announced that our captain, Captain J J Black, was to be promoted Rear Admiral. All the ship's company were delighted, particularly those whom he had delivered safely back from the Falklands.

After Nassau, we sailed to Belize. This was more a working than a social visit. The neighbouring country, Guatemala, has designs on Belize, so a sizeable British garrison is maintained to safeguard their recent independence. The sight of our Sea Harriers flying low over the jungle must have been a sobering sight for those viewing over the border.

Next on our Caribbean itinerary was Jamaica, where bananas grow like weeds and steel drums provide the music. We anchored at Montego Bay and soon established a boat routine to and from the shore. Jamaica was universally enjoyed, but perhaps best remembered for its friendly people and exquisite rum punches! [On the day of departure, two incidents caused some delay]. As dawn broke, it was very evident that the gash barge had sunk, for three days' accumulated rubbish was floating in [the sea off] Jamaica's premier resort! Divers quickly located the barge on the sea bed and raised it, much to the disappointment of the owner who had visions of a handsome payout. As if that was not enough for the Seaman Department, they had another surprise in store, when they came to weigh anchor, for it was soon realised that our cable had become fouled by one left on the sea bed by some previous visitor. After a number of unsuccessful attempts to lift it clear, the expertise of the Explosives Safety Officer was called upon. He grasped the unexpected opportunity of putting his training into practice and successfully severed the chain with a substantial explosive charge. The ship left Jamaica some six hours late and completed its passage to Barbados in something of a rush. ≫▸

> Our ten-day stay in Jamaica was essentially a 'Self Maintenance Period' and maintenance, in this context, applied as much to the ship's company as to the ship. With this in mind approximately 80 wives and girlfriends took the opportunity of exchanging the British winter for some tropical sunshine.
>
> [After this period of relaxation it was 'back to work']. We made our way to the US Naval Base at Roosevelt Roads, Puerto Rico to prepare for a busy week at sea on Exercise Readex. During this major USN exercise the ship was put through her operational paces with simulated air, surface and submarine attacks. On completion of the exercise, we turned eastwards towards Gibraltar. The passage provided two rest days when the aircraft were confined to the hangar and the flight deck became the venue for sports and kite flying competitions. A number of ingenious kites were produced, with the Regulators' entry looking a certain winner until some mischievous rival snipped their line!
>
> [One morning] I read, with some surprise and considerable interest, a signal requesting urgent dental treatment for a female patient from an RFA in company. She duly arrived looking somewhat agitated. Her routine pulpitis was soon treated and she was escorted to the sickbay to await her return [helicopter] flight.
>
> Some two hours later, I was summoned to the 'departure lounge' where it appeared that the patient had fainted. She quickly regained consciousness after I had separated her from a well meaning sailor, who was enthusiastically giving her the kiss of life. It was assumed that my ministrations had caused her problem, but on closer questioning she revealed her real fear. In order to return to her ship, which had no landing platform, she was required to jump out of the helicopter, dangling on the end of a wire!
>
> Our final exercise of the deployment was 'Springtrain', which takes place annually in the Gibraltar exercise areas. On completion of the exercise, the ship returned to Portsmouth, having steamed a total of 20,379 miles during our twelve week period away.

On 14 September 1983, Surgeon Rear Admiral (D) Philip Duly retired as DNDS, after what had been an eventful tenure of office. He was relieved by Surgeon Rear Admiral (D) F R B (Frank) Mathias, whom we have met elsewhere in these pages.

A Guy's Hospital graduate, Frank Mathias had qualified in 1952 and, after a year's house appointment at the Royal Sussex County Hospital, started his RN career at *HMS Raleigh*, the New Entry training establishment at Torpoint in Cornwall. After this initiation, Mathias quickly 'fell on his feet' with an appointment to *HMS Tamar* in Hong Kong in 1954.

Other appointments followed, including that to *HMS Centaur* and his involvement in the *Lakonia* disaster, recounted in the Prologue to this

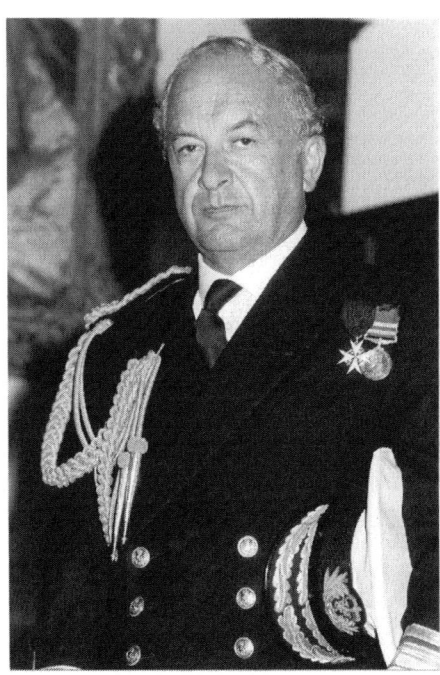

Surgeon Rear Admiral (D)
F R B Mathias OStJ QHDS

History. By the early 70s, he was Staff Dental Surgeon to the Flag Officer Malta, at the time that the Maltese Prime Minister, Dom Mintoff, chose to evict the British Armed Forces from the island. Having supervised the dismantling of the dental clinics and shipment of all equipment back to the UK, Mathias, found himself returning to Malta, when Mintoff's eviction order was rescinded, and when, once again, he had to go through the laborious process of re-establishing the clinics. Promotion to Surgeon Captain (D), in 1974, saw him hold the appointments of Command Dental Surgeon to the Flag Officer Naval Air Command, Assistant Director of the Branch and Command Dental Surgeon to C-in-C Naval Home Command.[65] Surgeon Captain Mathias was appointed Officer Brother of the Order of St. John of Jerusalem in 1981, the first RNDS officer to be appointed to this illustrious order and as Honorary Dental Surgeon to HM the Queen, in 1982.

The Exchange Programme with the US Navy Dental Corps, initiated in the 1970s, was continuing to roll forward, despite occasional sniping at its existence from both sides of the Atlantic. The first two RNDS officers to have participated in the programme, Surgeon Commanders (D) David Coppock and Ted Grant had both served at the Navy Graduate Dental School at Bethesda, Grant also doing time at the Washington Navy Yard Dental Clinic. Since then all RNDS exchange officers had served within the vast dental facility at the Norfolk, Virginia, Naval Base. The incumbent in 1983 was Surgeon Commander (D) John Hargraves. His first impressions of life as a newcomer on the other side of 'the Ditch', were published in the Branch Newsletter.[66]

Letter from America

From the moment the plane touches down, the first time visitor to the United States cannot help but be impressed by the vast scale of everything. Driving from Dulles Airport into Washington in the comfort of an air conditioned Cadillac, we had our first taste of the American Dream, vast freeways, choked with ➤

gas-guzzling automobiles – but to be truthful, there are a surprising number of Volkswagens, Datsuns and Hondas as well.

[After a weekend taking in the sights of Washington DC....]

The first Monday, I had to report to the British Defence Staff in Washington, for a briefing. This was followed by a visit to the Bureau of Medicine and Surgery, the headquarters of the [US Navy] Medical and Dental Corps, situated opposite the infamous Watergate Building. The Dental Corps has sixteen hundred officers and the headquarters staff is commensurate with a branch of this size. Having completed these calls there was time for a final dip in the hotel jacuzzi, before flying down to Norfolk [Virginia].

At Norfolk, the numbing acclimatisation continued. Again, the different scale of everything was very obvious. It is interesting to note that in the Tidewater area (Tidewater is comprised of the cities of Norfolk, Chesapeake, Virginia Beach and Portsmouth), there are 89,000 Navy and Marine Corps personnel.

Norfolk is referred to here as the Navy Capital of the World! Within this area, are homeported some 120 ships (23% of all US navy ships); there are 43 aircraft squadrons and 69 major shore facilities. These commands generate an annual 'take home' payroll of $2.55 billion!

When considering the above statistics, the size of the Naval Regional Dental Centre seems to be appropriate, although initially, it seems rather overwhelming. The new NRDC was officially dedicated on March 17 1981. The centre is 79,600 square feet and contains 113 operating rooms, 10 oral hygiene treatment rooms, a large prosthetics laboratory and administration offices. The Naval Regional Dental Centre is the regional headquarters and there are a further ten branch clinics throughout the area.

The United States Navy Dental Corps practises a multidisciplined approach to dentistry. That is to say, dental officers tend to specialise fairly early in their careers and then remain in one of the following specialties: oral surgery, prosthodontics, endodontics, operative (restorative), periodontics and preventive dentistry. There are also specialists in general dentistry and oral medicine. I am currently working in the prosthetics department, where I treat a very wide range of patients. At present, retired service personnel are treated in service facilities, as there is no national comprehensive dental care programme, to look after these people when they leave the Service. Initially I found it very strange to refer patients who required extractions for immediate dentures, or to endodontics, for overdentures, but interdepartmental co-operation is excellent and the only problem seems to be one of patients getting lost in the maze of corridors.

I was recently fortunate enough to go to sea, for a short period, in the *USS Carl Vinson*. The '*Vinson*' is the third and newest of the *Nimitz* class of nuclear powered aircraft carriers. Again, I was suitably staggered by all I saw and experienced. The '*Vinson*' is 1,092 feet long and displaces 95,000 tons and from »

> keel to masthead, she is 244 feet – equivalent to a 24 story building. The flight deck is 4½ acres and 256 feet from port to starboard. The complement of the '*Vinson*', with the air group embarked, is just over 6,000. The dental department required to support such a large ship's company, is suitably impressive.
>
> Normally, the dental complement consists of a senior dental surgeon and four dental officers. One dental officer is an oral surgeon and there is usually a prosthodontist. The other three are usually general dental practitioners, but there may be exceptions. There are twelve dental technicians (dental surgery assistants are designated "dental technicians" in the US Navy). There are also two dental laboratory technicians complemented.
>
> The clinic has six dental 'operatories'…. There is also a surgery for the dental hygienist and a preventive dentistry room. This compartment has six, small, partitioned basins for oral hygiene instruction and is equipped with a phase contrast microscope, linked to a wall mounted television monitor. This is used to demonstrate the components of plaque. The radiographic room contains an orthopantomograph machine, a standard intra-oral machine and a darkroom, equipped with an automatic processor, with a manual back-up capability.
>
> Additionally, there is a central sterilisation room, a spacious records office, a storeroom, an office for the SDS and a light, airy waiting area with closed circuit television. It was possible to watch flying operations on this and I became quite expert at evaluating F14 approaches.
>
> However, the facility in the department which impressed me the most was the comprehensive dental laboratory. [As well as a wide range of 'state of the art' equipment] ….there is even a small clean room for porcelain work [and] just to round off the inventory of this lavish department, is the installation of a computer terminal, this being used to record all the documents and a complete catalogue of dental stores items.
>
> Such a department is possible because the funding does not come from a hard-pressed medical or dental budget, but from the ship's budget. It would appear that front line ships such as the '*Carl Vinson*' command vast sums of money and the dental department expenditure, when compared to the overall cost of the ship – a staggering $1.3 billion – is a mere drop in the ocean.
>
> Needless to say, I thoroughly enjoyed the tremendous experience of my time in the '*Carl Vinson*' and I look forward to seeing other aspects of dentistry in the United States Navy during what is proving to be an exceptionally interesting and rewarding appointment.

It is interesting now to note Hargraves' amazement at the presence of a computer in the *Carl Vinson's* dental department – something unheard of at that time in any RNDS clinic.

In addition to the USN Dental Corps exchange programme, there were still other opportunities for RNDS personnel to experience life and work abroad and at sea. The Branch now had a permanent place on a secondment to the Royal Brunei Malay Regiment as Flotilla Dental Officer to the maritime cadre of the Sultan of Brunei's Armed Forces. This appointment was under the command of a senior RADC officer and RNDS dental officers on secondment to Brunei, wore army uniform and bore army rank. Nonetheless, over many years this arrangement has afforded numerous Royal Navy dental officers and their families the opportunity to experience the delights and challenges of that life in the tropical Far East which had, at one time, been so much part of many RN dental careers, when serving in Singapore.

The exchange programme with the Federal German Navy was also to continue until the late 80s. This too, enabled many RNDS officers to experience a different 'dental culture' as well as allowing the RNDS to welcome a number of FGN dental officers into its ranks.

Thus life at the 'coal face' continued to provide RN dental officers with an interesting and clinically rewarding career, together with increasing opportunities for postgraduate education and qualifications.

Junior dental officers were not the only ones to 'get in a bit of sea time'. In 1984, the Director, Surgeon Rear Admiral (D) Frank Mathias, sailed back from Gibraltar in *HMS Invincible*, on the last leg of the ship's passage home from the Far East. It was believed to be the first time a dental Flag Officer had been to sea 'on duty'! Sadly, life in the RNDS and indeed, the Royal Navy was not all fun and now it was, with the dust of the Falklands conflict well settled, new storm clouds were gathering on the horizon. Not this time a foreign enemy, but yet another review of the Medical and Dental Services, which was to threaten the autonomy and perhaps, the very existence of the RNDS.

In the early 70s Dr Henry Yellowlees had been a member of the Compton/Jarrett Committees in the then Defence Medical Review.

That review had, in fact, been of significant help to the RNDS at that time. At the beginning of 1984, the now Sir Henry Yellowlees was commissioned by the Secretary of State for Defence to conduct yet another review into the three Medical/Dental Services, with the brief to achieve significant savings through 'rationalisation'.

This review was to have far reaching and not always welcome consequences and was to become a cross which the Director, Admiral Mathias, was to find hard to bear.

This was to be yet another of the several studies which would recommend the further reorganisation of the Defence Medical Headquarters Organisation, which had commenced when Sir Clifford Jarrett produced his report in 1973, as described in Chapter Two of this History.

The Jarrett Committee offered 3 solutions for consideration, one of which included a Single Unified Directorate with a Surgeon General (SG) reporting to the Vice Chief of the Defence Staff (VCDS). Ultimately a less radical option was adopted, by a majority decision, which left much of the medical management structure intact; however, it was clear at that time, that the body politic would demand that something more radical be attempted, in due course. Further studies had followed in 1977, the Barraclough–Gober Report and the Stephens Report both of which produced variations on the themes proposed by Jarrett.

By this time it was recognised by the Central Medical Staffs that some change was inevitable and attempts to extend the interplay between the medical branches of the three services increased in non-contentious areas. The Defence Medical Services Postgraduate Council and its various tri-Service Specialty Boards had already ensured inter-Service discussion and a common purpose, towards improving the professional training of the specialist cadre of medical and dental officers. A few cross-Service appointments took place to take advantage of specialised courses run by each of the three Services such as Underwater and Aviation Medicine and this in some cases led to a reduction in civilian secondments. This tinkering, however desirable in itself, did little or nothing to bring about the savings in costs and posts which Ministers and, it has to be said, the Central Defence Staffs sought.

Implementation of John Nott's 1981 Defence Review recommendations was continuing, despite lessons learned during the recent conflict and the Medical Services had long been considered ripe for further scrutiny with a significant potential for yet more savings. The Cold War threat was gradually diminishing and concomitant adjustments in manpower and material assets were becoming a serious option. The Medical Services of the Armed Forces were at this time maintaining some 24 military hospitals and there were obvious signs that some significant rationalisation of resources could be achieved. It was also the view that there was great scope for post reductions and "star" savings amongst the staff of the medical, dental and nursing directorates, all of which had separate and similar empires in London.

The Falklands War had placed these matters on the back burner for a year or two, until 1984, when the then Secretary of State, the Right Hon. Michael Heseltine MP, reviewing the Services' medical organisation, stated that he could see scope for considerable streamlining particularly at the higher controlling and coordinating levels. In approaching Sir Henry Yellowlees to undertake a major review, the Ministry of Defence directed him to adopt a tri-partite study.

To some in the RN Medical and Dental Services, Orwell's predictions for the year '1984', were about to be realised!

Firstly, Yellowlees was to consider the medical headquarters structure. Secondly, he was to examine the arrangements for the use of MoD, NHS and private sector hospital resources and services, in particular as regards secondary care and postgraduate training, so as to achieve maximum cost effective use of all resources. Thirdly, his study was to consider the role of the Reserves in conjunction with civil medical resources, on the outbreak of war.

This was a massive task with, the almost impossible target date for completion by September that same year.

Sir Henry had been appointed Chief Medical Officer for England and Wales in 1973, a post which he held for a decade. Crucially he had also served on two of the previous committees which had reviewed the Headquarters organisation and was well aware of the complexities involved.

He had been an RAF pilot from 1941 to 1945 and thus had an insight into Service ways and had proved himself to be an outstanding administrator whilst serving in the Department of Health. He was said to be totally without status consciousness, genuinely non-discriminatory and always ready to give credit where it was due. He thus seemed to be eminently suited to conduct these studies.

However, it was always felt amongst the Central Medical Staffs that the final recommendations of the Part I study, the Central Organisation, were written before the study was conducted, a belief that was borne out by Sir Henry's changed views on the way that he wished to carry out the second part of his review – the hospitals' study. Nevertheless, it is likely that the conclusions for the reorganisation of the Central Medical Staffs would have been similar to his recommendations whoever had conducted the study. The need for change, however unwelcome to each single-Service Directorate, was inevitable and this is clearly evidenced by the drawing together of nearly all aspects of Yellowlees' recommendations by the Defence Central Staffs, which took place in subsequent decades.

The study commenced in March and Part I of the report was published at the end of June. The recommendations for the central staff were for a Surgeon General, in overall charge and under him to serve, two Deputy Surgeon Generals (Medical). Each Service was to be represented in the makeup of the three posts. There would also be a Deputy Surgeon General (Dental).

The next tier of management was to comprise six Assistant Surgeons General responsible respectively for:-

> **Organisation/Operations/Plans**
> **Service Hospitals**
> **Medical Supply**
> **Environment Medicine and Research**
> **Personnel & Training**
> **Nursing**

Beneath the Deputy Surgeon General (Dental) were to be two Assistant Surgeons General (Dental) again with each Service represented in the three posts.

The Surgeon General was to be appointed at three star level, the Deputy Surgeons General at two star and the Assistant Surgeons General at one star.

The Surgeon General and his staff were to be supported by a central Secretariat and Finance Department headed by a civil servant at Assistant Secretary grade. This latter structure mirroring what was already in place within the existing department of the Medical Director General (Naval).

These recommendations were accepted by the Secretary of State with the exception that Personnel Management would remain on a single Service basis under the control of the appropriate Principal Personnel Officer (Second Sea Lord in the case of the Navy). S of S also required these recommendations to be implemented by 2 January 1985. This left little time to implement such a radical change which also involved some relocation of staff. In addition, it was by no means clear how the new central structure would interface with the peripheral medical, dental and nursing services.

The tri-Service Defence Medical Services Headquarters was established at the end of December 1984. The first holder of the office of Surgeon General was Lieutenant General Sir Cameron Moffat who was Director General Army Medical Services whilst the senior dental post was filled by the head of the RAF Dental Service, Air Vice Marshal John Jones.

Several of the titles proposed by Yellowlees were dropped to conform more to Service convention and avoid the multiple use of the term "Surgeon General" amongst his deputies and assistants in the various starred posts. In the case of the dental services the three key posts were designated:

Director Defence Dental Services
Deputy Director Defence Dental Services (Organisation)
Deputy Director Defence Dental Services (Personnel & Training)[*]

---

[*] Much of the above description of the Yellowlees Study and its outcome was provided by Surgeon Commodore (D) Brian Robinson – Deputy Director Naval Dental Services, at the time of Yellowlees implementation.

The three single-Service medical and dental directorates had 'grouped up' and had moved to a new home at First Avenue House in Holborn, around 1980, when Admiral Mathias was the then Deputy Director of Naval Dental Services. There they had continued to lead their separate existences.

Thus, logistically, the formation of the new tri-Service Medical and Dental Directorates posed few problems. In terms of re-organisation, however, there were many bridges to cross. As recorded above, Air Vice Marshal John Jones, the Royal Air Force Dental Branch Director, was appointed as the first Director Defence Dental Services (DDDS). Surgeon Rear Admiral (D) Frank Mathias, whose post had been downgraded to one star (Surgeon Commodore (D)), was permitted to continue in post for the short term, but was to retire one year early in July 1985.

There is little doubt that, in pursuing the Government's sought after reduction in the number of 'stars' and the new dual hatted concept for the Directors of each single-Service branch, Yellowlees created many new problems, the interests of the single-Service branches being of necessity, pushed to the rear, whilst the work load placed upon deputies, who were also dual hatted, became, at times unmanageable. The situation was potentially particularly difficult for the Surgeon General and for DDDS, who, while remaining head of their own single-Service organisations, were supposed to exercise impartial control over tri-Service policies and their execution.

The outcome of 'Yellowlees II', the second part of Sir Henry Yellowlees' review, proved ultimately to be less radical in its proposals, and did not produce the dramatic savings which originally had been sought.

After some inter-Service infighting, which extended for the next two years and during which the roles in both war and peace of the Service hospitals were minutely examined, the Royal Naval Hospital Stonehouse (Plymouth) was spared (for the time being), balanced by the loss of one RAF hospital[67]. "Yellowlees III" was never completed and it is for conjecture that it was abandoned because Sir Henry was unhappy with the constraints placed upon him during the second part of his study.

Even before realising the savings achieved by Yellowlees, the effects of the 1981 Defence Review were also rolling on and shortly after assuming leadership of the RNDS, in late 1983, Admiral Mathias was obliged to announce other probable cuts pending, which were likely to affect the way in which dental officers in the clinics and the Fleet were able to do their jobs.

In an end of year message, published in the RNDS Newsletter, Admiral Mathias announced scrutiny into both the existence of the RN Dental Training School and the employment of (civilian) dental technicians, dedicated to the Royal Navy. With regard to the latter a blind trial was to be carried out, commencing in April 1984, at *HMS Drake* in Devonport, in which both the cost and quality of the RN dental laboratory and a contract laboratory would be compared.

An interim report was to be made to the Under Secretary of State for the Armed Forces, Lord Trefgarne, by September 1984. He also announced that the effect on dental officer manpower of the 1981 Review would result in a reduction from 102 in 1980 to 80 by 1988, with a consequent reduction in support personnel[68].

Yet another effect of the implementation of the 1981 Defence Review had been the announcement, in June 1983, that promotions to Surgeon Captain (D) would be reduced from once a year to one every eighteen months.

This did little to help the already low Branch morale and neither did it, two years later, when it was learned that Surgeon Rear (D) Admiral Frank Mathias would retire without the award of the CB, an honour which had been bestowed upon every Director of Naval Dental Services since 1956. This omission was regarded within the RNDS as an unnecessary insult to an able and dedicated officer and to the Branch.

These erosions to the prospects of career dental officers lead to a number of voluntary retirements, thus furthering the Government's policy of force reduction by 'natural wastage', rather than compulsory redundancy.

Whilst this upheaval was taking place at Directorate level, life at the 'coalface' continued much as before, with the ever present requirement to maintain a high quality of dental care for the men and women who manned and supported the Fleet.

As the RNDS progressed towards the last decade of the 20th Century, so this progress was punctuated occasionally and sadly by the passing of some of those distinguished dental officers who had contributed so much to both that progress and the Branch's reputation.

One of these was Surgeon Captain (D) W E ('Podge') Starkey, who died in May 1983. Podge had joined the RNVR about six months before the outbreak of WWII. At the end of the War, during which he served both ashore and afloat, he had transferred to the Permanent List, eventually turning his considerable talents to Oral Surgery.

After serving as Senior Specialist in the Royal Naval Hospital at Bighi in Malta, he returned to take up the post of Training Commander in the dental clinic at Victory Barracks, Portsmouth (now *HMS Nelson*). At that time few of the Branch oral surgeons had formal qualification in Oral Surgery and their appointments to RN Hospitals were based largely on experience. During their careers, most would chop and change between hospital and general service appointments.

Thus it was that Starkey found his final and long-term home in the RNDS, as the Director of Dental Training and Research at the RN Medical School (later the Institute of Naval Medicine in Alverstoke. Here, he continued the research into Strontium 90 levels in human teeth, started by Surgeon Rear Admiral (D) Bill Holgate*.

This research was regarded as highly important, by the Medical Research Council, which was, at the time, conducting broader studies into the medical effects of atmospheric nuclear weapon tests. Starkey's achievements were recognised by the award of the OBE in 1964.

Towards the end of his naval career, he undertook part-time duties at the Department of Dental Science at the Royal College of Surgeons of England, this leading, upon his retirement from the Navy, to an MRC research appointment at Bristol University.

This talented man was also known, throughout the RNDS, as a raconteur and as a most entertaining lecturer. On the regular occasions on which he was persuaded to talk to an audience of dental officers on a topic 'of the moment', he always attracted a full house. Starkey had, not only completed a distinguished career in the RNDS, but had also managed to continue in an active research post after his retirement from the Navy.

All RNDS officers and ratings were, however, saddened by the news of the passing of Surgeon Captain (D) A A (Alan) Davies, whilst still in service, in December 1984. Qualifying at the Turner Dental School in Manchester in July 1952, Alan Davies joined the Navy in February 1953, after completion of a house appointment. The early part of his career was spent at sea in the cruisers *HMS Gambia* and *HMS Jamaica*, moving on to serve some hospital appointments and then as a 'general service' RN dental officer. A quiet and unassuming man, he was liked and respected by his colleagues, both as a skilled dental surgeon and for an astonishing list of 'extramural' talents. He was an experienced yachtsman and as such, became an offshore examiner for the Royal Yachting Association. He was also Chairman of the Plymouth branch of the Royal Naval Sailing Association.

Alan Davies was also a skilled mountaineer and rock climber and was responsible for the setting up of the Station Mountain Rescue Team at the Royal Naval Air Station, Lossiemouth.

As if these activities were not enough to keep him occupied, Alan Davies was also a very talented musician. As a student, he had performed with the Hallé Choir and was an accomplished wind instrument player – most notably, the French horn.

---

* See both Volume I of this History and Appendix I of this volume.

His senior appointments included Director of Dental Training and Research, Staff Dental Surgeon to Flag Officer Submarines and Senior Dental Surgeon at both *HMS Drake* and *HMS Nelson*. As a Surgeon Captain, he was appointed as an Honorary Dental Surgeon to Her Majesty the Queen.

One appointment which he particularly enjoyed was as Officer in Charge of the RN Dental Training School.

During his time at RNDTS, he developed an affection and respect for the dental support staff and this was recognised when his widow, Irene, endowed the Alan Acton Davies Memorial Prize; awarded annually for excellence by Dental Surgery Assistants and Dental Hygienists. Alan Davies' untimely loss to the RNDS was widely mourned[69].

Despite the threat hanging over the RN Dental Training School, the service it provided to the Branch continued to evolve.

A five-day Senior Rates' Management Course was introduced in mid 1984[70] and in September, the School ran its first Dental Hygienist Refresher Course[71]. The Dental Training School also became involved in the Government's recently introduced Youth Training Scheme, taking on five, seventeen year old, school leavers for training as Dental Surgery Assistants.

Another first for the RNDS at this time was the award of Membership in General Dental Surgery to Surgeon Commanders (D) J G (John) Iles and D C C (David) Alexander. These were to be the first of a significant number of MGDS passes obtained by RNDS personnel.

Proficiency in dentistry is not the only requirement for RN dental officers. There may be occasions when medical or casualty situations have to be dealt with, either in the absence of a medical officer, or when a mass casualty situation overwhelms the medical staff available. A graphic account of Surgeon Lieutenant (D) G J (Graeme) Lumley's experience of the latter is copied below from the RNDS Newsletter[72]. Such incidents do not only occur during combat. Life at sea can always be hazardous. Lumley had joined *RFA Olwen**, as dental officer to a South Atlantic task group. After an easy voyage as far as the Ascension Islands, the weather began to deteriorate and the ships of the task group were battered by Force 9 to 10 winds and heavy seas.

> ### *Casualties!*
> After five days beating into the storm, the weather began to ease off and it was decided to send a party on to the forecastle to inspect the quite considerable weather damage. The ship slowed down and a party of twelve were sent out. ➤

---

* Royal Fleet Auxiliary (RFA) ships are merchant ships which accompany and support RN Warships. Their traditions and terminology are those of the Merchant Navy and they fly the Blue Ensign. They often carry additional RN personnel and RN helicopters with aircrew and support crews. When operating in combat zones they may be armed.

At about 1130 the ship ran into two freak waves, the second breaking right over the forecastle, sweeping the men off their feet into the deck fittings.

On hearing the pipe [broadcast] closing up the stretcher parties to deal with casualties…, I made my way down to the hospital, arriving just as the first casualties were brought in.

The first two brought in, were both soaked through and badly shocked. As I was sorting out first-aiders to deal with them, the more seriously injured started coming in. The first stretcher was carrying [a man] who had a crush injury to his left temple. The back of his head was blood-soaked and his lips were blue. He had no pulse and was not breathing. With assistance, I started cardiopulmonary resuscitation, whilst questioning the stretcher bearers on the numbers of injured and their condition.

Learning that there were another three or four badly injured, I left the first-aiders to continue to work on this man and went to look at the next man who had been brought in.

Two further casualties were being looked after in the hospital and another stretcher was coming through the door. With the hospital crowded, I instructed that he be taken to the Officers' Lounge, where I examined him.

He was not breathing and had no pulse; cardiopulmonary resuscitation was therefore started and further examination revealed a large hole in the upper left thigh and a field dressing was placed tightly over the injury. I had just finished this when further casualties were brought in.

The most serious had a simple fracture of the left forearm, a possible fracture of the left femur and what appeared to be compound fractures of the right femur and pelvis. The open wounds were dressed and morphine administered, first-aiders being left to place a temporary splint on the left forearm. The other casualty was very shocked, but apart from a large swelling medial to the left scapula, he appeared uninjured.

In the hospital I found the first patient with a simple fracture of the left forearm and a compound fracture of the left femur. He also had a full thickness laceration to his left cheek, with other cuts on his chin. He was bleeding from the left ear.

Morphine had been given him by the RFA doctor and his pulse and breathing were strong.

The other casualty was in great pain from his chest. He had no external injuries, but the left side of his chest was very tender to palpation and sounded slightly dull. I was sure that he had fractured ribs on this side and probably had a pneumothorax. He was lying on his back and his breathing was strained. I administered 15 milligrams of morphine, to reduce the pain enough to allow us to sit him up and give him oxygen. He appeared to be breathing easier, so I left the Second Officer to watch him, with instructions to call me if there were any change, and returned to the Lounge. »+

The resuscitation efforts were not proving effective; however, the less seriously injured were looking more cheerful. I did a quick check of the remainder of those who had been on the forecastle and then assigned them simple tasks to prevent shock setting in. It was now about 1215 and the medical officer from *HMS Broadsword,* Surgeon Lieutenant Alec Goodwin, arrived [by helicopter]. I gave him a rapid brief on the situation, the state of the injured and the treatment we had carried out so far.

The second serious casualty was pronounced dead, as the resuscitation efforts had been in progress for thirty minutes with no effect. We then went round the injured. All were re-examined and injuries confirmed. About 1230, Surgeon Lieutenant Malcolm Scott arrived from *HMS Birmingham* and he was briefed on the situation. Whilst the doctors worked on the two casualties in the hospital, I put up an IV line on the patient with limb fractures and made him more comfortable in the lounge. With both femurs and his pelvis fractured, heavy blood loss was estimated, so two units of Haemocel were run in rapidly, then another more slowly. I then went round to check on the cases of shock. All were doing well and a snack of soup and bread were provided for them from the galley.

In the hospital, a chest drain had been inserted for the chest injury man; however, it was now obvious that there was a flail segment on the left side.

Problems were experienced in placing an IV line and [after two attempts] a line was finally placed in the left cubital fossa above the fractured forearm. The flail segment was now causing concern and so sutures were placed through the intercostals muscles of the segment and then secured with rubber bands to the edge of the bunk.

With all the seriously injured now stable, it was time to sit down and take stock. Full notes were written for each patient, along with fluid balance charts and drug administration records. Those with minor injuries were examined by the doctors and left in the care of the first aiders.

It was decided to bring over [a member of *Broadsword's* medical staff] to assist in the nursing care of the injured and to stabilise the fractures and arrange CASEVAC to the British Military Hospital Stanley (BMH), as soon as possible. We worked on each of the injured as a team. The forearm fracture was reduced and a backslab [splint] placed. The compound fracture of the leg was [partially] reduced and a 'Jet Splint' placed.

This later proved to be inadequate … and the injured leg was splinted to the sound right leg. I carried out a more careful examination of the facial injury. The left maxilla was completely smashed and I removed [the upper left premolars] which had been completely evulsed. Bruising around both eyes and bleeding from the ear indicated the possibility of a Le Fort III fracture and so, appropriate antibiotic cover was instituted. ➺

> Examination of the mandible was made difficult by the severity of the soft tissue damage and resultant oedema. I was reluctant to examine intra-orally too far as I did not want to jeopardise the airway. X-rays taken later at BMH showed that the mandible was in several pieces. An early attempt to reduce the leg fractures had to be abandoned, as it was causing the patient too much pain. A subsequent attempt was successful when I obtained adequate analgesia using IV Pethidine and Valium.
>
> [Our sister ship] *RFA Olna* had sailed from Stanley. She was to sail north and then fly off the Sea Kings. The intention was to leapfrog the Sea Kings from us to *Olna* and then on to Stanley, where BMH had been alerted.
>
> We finally finished working on the injured at about 0130 and I snatched a couple of hours sleep. The next morning was spent clothing the injured for a long, cold trip. We pinned as much clothing as we could around them. They were then placed in sleeping bags in air-portable stretchers, which were then wrapped in plastic shower curtains. It was decided that the two doctors would travel in the first helo, with the casualty who was causing the most concern. They would take the only walking casualty we had, as well. I was to go in the second helo with *Broadsword's* Petty Officer Medical Assistant and the other two casualties.
>
> All went as planned. The trip to Stanley took several hours with a brief stopover on [*RFA*] *Olna* to refuel. All the injured arrived at BMH alive and stable. We handed them over to the hospital staff who worked overnight in theatre. We were returned to our respective ships the following day by helo. The injured were all CASEVACed to UK, over the next couple of weeks. All have now made a complete recovery and are out of hospital.
>
> [N.B. "CASEVAC" is the Service abbreviation for "Casualty Evacuation"]

The above, slightly abridged account, describes one of the most extreme casualty situations encountered by a Royal Navy dental officer in war or peace. It demonstrates well, however, the sort of situation for which RNDS personnel must be trained and prepared, when they are deployed to sea. It is not all 'filling and drilling' by any means! Lumley was a 'graduate' of the Combat Casualty Care Course and had done a resuscitation course prior to embarkation. He had clearly learned his lessons well.

For some years the RNDS had been involved in making a series of films on Oral Health and Dental First Aid for non-dental personnel such as doctors and medical assistants at sea, and the cox'ns of small ships and submarines which carried no medical staff. During the previous year, the latest effort, titled "A Hole in One – Management of Dental Emergencies by Non-Medically Trained Personnel" had been entered for the 1984 BMA Film Competition. This film was memorable for its opening sequence, starring Surgeon Captain

(D) D A (David) Coppock, by 1985 the Assistant Director Dental Services (Navy) – ADDS(N), sinking a putt on the golf course. This sequence was followed by a close up of a ball of dental cement being swept from a glass slab by a 'plastic' dental instrument very much the same shape as the putter and emulating the same action!

The announcement that this film had won the Gold Award was met with great delight [73]. Both Gold and Silver Awards had been previously won by RNDS training films.

Another cause of great pleasure within the Branch, was the admission to the Grade of Officer (Brother) in the Order of St John of Jerusalem, of Surgeon Commander (D) G H A (George) Rudge. His appointment to this honour was principally in recognition of his work during the Falklands Campaign. George Rudge was the second RNDS officer to be thus honoured.

January 1985 saw the implementation of the new Yellowlees structure, with Surgeon Rear Admiral Mathias taking on the new title of Director of Dental Services (Navy) – DDS(N). He also wore a second (tri-Service) hat as Deputy Director Defence Dental Services (Organisation) – DDDDS(Org).

Early 1985 also saw the appointment of Surgeon Captain (D) C T (Clem) Stacey, then serving as Fleet Dental Surgeon on the staff of C-in-C Fleet at Northwood, Middlesex as an Honorary Dental Surgeon to HM the Queen. On Friday 10 May 1985, the third Wood Lecture and Clinical Day was held at the Institute of Naval Medicine, the key lecture being given by Professor Sir Paul Bramley. Although an oral surgeon himself, Professor Bramley chose to speak on the non-clinical subject of 'dental politics', lifting the veil on a (within the RNDS) little understood, but fascinating aspect of our profession, with a glimpse of his view of the future of dentistry in the UK. Prior to the 'main event', a number of RN Dental Officers had treated their audience to a variety of high quality presentations on matters of both clinical and general interest. The proceedings at INM were followed by the Director's Dinner, held in the Wardroom at *HMS Dolphin* and attended by 112 serving, reserve and retired dental officers[74].

At the Dinner, the Harvey-Fletcher Medal and Prize was presented, by Admiral Mathias, to Surgeon Lieutenant Commander (D) A M (Andy) Prosser.

We have met Andy earlier in this History, in his accounts both of his experiences with 40 Commando Royal Marines, during the Falklands Campaign and on the British Joint Services Hovercraft Expedition to Peru. In his citation, Admiral Mathias commended Prosser for his prowess in passing the All Arms Commando Course, no mean achievement in itself and in addition to the above mentioned achievements, his service with the Commando in

South Armagh, Northern Ireland. He also praised the manner in which he had more recently dealt with serious illness, commenting that his dedication and bravery had earned him the highest respect of his colleagues and had enhanced the reputation of the Dental Branch. Prosser was about to leave the Royal Navy on completion of an eventful Short Service Commission[75]. Sadly, within a year of his leaving the RNDS, Andy Prosser was to succumb to a recurrence of his illness.

May 1985 also saw the retirement from the Royal Navy of Surgeon Commander (D) G B (Geoff) Keeble. Keeble, an oral surgeon, had served in *SS Uganda* during the Falklands campaign, which had interrupted his last appointment as Officer-in-Charge of the RN Dental Training School.

The long established post of Director of Dental Training and Research (DDTR) at the Institute of Naval Medicine in Alverstoke (INM) had in 1982 been combined with that of INM's Head of the Training Division. The appointments had been combined, following negotiation by the then incumbent, Surgeon Captain (D) Brian Robinson, to provide the measure of responsibility needed to justify the appointment of a Surgeon Captain (D) at a time when there was continuing downward pressure on senior manpower billets, both at INM and in the RNDS.

In addition to the traditional tasks of supervision of training and research within the Branch, DDTR now held departmental responsibility for all training courses provided by INM, including all radiation protection courses and the training of medical staff in nuclear powered submarines.

The latter, were not only required to provide seaborne medical support to personnel in these boats, but were also trained as specialists in nuclear health physics, able to provide the commanding officer with advice on radiation problems and the monitoring of the nuclear environment within the boats.

In addition, DDTR was also responsible for the organisation and running of all conferences and symposia at INM and, again as Head of Training, the running of New Entry Medical and Dental Officer Courses, including the Combat Casualty Care Course, which by now included all newly entered medical, dental, medical services and nursing officers.

Add to the above the continuing editorship of the RNDS Newsletter and the administration of a training staff of some size and DDTR found himself with a demanding but intensely interesting job.

Although not directly involved in Radiation Protection training and the training of Medical Assistants in submarines (MA(SM)), the proper execution of his duties required the acquisition of a broad understanding of the role of both ballistic missile and hunter-killer submarines in the Cold War environment.

Robinson was relieved in the DDTR post by Surgeon Captain (D) T J C (Timothy) Hall who was, in June 1985, himself relieved by Acting Surgeon Captain (D) S N (Stewart) Bussell. Both officers had carried forward the combined appointment, taking particular interest in the Combat Casualty Care Course – still regarded, with pride, as an RNDS achievement, despite the participation of officers from the medical branches.

On 2 July 1985, Surgeon Commodore (D) David Coppock MSc BDS, relieved Admiral Mathias as DDS(N). David Coppock was the first Director to be appointed in the one-star (Commodore) rank. He was later to be promoted Surgeon Rear Admiral (D) on appointment as Director of Defence Dental Services and would be the last RN dental officer to attain two-star rank within the span of this History. The photograph below shows him in the higher rank.

He had joined the Royal Navy in 1955, soon after qualifying from Guy's Hospital. His career had included sea time in the aircraft carriers *HMS Eagle* and *HMS Hermes* (the latter appointment including operational involvement in the Suez crisis of 1956), overseas shore appointments in Hong Kong and Gibraltar and he had been the first RNDS officer to serve on exchange with the US Navy Dental Corps. His non-clinical appointments had included Director of Dental Training and Research and Command Dental Surgeon to C-in-C Naval Home Command.

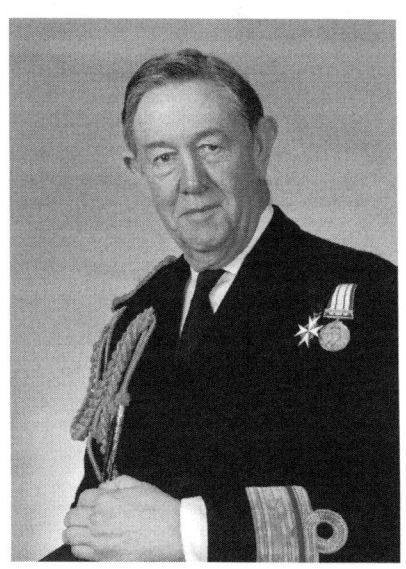

Surgeon Rear Admiral (D)
David Coppock CB OStJ QHDS

In common with many of his RNDS colleagues, David Coppock had participated frequently over the years in Royal Navy thespian activities with some success, both as an actor and producer. He was also a talented and amusing raconteur, being much in demand as an after dinner speaker. It was probably serendipity which found this man of great humour and charisma appointed head of the RNDS early in the History of the Defence Dental Services Directorate.

He would need all his skills and experience to steer Naval Dentistry through the difficult times ahead.

The evolution of dental records within the Defence Dental Services (DDS) had continued and at the beginning of 1985 the new record folder (F Med 271) was introduced.

This had room not only for treatment notes but for radiographs, a medical History form and the newly introduced Periodontal Index for Treatment (PIT). The latter had been devised following a collaborative research programme carried out in 1981, between the RN Dental Training School and Professor R D Emslie of Guy's Hospital as part of a wider World Health Organisation research project. The PIT anticipated, by around two years, the introduction of a similar, but more complex, and internationally accepted index into the General Dental Services of the NHS. Its introduction served two purposes. It heightened the awareness of dental officers to the importance of the diagnosis and control of periodontal (gum) disease and provided a simple guide to treatment planning of these conditions.

Coincident with the reorganisation of Service dentistry, a new system of fiscal responsibility had been introduced into the Armed Services, with budgets being devolved downwards from Top Level (Commands) to establishments (ships were initially exempt from this measure). Thus each establishment commanding officer held an Establishment Responsibility Budget (ERB), for which he had to bid each year.

October 1985 saw a modification of the colour coding system of the dental status of each service man and woman. At around the same time, Surgeon Captain (D) Brian Robinson, by now Command Dental Surgeon to C-in-C Naval Home Command, introduced a Clinical Profile Monitoring System[76]. The CPMS was built around some simple 'Performance Indicators' (PI), which themselves enabled both Commands and those who held the purse strings in the MoD, to determine whether they were getting value for money from the RNDS. Robinson devised a set of PIs for the clinics within Naval Home Command. They included Fitness Levels; Waiting Times for Treatment and Numbers Out of Date for Inspection. The results from each clinic could be aggregated to give an objective view of the clinic's efficiency and could inform Command and MoD reports of performance against previously set targets.

CPMS was a useful tool. It soon identified which clinics were stretched and which were overmanned. Commanding officers liked it, because it gave them easily understood management information. Eventually it was adopted by most other commands[77].

In July 1985, Surgeon Commander L C (Clive) Langan, joined the newly commissioned *HMS Ark Royal*, the last of the three *Invincible* Class aircraft carriers – a welcome additional sea-going appointment for an RN dental officer.

Adventure and exercise was not only the prerogative of RNDS personnel serving at sea and abroad. Despite, or perhaps because of, the pressures of work within the busy shore-based dental clinics, senior RNDS officers encouraged the occasional 'time out' for adventurous training.

The Spring 1985 edition of the RNDS Newsletter carries an account of one such 'exped', undertaken the previous winter and led by the Senior Dental Surgeon at *HMS Cochrane* at Rosyth in Scotland[78]. An abridged version of the *Cochrane* team's adventures is given below.

> ### *'Fun' in a Cold Climate!*
>
> There was a mixed reaction when the Senior Dental Surgeon Announced that he thought it was time for the *Cochrane* dental team to "get away from it all" for a relaxing winter long weekend in the Cairngorms.
>
> Thus it was, on a Friday at the end of November, the enthusiastic and the reluctant could be seen cramming themselves into a hired red minibus, together with a mountain of personal gear, sleeping bags, long johns, knitting, etc. The convoy headed north, lead by Petty Officer PT Instructor Henry Gibson in a Landrover, also crammed to the gunnels with ropes, climbing equipment and food, food and more food!
>
> Pine Cottage is situated in the village of Newtonmore, about 15 miles south of Aviemore. It is owned by *HMS Cochrane* and provides a first class base for adventurous training activities in the Cairngorms area. Friday night was St. Andrew's Night and the party, en masse, repaired to a local hostelry where, it was advertised, a Ceilidh (Gaelic for Rave Up) was to take place. The music was certainly Highland in nature (strangled cats etc.), but there was not much flinging going on. As soon as the music gathered a bit of momentum and hands and feet started to tap out the rhythm, we, the audience were severely admonished by the MC (who also doubled up as cat-strangler-in-chief). "Be quiet!" we were told, "This is a seerrrious occasion!"
>
> Bright and early Saturday morning, the party piled into the minibus and we headed for the hills.
>
> Half an hour's drive found us in the car park at the foot of the Cairngorm ski complex, where we divided into two teams. The 'Young and Energetic' following 'clubswinger' Henry Gibson and the 'Golden Oldies' led by Iain Burton and his wife Janice. Iain, an experienced mountain man, is the Captain's driver at *HMS Cochrane*. The plan was for each team to assault the Cairn Gorm by a circular route, from a different direction, meeting in the middle and completing each circuit back to the car park. As we set off the weather conditions were clear and dry. Visibility was excellent and, apart from a few innocent looking white patches, high above us, there was no snow.
>
> The Clubswinger's team set off to make the direct assault, up the ski-runs to the South-West.
>
> An initial fast pace slowed fairly rapidly and several Wren DSAs exhibited hidden talents as 'heavy breathers', by the time the Ptarmigan Hut was reached. »

Thinking herself at the summit, Bindy Southey suffered a mild sense of humour failure, when told they were only half way up! Meanwhile, Hare and Tortoise style, the Golden Oldies were making good progress on the gentler, but longer ascent towards Cairn Lochan, the only obstacles being frequent burns in spate, which had to be leapt across.

By midday the Oldies were walking the ridge above Coire an Lochain, looking down at 'Jean's Hut' far below. It was here that the 'innocent white stuff' seen from below, turned out to be hard, frozen snow, which, in the steeper parts, presented quite a problem as we did not have crampons. Iain Burton made the ascent somewhat easier, by cutting steps with his ice axe. It was also here that Bindy Southey, Sandra Foster and Jennie Richards, in the other team, travelling west-about, made a spectacular and rapid descent on the broadest parts of their anatomies!

The two teams met up on the ridge above Coire an Sneachda and after a brief breather, continued on their respective ways. The views, by now, in all directions, were breathtaking. Loch Morlich and Rothiemurchus could be clearly seen below us, to the North. To the South, only three miles distant, the peak of Ben Macdhui, at 1309 metres, the second highest in Scotland. Closer still was Loch Etchachan, one of the highest mountain lochs. At the foot of the final ascent to Cairn Gorm, the 'Oldies' split up; Jennie Burton, Leading Wren Janet Gill and Chief Wren Eleanor White, making the direct descent to the car park via Coire Chais. Iain Burton, Surgeon Lieutenant (D) Steve Liggins, POMA Dave Wilson and the SDS (Surgeon Commander (D) Ted Grant), making the final assault on the peak (1245 metres). It was whilst surveying the view from the top that the first snow flakes fell. By the time the 'Oldies' were reunited in the warmth of the car park cafeteria, near 'white-out' conditions prevailed. Forty five minutes later the vanguard of the 'Young and Energetic' loomed out of the blizzard! Sense of humour once again restored by hot drinks and food, we left the snow-covered car park to find it raining back at Pine Cottage.

On Sunday, most of the party drove north to Kingussie, where Iain Burton led us on a brisk 20 minute climb, to some crags, several hundred feet above the village. The view was unbelievable, with a white blanket of mist filling the Spey valley below, across which could be seen the snow covered peaks which were the scene of our previous day's exertions.

The object of this day's exercise was to introduce us to the joys of rock climbing. Led, once again by Iain Burton, we assaulted various precipitous rock faces, from both above and below. Surgeon Lieutenant (D) Nick Poppelwell gave fair imitations of a fly, with Chief Wren (DH) Eleanor White not far behind him in speed of ascent. Bringing up the rear, Steve Liggins and the SDS were more than somewhat slower, but made it to the top, despite fingers freezing to the rock face. It was the latter two who entertained the rest of the party with their efforts at abseiling down! Steve Liggins got his moleskin britches in a twist, when ⇒

> he lost contact with the rock face, half way down.
>
> SDS lost his footing at the top and, giving a fair imitation of a pendulum, met the rock face going the other way, the point of contact being where the van keys were in his pocket. The result was a spectacular key-shaped bruise in a place where he was far too bashful to show it off!
>
> The weather having clamped down on Monday, on Tuesday we returned to *Cochrane*, amid (to the surprise of SDS) cries of: "When can we do it again?"

In the new tri-Service Directorate, life was not at all a 'bed of roses'. The task of interweaving, the traditions, objectives and ambitions of those at the top of the three Service Dental Branches, was, of necessity a delicate one, requiring a high degree of tact and sensitivity by all concerned. This was not always forthcoming.

The new Director, Surgeon Commodore (D) D A (David) Coppock, quickly found himself embroiled in some of the in-fighting which was to characterise the next few years within the Directorate.

Shortly after assuming the post, he felt constrained to write a brief message in the Branch Newsletter.[79] The message gives a flavour of the times and is reproduced below.

> ### *Message from the Director*
>
> This is a brief message from your new leader to inform you that the dust is slowly settling following the departure of Surgeon Rear Admiral (D) Mathias.
>
> Although I served in the same building as Deputy [Director], for three and a half years, not so long ago, I can assure you that things have changed dramatically. No longer are our pin-stripe suits dark blue. We mingle with our colleagues from the other two Services, as we struggle to set up an efficient combined Directorate. There are naturally many problems to overcome and long held prejudices to suppress, but slowly things are beginning to take shape. We have a common aim, so we shall succeed, given time.
>
> I cannot claim any major achievements during my short time here. There are daunting challenges ahead and some of the solutions are unpalatable, but, be assured, my Deputy and I are constantly fighting for your best interests. Common Terms of Service are one of our long term aims; a simple enough arrangement to achieve, you might think. It is only when one looks beneath the surface that the snags and pitfalls appear and my original over-simplistic views will have to be modified.
>
> Although we are under constant surveillance, or perhaps because of it, I am anxious to direct our measurement of efficiency away from the outdated

> piecework priority, which has dogged the entire profession for too long. The new clinical profile is a step in the right direction and I intend to go further down the path to ensure fighting fitness for our patients, based on high quality dentistry and a scrupulous clinical assessment of their true needs.
>
> It has never been more important to keep the lines of communication open in both directions. Whilst I cannot burst into print on some of the more delicate issues, I intend to hold regular meetings with my senior management officers, so that what information I can leak will be quickly disseminated. I also hope to get around the parish in the coming months to maintain the personal contact, which I rate highly.
>
> In the meantime, I must stick to generalities. "Value for Money" are the watchwords, so be sure you all give it.

Coppock mentions in his message, the particularly sensitive problem of "common Terms of Service". These had, historically, evolved differently within the three Branches. The RNDS, being the smallest of the three, had far less room for manoeuvre. For instance, retirement age for dental officers reaching the rank of Captain, or equivalent, differed; being 57 in the RNDS and 60 in the Royal Army Dental Corps and the RAF Dental Branch.

Within our smaller organisation, an immediate move to the higher retirement age, would lead to an unacceptable blockage in promotions for those lower down, since it was unlikely that the Branch would be granted additional senior billets.

An even more difficult problem was also to do with promotions. Within the RNDS, promotion to senior rank (Surgeon Commander (D) and Surgeon Captain (D)) was by selection on merit and was subject to scrutiny by the 'Big Navy' in the person of the Second Sea Lord (Chief of Naval Personnel).

The number of 'billets' within each rank band, was also strictly controlled by the Director General Naval Manpower Planning. At an individual level, promotion not only opened up further career opportunities but brought increased pay and, ultimately, increased pensions. In the RADC and the RAF Dental Branch, promotions to Commander and Captain equivalent, were made generally on time served. Some were selected for earlier promotion on merit, but most would achieve senior rank within a full career.

Also, within the RNDS rating structure, it was not possible for Wren Dental Surgery Assistants and Dental Hygienists to achieve rank beyond Chief Petty Officer and those who were selected for promotion to officer rank, were obliged to leave the Branch and take promotion in another category, since there were no dental support officer billets in the RNDS.

Another, lesser problem was that of leave allowances. Once again the RNDS was the 'poor cousin'. It was to take many years and another major structural review of the Defence Dental Services, before most of these problems could be properly addressed.

In his message, Commodore Coppock also mentioned the setting up of a "regular meetings with my senior management officers". These meetings of 'Command and Staff Dental Advisers', or 'RNDS Managers' Meetings' as they became known, were to become a regular feature of Directorate routine and worked well, enabling, not only the dissemination of information from 'above', but also, discussion of feedback from the 'coalface'.

The first Managers' Meeting, held in the tri-Service Directorate at First Avenue House, addressed mainly the manpower problems rolling on from the 1981 Defence Review.

Although the numbers of dental officers had almost kept pace with the overall numbers of naval personnel, the meeting recognised that there was a worrying shortfall in Dental Surgery Assistant (DSA) numbers.

In order to address a rising rate of unemployment amongst school-leavers, the Government had recently set up a Youth Training Scheme (YTS) and the Armed Forces had agreed to accept one-year YTS 'recruits' for training in various categories. It was hoped that this might include the DSA category, thus alleviating some of the manpower stretch.

Another matter which would have longer term implications for the Branch, was the decision by the General Dental Council to introduce a period of Vocational Training (VT) for new dental graduates. Following discussion of this scheme by a committee set up by Surgeon Captain (D) S N (Stewart) Bussell, the Director of Dental Training and Research, it was decided that the RNDS would run a pilot scheme in early 1986. The scheme would run for twelve months and would initially involve two New Entry Dental Officers. The course would include the Combat Casualty Care Course, Resuscitation Training and general postgraduate clinical training[80].

Amid all the 'gloom and doom' at Directorate level, there were still opportunities for RNDS personnel for travel, adventure and recreation. Surgeon Lieutenant Commander (D) Stephen Lambert Humble gives the following account of sporting endeavour in Hong Kong[81].

Enter the Dragon

The madness begins just after Easter. Suddenly about 40 men and not quite so many women leap into jogging outfits and can be seen at all hours of the day and night, running round the perimeters of the Naval Base at *HMS Tamar*. ≫▸

They are beginning to train for that one-day event, known as Tuen Ng. Any wiser? Well, of course, if you have been fortunate enough to serve in *HMS Tamar*, you will know that this is the Dragon Boat Festival.

The Festival of the Dragon Boats is held on the fifth day of the fifth moon, which for those who don't follow the Chinese calendar is early to mid-June. It is also known as Poet's Day and commemorates the death of the poet Ch'u Yuen, who drowned himself in the Mi Lo River in Hunan Province, in protest against the corrupt and decadent government of the day. It is said that a rice dumpling was thrown into the water, to feed the fish which would otherwise have eaten his body and the water was beaten with paddles to scare off evil spirits and other fish. Nowadays, the dumplings are still made and eaten by the celebrants and, narrow, gaily decorated boats, with the head and tail of a dragon, race against each other, paddling furiously to the beating of large drums on the boats.

Back in *Tamar*, six weeks away from the races, the prospective team members take to the water – of the swimming pools, that is! The training is vicious. They swim up and down the pool, getting out at each end, doing ten press-ups and back in again. This is repeated, non-stop, for about 20 minutes. My surgery window overlooks the pool and, at the end of the session, I am exhausted, just watching! The fun bit now comes. They practice paddling surf boards up and down the pool, kneeling upon them and, amid much laughter, falling off them. Next, to get their rhythm going, they kneel along the side of the pool, each with a paddle and attempt to paddle *Tamar* itself, half way up Hong Kong harbour.

At last they are ready to take to the boats, for real; and now for the real sorting of the men from the boys – and the women from the girls! Some fail to make the team and the rest fight to be in the front half of the boat, where the best oarsmen and women will be. My interest, naturally, polarises around the *Tamar* ladies team, not least because Leading Wren (DH) Karin Evans has made the team and has gained considerable kudos, by being [chosen as] port side bow (stroke) oarswoman.

The day of the race dawns. It is blisteringly hot – with temperatures in the mid-90s and no wind. The men's' team had left *Tamar* at 0600, in order to 'stake out' the best position on the water. Amidst great excitement, lots of San Miguel (drunk by the supporters) and a tremendous cacophony of noise, the races begin and last all day. At the end, the men's team finishes second, but the ladies' team succeed in winning the trophy. Well done Karin!

RNDS personnel have always taken great pride in the standard of their work, which so often goes unappreciated by the majority of their clients. It was thus, with pleasure that a letter was received in late 1985 at the dental clinic in *HMS Cochrane* at Rosyth. It read as follows:

"Dear Sir, I just thought you might be interested that today my husband is having extracted, a molar which he had filled at Rosyth in 1941! It has never been touched since, the filling still being intact; the tooth has almost worn away! He maintains it was filled with a bit of a battleship, but it speaks well of the Royal Navy dental surgeons and he wishes he could have come back to Rosyth, to allow the RN to finish the job it started 45 years ago!

Yours sincerely, B M White (Mrs)"

A reply was sent to Mrs White which read as follows:

"Dear Mrs White,
We are really thrilled to hear
your very welcome news.
The tooth which at Rosyth was filled
Has taken years to lose.

We Naval 'Toothies' work so hard
So Jack can without problems dine
And ever help his country guard
In Senior Service still so fine.

We're oft' forgotten, seldom praised
But, Madam, you have filled our cup.
Our flagging spirits you have raised
Dear Mrs White, you've cheered us up!"

Despite the longevity of such conservative treatment, there was now a definite movement within UK dentistry away from 'drilling and filling' and towards a more preventive approach – a philosophy long held by many within the RNDS and indeed within our sister Services, the three Service dental branches having lead the way, nationally, with the training and employment of dental hygienists.

In 1986, a number of papers from both Government and from within the profession would point in this direction and, in order to ensure that the RNDS remained 'ahead of the game', the Director, Commodore Coppock, set up a 'think tank' of his senior officers, named the RN Dental Strategy Review Group. This group was to meet regularly over the next several years, not only to discuss the matter of Preventive Dentistry, but to 'brainstorm' various issues and problems, as they occurred and to advise the Director on the way forward in each case.

Another, almost inevitable, casualty of the economic and political climate in 1985 was the much respected Royal Naval Dental Training School

(RNDTS). Occupying, as it did, part of an old Edwardian drill hall within the perimeter of *HMS Nelson,* a new build had been on the cards in 1981, when Portsmouth City Council had proposed widening the road next to the school.

This event would have meant moving out of the building. The Council proposal had included provision of some money to help provide new premises. Sadly, what had looked like an affordable scheme had been quashed by John Nott's Defence Review and RNDTS had been under threat since that time. Both of the sister branches had modern training facilities and there were no longer either the funds or the political will to provide the same for the RNDS. Thus RNDTS closed.

The school so ably launched by Philip Duly, had for the past twenty years, trained many hundreds of Dental Surgery Assistants, Dental Hygienists (including civilians), Medical Assistants (Dental) and had run both qualifying and advancement courses for all RN dental ratings. It had also provided post-graduate refresher courses for dental officers and dental first aid courses for non-medical personnel in small ships and submarines. The school's reputation for first class training and efficient administration was no longer a defence.

Losing its 'Direct Command' training establishment status, a new department was set up within *HMS Nelson* under Surgeon Commander (D) A J (Alan) Woodman, the last Officer-in-Charge of RNDTS and now designated Commander Dental Training (CDT).

Dental Hygienist training was transferred, initially to the Institute of Dental Health and Training at RAF Halton, but was later moved again to the Royal Army Dental Corps Training Centre in Aldershot. There the staff included one Chief Wren Dental Hygienist, who also fulfilled the role of Divisional Officer to the WRNS personnel. All other training originally carried out at RNDTS, was continued in the new department.

John Nott's legacy lived on!

*****

Chapter 6

Changes and Challenges
1986 – 1989

In addition to the changing scene in dental treatment planning philosophy, another 'revolution' was beginning to impinge upon the working lives of all in the RNDS. Computers had been around in one form or another for many years, but the majority of these were mainframe computers, based in and used by universities, large commercial organisations and industry. Now, in the mid to late 1980s, personal computers (PCs) were beginning to come within the affordable range of individuals – albeit, as yet, with little memory and power compared with those available today and far less 'user friendly'. The RNDS Newsletter of Summer 1986 (written on an Amstrad Word Processor), carried an editorial which acknowledged the potential for the use of computers within the RNDS [82].

This issue also carried articles on the use of computers within the clinics for such purposes as appointment systems, patient records and the recording of dental treatment. Chief Wren DSA Sally Rowe reported on a course on 'Microcomputers for Administration', which she had attended at Exeter University. The course had included word processing and the storage and retrieval of records (databases). It should be remembered that although software design was advancing rapidly, that available for office use at that time, did not include the graphic interfaces such as Windows and production of a word processed document or the use of a database, required the user to learn a series of 'command codes'.

The first RNDS Managers' Meeting of 1986 addressed the issue of simplifying the work returns from the clinics and of developing a new computerised system which would enable the Director to provide quick answers to the many 'efficiency' and 'cost effectiveness' questions asked of him. At the same meeting, managers were informed of the progress of a MoD enquiry into the employment of dental technicians in the Armed Forces [83].

Despite some early difficulties, there were those in the Branch who were bitten by the computer bug from the start and who made it their business fully to understand computers and their potential application to our business.

Foremost among these was Surgeon Commander (D) Stephen Lambert Humble, who was in due course, to become Adviser in Information Technology to the Medical Director General (Naval) and who, within the next decade, was to be instrumental in bringing about the introduction of a full clinical support IT system into RN dental clinics, this same system, being taken up eventually by the sister Branches.

Another RN dental officer who was, at that time, developing 'specialist' interests, was Surgeon Commander (D) D C C (David) Alexander. Alexander, an experienced clinician, was now showing himself to be equally talented in the field of research. In mid-1986, he published a paper on caries activity in a sample of 25 year-olds [84]. In following up this line of research, Alexander was to become a self-taught and nationally acknowledged authority on nutrition. Employed in a specially created research post as Head of Oral Research at the Institute of Naval Medicine, he published a series of papers on the nutrition and diet of sailors. Eventually, moving away from the links between diet and dental disease, he led a large research project on the dietary needs of Royal Marines.

It was around this time also, that health care workers of all disciplines were beginning to be aware of the dangers of cross-infection with special regard to Hepatitis B and HIV/AIDS. The Defence Dental Services were quick to react to these issues and all clinical staff were to adopt the use of facemasks and disposable gloves when treating patients. The more complex issues of conducting sound infection control procedures when using chairside equipment were also addressed. The impact on our clinical assistants was reflected in another Newsletter article by PO Wren DH Yvonne Evans [85].

Also in early 1986, DNDS was able to announce the launch of the memorial prize in honour of Surgeon Captain (D) Alan Davies, whose death, whilst in service, two years previously, had been greatly mourned within the RNDS. Thanks to a generous donation from his widow, Irene Davies and additional donations collected from RNDS personnel of all ranks, a prize fund was set up to award the annual Alan Acton Davies Memorial Prize to the RNDS rating judged to have contributed the most to the Branch and its reputation during each year. The Prize would consist of a medallion, an inscription on an honours board and a cash prize.

Another 1986 innovation was the launch of the Dental Surgery Design Steering Committee, under the Chairmanship of Surgeon Captain (D) Brian Robinson whose objective was to avoid some of the costly procurement mistakes of the past. Surgeon Commander (D) M W (Mark) Weston was designated team leader. He proved to be a very capable organiser and the benefits of his design skills and those of other team members, soon became apparent.

The dental care of all RN personnel, working in the many MoD departments in London had, for many years been vested in the Naval Dental Clinic (NDC) in the Empress State Building at Earls Court. The NDC staff consisted of two dental officers, three Wren DSAs and a dental hygienist. The clinic's 'parish' also included the Royal Naval College Greenwich, the Royal Marines School of Music at Deal in Kent and, somewhat more exotically, the NATO Base at Naples in Italy. The three latter commitments were covered by periodic visits from the main clinic staff. In Naples there was a permanent billet for a Leading Wren Dental Hygienist. The incumbent in this post was able to offer dental hygiene treatment to all British Armed Forces personnel on the Base and their dependants, including oral hygiene classes for the mothers and children[*]. She also provided dental first aid for 'pain cases', arranging treatment with the dental department at the US Navy Hospital, when required. During the three-monthly visits of the dental officer from Earls Court, she acted as Dental Surgery Assistant, arranging his appointments in the interim.

In Winter 1986, the RNDS Newsletter carried an amusing account of one such visit to Naples by Surgeon Lieutenant Commander (D) D L (Lynford) Thomas, the assistant dental officer at NDC at that time[86]. An abridged version of this is shown below:

> ### *Movers & Shakers*
>
> "Did the Earth move for you too?" – Not a normal conversation between dentist and dental hygienist, I know, but this is Naples and we are discussing the events of the previous night. Stop sniggering at the back! It was another earth tremor.
>
> For the past couple of years, I have been in the Naval Dental Clinic, Empress State Building, with its panoramic vista of the Earl's Court car park. When this pleasure begins to pall, I jet-set to our branch practice, just outside Naples, where my trusty dental hygienist has long awaited my return.
>
> She has prepared a gathering in my honour. The waiting room is FULL of pain cases!
>
> The dental surgery is in the British Services sick-bay, which is itself situated in a large NATO base five miles from the centre of Naples. The patient load is approximately 550, comprising servicemen of all three services, plus families. The NATO base is very near to the town of Pozzuoli, which has been the epicentre of the tremors which have caused considerable damage to buildings in the area during the last few years. Many buildings in the base have been comprehensively shaken and the sick-bay is no exception. A full modernisation is in progress, which is why this article is being written with the aid of a cup of instant coffee in Fulham and not with a cappuccino at the base swimming pool in Naples! ➤

---

[*] At that time the General Dental Council directed that all dental hygienists must work under the direct supervision of a dental surgeon. However, in recognition of the peripatetic and sometimes isolated nature of their practices, RN dental hygienists were given 'special dispensation' to practice unsupervised, albeit always to the prescription of a dental officer.

Picture a quiet evening in Naples. An underground train is heard in the distance. It gets closer and closer. Strange – we're nowhere near an underground line! The tiles on the floor start to ripple; the light fittings swing; that damned underground train is passing right under the house! If the base happy hour was yesterday, then this must be a tremor. In fact, the tremors have been quite minor for the past year, with some experts seeing this as the calm before the proverbial 'big bang'.

[Because of the tremors] all the British families have had to move to an area outside a 10 km. radius of the base and the drive to work every morning has a superb view over the Bay of Pozzuoli, with Vesuvius in the background. It also stinks, due to the hydrogen sulphide being given off in clouds of steam near the base. The longish journey to the base plus the traffic problem, often means that patient timekeeping for appointments is 'variable'. Visits to the British primary school of 90 children, are made twice yearly for inspections and the dental hygienist also visits to arrange dental health education projects.

Now let me, in no particular order, give you a sample of the flavour of Naples. It is dirty, noisy, crazy, dangerous on the road, frustrating, but always interesting. Many Brits are less than ecstatic about Naples, but the few that do like the place are enchanted by it. I will admit to having failed to fall prey to her elusive charms.

The hygienist lives above the shop – literally. Wrens' Quarters is above the sick-bay. This, plus the Italian plumbing, leads to some interesting problems and I am developing a fetish for wading, ankle deep, through Wrens' cold bathwater in the clinic. Added to this are numerous unexpected power cuts and water shortages.

The buildings are dirty and unkept on the outside, but often plush inside. The Italians dress with some style and have a happier disposition than we Brits. They are an outgoing gregarious lot, who go as far as to display their emotions in public. It is the only place I have ever seen young lads openly admire a baby!

Most Brit families live in large houses or villas, which are pleasant in summer but cold in winter due to insufficient heating. Power and water cuts are frequent. Refuse collections are few and rubbish is often dumped at the roadside, with numerous dead dogs thrown in for good measure. There are rumoured to be Mafia connections with the landlords and petty crime is endemic.

Most Brits have been burgled, relieved of wallets and jewellery, had cars broken into or stolen or a combination of these. The thieves are very open about it and will wait in their cars and watch until people leave home. In order to get a good night's sleep, many families will get a guard dog. These muts will invariably bark all night in competition with neighbouring muts. Therefore no-one gets a good night's sleep and, since they are awake anyway and can hear burglars, it defeats the object of having a guard dog. ➻

> Driving in Naples .... is in another dimension. Forget everything you ever learned about driving. Red lights, lane discipline, one-way streets – they are all extremely optional. It is not unusual to see a family of four on a Lambretta scooter.
>
> Having said all that, after the sheer terror of the first few days, driving in Naples soon becomes second nature and the difficulty comes with adapting to UK road conditions when I come back.
>
> Food – [Apart from pizzas and pasta], one of the highlights was being presented with a dirty great octopus, reposing languidly in a plate of tomato sauce, when all I wanted was a piece of grilled fish. No my Italian is not fluent!
>
> Travel – Playing tourists is very easy around Naples. Rome is not far. Pompei, Herculanium, the islands of Capri and Ischia and the Amalfi Coast are closer. As much History, culture and sightseeing as one could wish. One of the perks of the job is the odd visit to Rome by the dentist and hygienist, to carry out inspections on the servicemen and families based there. This can, of course, be combined with some time in the Eternal City, which really is a pleasure. A recent visit to the Vatican Museum was mind boggling! In the summer months, there are the pleasures of the base swimming pool and the NATO beach. The [water quality] is rigorously monitored by the Americans and should any pre-set limits be exceeded, the water is declared out of bounds. While the Americans are busy going through the motions of applying these public health measures, on either side of the NATO beach, the Neapolitans are busy just going through the motions!
>
> The NATO base is built in an area which the Romans called the "Burning Fields", due to the release of fumes from the ground. For the past few years, a bulge of 15 km in diameter has been swelling in the bay near the base. The uplifting of the area by a few metres has been accompanied by the aforementioned tremors. If the pressure is released on land, the damage is not expected to be catastrophic. If, however, the molten magma erupts under water, the sudden flashing into steam will cause an enormous explosion with no warning. As things have been quiet for many months now, some experts are predicting interesting developments. Volunteers for the Naples job – one step forward please!

In January 1987, Surgeon Captain (D) T J C (Timothy) Hall was appointed Assistant Director Naval Dental Services (ADNDS) and Surgeon Captain (D) Brian Robinson became Command Dental Surgeon to the Commander-in-Chief Naval Home Command.

1987, sadly, was to see the passing of three stalwarts of the Dental Branch, each of whom had seen service during World War II. Surgeon Captain (D) J B (John) Inverdale, who died in January 1987, had joined the Service in 1937.

During a long and distinguished career he served in many parts of the world, starting the war in the depot ship *HMS Maidstone* and finishing it in the Royal Naval Hospital, Bermuda. As well as qualifying as a Specialist in Dental Surgery and serving shortly thereafter in RNH Plymouth, he spent some time with the Royal Marines and eventually served, by then as a Surgeon Captain (D), in three Command Appointments, with Commander-in-Chief Far East Fleet, in Singapore during the 'Confrontation' with Indonesia; with Commander-in-Chief Portsmouth (and as Fleet Dental Surgeon to C-in-C Western Fleet) and with Commander-in-Chief Naval Home Command. Outside of his professional career, John Inverdale's great enthusiasm was for Rugby football and, for a period during the 60s he was Chairman and selector for the Joint Services Rugby Team. His interest in sport was clearly passed to the next generation and his son (also John), is currently one of the senior BBC sports 'anchormen'[87].

Surgeon Captain (D) K E J (Ken) Fletcher, who died in March 1987, was the son of Surgeon Rear Admiral (D) E E Fletcher, the 'father' of the RNDS.

Qualifying at Guy's Hospital in 1934, he joined the Navy in 1935 and in 1936, found himself on the China Station in the cruiser *HMS Cumberland*. During the War, Ken Fletcher was appointed as Naval Liaison Officer, New York*. Whilst there, he met and married a Canadian Wren, Georgina.

His post war appointments included several in New Entry Training Establishments and after his promotion to Surgeon Captain (D), he relieved John Inverdale as Fleet Dental Surgeon to C-in-C Far East Fleet, in Singapore. His final appointment was as Command Dental Surgeon to C-in-C Plymouth and he retired from the Royal Navy in 1967, to work in the Dorset Schools' Dental Service[88].

It is poignant to note that both the above officers were predeceased by their wives, but died within less than a year of their loss.

The third retired naval dental officer to die in 1987 was Surgeon Captain (D) K A ('Johnny') Johnson, who passed on in June of that year. Joining the Navy in 1939, his career also took him around the world, including a period in Hong Kong and, coincidentally, also to Singapore as Fleet Dental Surgeon, where he relieved Ken Fletcher[89]. He was a large and ebullient man and, as a Surgeon Captain (D), could seem somewhat intimidating to a young and junior dental officer, as was the author when serving his first RNDS appointment at *HMS Ganges,* where Johnson was Senior Dental Surgeon. Beneath this stern exterior, however, it soon became evident that 'Johnny'

---

* History does not relate whether this appointment involved dentistry, or whether it was purely a staff appointment, but it is known that he also served in the dental clinic at Asbury Park in New Jersey, a holding facility for RN personnel joining the US built 'Liberty Ships'.

Johnson was a kindly and caring man and a wonderful mentor to someone just embarking upon a naval career.

It has been the author's privilege to serve with all three of the above distinguished RN dental officers.

June 1987 saw the appointment of Surgeon Captain (D) S N (Stewart) Bussell as Commanding Officer of the RN Medical Staff School at Haslar. This was a 'non-dental' appointment, the school being responsible for all initial professional and the advancement[†] training of Medical Assistants in the RN Medical Services. Bussell was relieved at the Institute of Naval Medicine by Surgeon Captain (D) E J (Ted) Grant, as Director of Dental Training and Research and as Head of the Training Division at the Institute.

June 1987 also saw the retirement, after 34 years in the RNDS, of Surgeon Captain (D) Alan Moore, the then Fleet Dental Surgeon at Northwood. During his time at the Fleet Headquarters, Alan Moore had been appointed as an Honorary Dental Surgeon to HM the Queen.

Little has been said, thus far in this History, about the Royal Naval Reserve Dental Branch. This omission does not reflect the high value placed by the RNDS on the contribution made by its RNR colleagues. The RNR is a force of part-time volunteers, who train in peacetime for a variety of sea and shore tasks, which they would carry out in times of tension or war[90].

An insight into the invaluable support given by dental reserve officers, is given in an article by the Principal Dental Officer (Reserves – (PDO(R)), Surgeon Commander (D) H (Hugh) Cannell RD RNR, in the Spring 1987 issue of the RNDS Newsletter. It is reproduced below, in abridged version[91].

The RNR Dental Branch

Why do we require 32 trained officers as a Reserve for a Regular Branch of only just over twice that number? It does seem paradoxical that whilst the professional career men in the RN, have been cut in numbers, the Reserves are said to be expanding overall. Cost effectiveness seems to be the reason. From the Treasury's point of view, it is much cheaper in an emergency to draw upon trained men, supplied from civilian sources, than to pay for regular forces who [include] within their own numbers, their wartime enhanced manpower requirement.

[However], the number of officers in the Reserve Dental Branch is not expanding; unlike the remainder of the RNR. Indeed, the Reserve (D) has reduced its number by about three per cent.

The cuts in the Regular Forces have already strained the dental services in the RN. In addition, the successful efforts of the profession as a whole, in improving ➤

[†] Promotion.

the dental health of most within the UK, has also lead to increased expectations within all patient groups. It is no longer acceptable for an extraction to be the outcome of a treatment episode.

The higher expectations of our patients, placed together with the existing excellent standard of treatment provided for the RN, is something of a rod for our own backs. Yet it is a professionally satisfying, albeit strained, situation. The Reserve Dental Branch is of help here. To allow for leave periods, sickness and absence on courses, the RNDS must have some locum cover.

Traditionally, the comprehensive range of dental skills within the Reserve has been of importance to the RN Dental Branch. Those of the general dental practitioner, being the most sought after as locums.

Here though is a problem, independent of anything that the RN can do. It is the problem of [the general dental practitioner's] civilian status as self-employed. Although contracted to provide NHS treatment to the local [health authority], he has to employ his own ancillary and lay staff.

[Whilst undertaking an annual period of Service], the RN grants him naval pay. Unhappily, this may not be sufficient for him to recoup his wage bill. Increasingly, the RNR [dentist] uses his vacation time to do his annual two weeks with his Regular colleagues. Increasingly too, dental practices worry about releasing their Principals to act as Reserves to the RN. [As a result of this] more and more Reserve officers are coming forward from within the salaried [sector], rather than from the self-employed areas of civilian practice.

The critical mass problem and the reduction of the number of bases abroad, has resulted in fewer opportunities for the training of oral surgery specialists in the RN. The RNR can also help in this field. There are seven oral surgery-trained Reserve officers. Six of these are civilian consultants. The [availability] of these to the RN, depends upon their skill in obtaining release from their hospitals. Usually this annual training commitment is undertaken as an addition to their civilian annual leave entitlement. Within the last year, the normal pattern of carefully arranged locums at the RN Hospitals at Haslar, Stonehouse and Gibraltar has been carried out and the oral surgeons [may also] turn their hands to [the] part-time [general] dental surgeon role.

How then can we understand these RNR 'toothies' better? Certainly by knowing the restraints imposed by their civilian jobs. Perhaps also, by recognition that they are truly volunteers. [So] what do we get out of it?

The older RNR officers will know that their most long lasting and firm friends have come from their contacts with the RN. Often, a civilian practitioner may feel isolated in his practice. [Thus] it is with a sense of relief that he comes for a while to work as a member of a team of skilled and friendly dental surgeons. The faint chance, at least for the younger officers, to get to sea; to wear the uniform and be proud of it; to learn how to make do in the best traditions »▸

of the Service; to get out of his surgery and work somewhere different; to take part in the semi-mysterious camaraderie and language, with such terms as "pier head jump", "RPC" or "run ashore"; to be able to grumble [when attempting] a filling in the Bay of Biscay, or [about] a Senior Dental Surgeon, who insists that the day starts at 0700.

To remain in the RNR does demand a high degree of motivation. It is not easy to arrive at [the local RNR unit] feeling fresh and burning with energy, after a long day at civilian duties. Duties at [the unit] to which the RNR toothie is attached, vary. Within the two hours, once a week, may have to be packed, charting and inspection of all new recruits, general recruiting duties, and perhaps [sport]. At [an RNR unit], each evening's drill commences with formal Divisions and prayers. Thereafter, the dental officer performs the standard dental inspections. No treatment other than real emergencies is undertaken. Not all Divisions have dental surgeries or the space for them.

The RNR toothie is much more likely to be employed in his Division as an officer using his generalist skills, but [may be employed in non-dental tasks such as] public relations, interviewing or administration. Many are the Recruiting Officer for the Division. Others not only run the Wardroom wine books, but double up as Boat Officers, New Entry Admin. Officers, University Liaison Officers, or that officer whom the CO always needs to help man an official function or parade.

Several RNR [dental] officers have obtained watch-keeping certificates and are proud to be on their Division's strength as part-time 'fishheads'. Their dental duties remain their primary task. [Most RNR dental officers have a commitment to] attend at the RNR Division, one evening a week. [However, those] who have been given duties of special importance to the Division, may opt to go on 'List 3' and attend two evenings a week. Their commitment becomes an exacting one and is something more than a hobby.

All RNR officers and ratings, if their attendance and annual training commitment is satisfied, qualify for a tax-free bounty each year. In the case of a List 3 officer, this amounts to several hundred pounds. [Travel costs and an attendance allowance are also paid]. [The] tax-free bounty is a recent benefit and attendance payment, a very new perk. Most of the older officers still seem somewhat embarrassed by this largesse.

The *esprit de corps* is also a force to be reckoned with. It exists because of the tight knit groups of officers who get together on drill nights. The Wardroom is, of course, the hub. The RNR is proud of its hospitable traditions.

Some of our Branch are temporarily or semi-permanently attached to Royal Marines or Royal Marines Reserve units. We have several officers who have achieved the coveted Green Beret.

> Up to four years ago, some RNR Divisions had Dental Surgery Assistants on their strength. [However], the DSA's WRNR programme fell into disuse, due to a number of related events. The Royal Naval Dental Training School, on which we relied for courses for our DSAs, was disestablished. Also, the blandishments of other branches, with more exciting life styles, attracted our Wrens. [This] situation is about to change for the better. The Command Dental Surgeon is about to reinstitute the DSA's RNR.
>
> The RNR 'toothwright' is, we admit, something of an anomaly. In short, he or she is there to back up your efforts in the RN. Now we have a defined role, you will find that we can integrate with the RN, without upsetting things too much. Above all, it should be remembered that we are happy with our lot and … rather proud of it!

By now Vocational Training for newly qualified dental officers had been adopted within the RNDS as well as in the other Service branches and civilian dentistry. Newly qualified dental officers would spend their first year in the Navy under the wing of an accredited trainer. The trainer, usually the Senior Dental Surgeon of the clinic to which the new officer was attached, would supervise all aspects of his or her clinical work. Additionally, time was built in for day release to attend local 'study days', under the auspices of civilian vocational training organisations.

Vocational Training was defined as a period of guidance, during which the skills learned as an undergraduate are moulded and adapted to the most appropriate treatment for the patient, within the capabilities of the clinician. The introduction of Vocational Training was part of a general movement within the dental profession, to ensure clinical professional development throughout dental careers.

The dental branches of the Armed Forces could not afford to be left out of this process and, as well as this supervised training early in the RN dental officer's career, greater emphasis was now being placed upon post-graduate academic and clinical training.

Master of Science (MSc) qualifications and Membership in General Dental Surgery (MGDS) of the various Royal Colleges had now become sought after goals by many RN dentists. The MSc courses, in a number of different dental disciplines, were allocated by selection, usually at a rate of two officers a year. They were full-time courses, which lasted for one year and were usually, but not always, conducted at the Eastman Dental Institute in London. Upon graduation, dental officers were appointed, in due course, as local advisors in their particular disciplines. They were expected to give at least five years 'payback' of service to the Royal Navy.

Where appointments provided enough stability, other dental officers had begun to study for and sit the MGDS examinations. These were undertaken by dental officers of some clinical experience, who combined a clinical appointment with day, and occasionally, week, release courses. A great deal of dedication and application was required of these officers, to meet the requirements of both a busy clinical job and the not inconsiderable demands of the MGDS course.

Early in the 1980s, the new Faculty of General Dental Practice (UK) had been established at the Royal College of Surgeons of England. The new Faculty sat alongside the long-established Faculty of Dental Surgery, the English academic home of Oral and Maxillofacial Surgeons. Once established, the Faculty launched a new clinical qualification, aimed at dentists around two to three years on from completion of Vocational Training. This was the Diploma in General Dental Practice and was the first of a progression of such qualifications aimed at different phases of dental careers. At the launch of the DGDP, several senior RN dental officers, who had been involved in clinical training, were awarded an honorary diploma.

Following on from the Falklands conflict, it was still an important requirement that the RNDS select a regular supply of young (and fit!) dental officers to undertake the very demanding All Arms Commando Course at the Commando Training Centre Royal Marines, Lympstone. Not all of those who embarked upon this endeavour, were able to complete the course and achieve the award of the coveted Green Beret. Those who did, were appointed to Commando units and found themselves serving in some challenging environments.

The Cold War was at that time, the driver for much UK and NATO defence policy. With the assumption that attack, when it came, might be from the northern borders of the Eastern Bloc countries, the Royal Marines had become NATO's front line experts in Arctic Warfare. To hone their skills in this area, annual exercises and training were undertaken in northern Norway.

At the same time, the UK Government had a serious security problem much closer to home. The 'Troubles' in Northern Ireland had been festering on since around 1970 and the Royal Marines were expected to take their turn with British Army units, providing security and "aid to the civil power" on the streets and in the countryside of Ulster.

Where the Royal Marines units went, so did their dental officers. Surgeon Lieutenant (D) M R C (Mike) Gall had only recently returned from the Arctic, when his unit was deployed to Ulster. His short article in the RNDS Newsletter gives a flavour of life before and during his deployment[92].

Troubles!

Preparation for the tour began on return from post-Norway leave. Arctic patrol techniques had to be forgotten and the intricacies of urban street patrolling learnt. During the brief period [back at] *HMS Condor*, I considered buying shares in Stabilok [a much used, pinned tooth restoration system]. The perennial problem of fractured cusps resulting from Arctic Rolls and 'deep frozen' chocolate bars, seemed never ending. Clinical dentistry, however, stopped for the two-week Northern Ireland training package at Lydd and Hythe on the south Kent coast.

The extensive ranges were far removed from those at Lympstone or Tregantle Fort, fondly (?) remembered from the Commando course. Basic weapon handling revised and sights zeroed, we moved onto stances directed at firing safely in a built up area. The realistic ranges took the form of sangar shoots and street scenes, some with friendly, talking dummies, along with the remote-controlled snipers that provided targets for the observant. Booby traps were also laid for the unwary medical and dental officers. Training culminated with three days in Ryde Village, a full-scale model village, complete with a secure company location and surrounding patrol area. On the streets, cordoning of suspect cars, contact reporting and public relations were practised under the ever-watchful video camera.

The movements of personnel in the Command location came under the same scrutiny, as we dealt with proxy bombs and mortar attacks in the course of running patrol programmes. As ever 'Royal' took his training seriously, not least when fighting in controlled (?) riot situations. Sickbay staff were kept busy suturing, making referrals for X-rays and removing fractured teeth from swollen lips! Visiting RUC [Royal Ulster Constabulary] were left wondering what would happen in the event of a real riot, in view of the enthusiasm shown for assaulting each other.

With fine weather on 2 July, the RAF flew us to Aldergrove to start our eighteen week tour in the predominantly Catholic west side of Belfast. The three fighting companies were split up: 'X-ray' going to North Howard Street Mill, 'Yankee' staying with the Echelon at Musgrave Park and 'Zulu' going to Fort Whiterock. The Command moved to the joint RUC/military operations room at Springfield Road.

Just as at sea, I encountered the problem: "Where do we put the dentist?" No room in the sickbay and bunk spaces at a premium. The military wing of Musgrave Park Hospital appeared the obvious answer. Surgery facilities were available in the little used oral surgery department, as it was used only three days a month by a visiting RADC consultant. The hospital was even able to offer me the professional services of a DSA.

While the facilities were excellent, making the *Condor* surgery look antique,

> the problems of moving patients led me to set up the portable dental unit at each of the company locations. A Gemini [a rigid/inflatable boat] or a jackstay transfer is easier to arrange than finding an uncommitted, armoured vehicle, to move dental patients in Belfast.
>
> In addition to dentistry, I found myself in the Joint Ops Room at Springfield Road, between midnight and four, doing the 'doom' watch every six days.
>
> Ninety-five per cent boredom, I was warned, nothing to do but log relevant radio transmissions and drink coffee. My first watch, on the anniversary of Internment, showed me the other five per cent!
>
> Fortunately, everybody expected a busy night and came to my rescue when I pressed the panic button. I was coping well enough with the stoning and petrol bombing, but the sniping attack on a patrol had me looking for help. Trying to log times and events, inform Brigade and keep a clear picture of who was moving into the area, following the contact report, had us all at thirty thousand feet, with the Ops Officer some ten thousand feet higher!
>
> Four o'clock came and went as I scribbled furiously, wondering how control could ever be kept during a prolonged exchange of fire. On the eventful journey back to the Echelon, I got a taste of what it had felt like for the patrols on the ground. We were still being bricked and petrol bombed by gangs of youths, at five in the morning, as we drove around the burning cars on the Falls Road. Needless to say, all my subsequent watches have been spent putting Ireland to rights, over coffee with RUC watchkeepers.
>
> After this, what next? Leave, mountain training and back to Arctic Norway for ten weeks!

Just another day or two in the life of a Royal Navy dental officer!

In July 1987, the fourth Wood Lecture and Clinical Day was held at the Institute of Naval Medicine. The keynote lecture was given by Dr John McLean, both an eminent clinician and a recognised dental materials scientist. He was ably supported by presentations, both clinical and those describing the travels and experiences of those RNDS officers, still managing to see quite a bit of the world. During the break for a buffet lunch, those attending were able to 'browse' a supporting dental trades' exhibition. The day was rounded off with the Director's Dinner, held in the Wardroom Mess in *HMS Dolphin*, at which both Dr McLean and Air Vice Marshal Jones, the Director of Defence Dental Services, were guests of honour.

Following on from the trial, detailed in the previous chapter, to determine both the cost effectiveness and the quality of contract dental laboratory work, *vis à vis* the RNDS in house, civilian dental technicians, the Ministry of Defence had now decided that the 'home grown' solution was no longer sustainable.

The final decision was based partly on cost grounds, but mainly because, as civilians, the RNDS technicians had no identifiable war role, unlike their uniformed Army and RAF counterparts. A bitter dispute took place within the Defence Dental Services Directorate, the outcome of which was that the views of the RAF prevailed, to retain all its uniformed technicians, by filling the identified war role posts for both their own service and that of the Navy. Thus, with great sadness, the Branch said farewell to its small but loyal and, in many cases, long-serving cadre of dental technicians[93].

Late 1987 also saw the retirement of one of the stalwarts of the Branch, Chief Wren Dental Hygienist Eleanor White, after a career spanning 23 years. Eleanor White, a Scot, served, not only around the UK, but in Gibraltar and Singapore. She had also served as the Senior Dental Hygiene Instructor at the RN Dental Training School. Her final draft was in *HMS Cochrane* at Rosyth; close to where she had joined the Wrens.

Another retirement in January 1988 was that of Air Vice Marshal John Jones, the Director of Defence Dental Services, who was succeeded by DNDS, Surgeon Commodore (D) David Coppock, promoted to Surgeon Rear Admiral (D) in his place.

The Branch took great pleasure in the re-establishment of the two-star rank, albeit for the time being. Admiral Coppock's promotion, however, brought a number of new problems.

Since his duties were, from now on to be mainly tri-Service, the day to day running of the RNDS devolved mainly to the Deputy Director, Surgeon Captain (D) Brian Robinson, this, in turn creating greater stretch amongst other supporting senior staff.

The RNDS Strategy Review Group continued to look at the future of the Branch and during 1988, proposed a policy of regionalisation which, it had calculated, would produce financial savings of 10%, whilst remaining able to respond to the present and future needs of the Royal Navy.

This proposal was a response to the Government's relentless pursuit of reductions in public spending and more specifically, reductions in uniformed personnel across the Armed Forces. However, early in the year, the Deputy Chief of Defence Staff (Personnel and Plans) directed that the Defence Dental Services should justify their manpower numbers and look at ways and means of replacing uniformed personnel with civilians. A well researched paper, in reply to this directive concluded that no changes were necessary to the substantially uniformed service[94].

Inevitably, the Principal Personnel Officers (PPOs), Second Sea Lord and his colleagues in the other two Services, were not convinced. It was made clear that "No change was not an option" and the wheels were set in motion for the Head of Management Services (Organisation) (Man S Org) to conduct an external 'independent' study on the Defence Dental Services – of which, more later.

An event which caused great sadness throughout the RNDS, was the news of the untimely death of Surgeon Lieutenant Commander (D) Andy Prosser. We have read of his exploits during the Falklands conflict and with the British Joint Services Hovercraft Expedition in Peru. Readers will remember that, shortly before completion of his eventful Short Service Commission, he had been awarded the Harvey-Fletcher Medal and Prize for his meritorious service in the RNDS. At the time of his retirement from the Service, he was already suffering from the illness which was to lead to his death. After leaving the Service, he went into practice in Bristol and, true to the determination with which he had approached various challenges in his all too short life, he continued working almost to the end[95].

All three Services had over many years, attempted to provide primary dental care as close as possible to the front line, in order not to disrupt manpower requirements in operational situations. In the RNDS, two types of equipment had evolved: one being the Frigate Portable Dental Unit (FPDU), referred to in previous chapters of this History; the other being the development of mobile dental surgeries, both towable and self-propelled.

In the Spring 1988 issue of the RNDS Newsletter, Surgeon Captain (D) Brian Robinson produced a well researched History of the evolution of these equipments[96]. An abridged version of this is reproduced below:

Dentistry on the Move

The Armed Forces have been in the mobile surgery game since WWII. Certainly, the Royal Air Force operated dental trailers from 1942 in North Africa with considerable success and the Army made extensive use of caravans, during the invasion of Europe. Reference to the RN use of mobile vehicles is sketchy, but there are reports of the Navy using mobile caravans, borrowed from the Army, in 1944. One of these started in North Africa and travelled through the full length of Italy as far as Venice, under the general direction of the Fleet Dental Surgeon to C-in-C Med. Towards the end of WWII, a mobile dental unit was constructed and built on a trailer by Royal Marine engineers in Australia. This had running water, electric power and was mosquito proof!

After the War, the RNDS wished, quite naturally, to keep up with its sister branches and, logically sought a maritime solution. As a newly-entered Surgeon Lieutenant, I recall hearing stories of plans for a dental surgery, mounted on a barge, which would be secured alongside the vessel due to receive treatment. ➢

Fortunately, sanity prevailed before dental officers were required to pass the Ship Command Examination and the Branch embarked upon its long flirtation with caravans.

The RAF was again in the van (no pun intended!), with the development of 'prime movers'[self-propelled dental facilities, constructed on the back of a truck], for whilst the Army stuck to caravans throughout the War, the Second Tactical Air Force was equipped with 32 mobile dental units, all based upon a Fordson chassis.

The RN Prime Mover system was to develop much later. This motorised mobile unit, essentially a dental caravan body, secured to a Bedford truck chassis, first appeared in 1977. The late Surgeon Captain (D) Alan Davies did much to bring the project to fruition. His design has proved very successful and its replacement is taking place only now, because the tractor unit has reached the end of its planned working life.

The origins of the Frigate Portable Dental Unit are more obscure. Shore-based portable equipment was used by the RN as early as 1940, when *HMS Glendower* [a new entry establishment], commissioned.

It is recorded that three dental officers were drafted with portable equipment and set up their surgeries in bell tents. Apparently the shortage of equipment and staff rendered it impossible to meet the demands made by a continuous intake of 300 recruits per week.

An RN mobile dental unit also functioned around the Suez Canal area, operating out of Alexandria in 1942/43, whilst a less fortunate dental officer, used a portable dental surgery and laboratory equipment, to operate on a circuit which included an Auxiliary Naval Hospital on the Kola Inlet, Moscow and Archangel!

The first reference to a seagoing system comes in 1946. As the war with Japan reached its climax, the British Pacific Fleet numbered some 237,000 officers and men. Whereas the major units of the Fleet were well supplied with dental officers, (i.e. battleships, aircraft carriers and cruisers), a continual problem was how to bring treatment to destroyers and escort vessels in the forward screen. Whilst desperate cases could sometimes be transferred to the large ships, most pain cases had to wait for weeks, until the ship reached Australia for its R and R period. Approval was eventually obtained to carry dental officers with mobile equipment in these small ships, but before it could be implemented, the Japanese capitulated. The Royal Australian Navy was quicker off the mark, however. To quote a report of the time: "It has been demonstrated that a dental officer can work effectively in a destroyer under operational conditions in the tropics. *HMAS Napier* has been at sea 35 days of the 40 that the dental officer has been on board".

Photographs exist from 1952 of portable units employing an electric engine, ⟫⟶

> with cable drive and custom made instrument and stores cabinets. The FPDU as we know it today, with an air turbine, would appear to have materialised in the mid sixties. The introduction of this excellent concept to the Fleet, allowed dental officers the opportunity to practice routine dentistry in small ships for the first time. [Robinson then continues by giving a list of all previous marks of dental caravans, prime movers and portable dental units, together with details of where they were built.]
>
> The RN will [now] take delivery of four Mark V caravans in January 1988. These have been constructed by Locomotors of Andover.
>
> The design specification was hurriedly completed at the end of 1985, without having had the benefit of working experience with the Mk IV vans. Some deficiencies were apparent, however, and hopefully, these will have been eliminated in the new vehicle. The Mark II Prime Mover is well under way, with construction being carried out at the RN MT Workshops, Portsmouth.
>
> The Project Officer, Surgeon Lieutenant Commander (D) Mark Weston, has been responsible for its evolution and, with the benefit of experience during the Mk V caravan build, this unit should be of even better design.
>
> Developments in the portable dental field are being progressed by a joint Army/Navy venture with Tridac Ltd. The company is developing three prototypes based upon [their existing static models] with fibre optic, high speed handpieces. The unit will be fitted into a standard Lacon [sea and air transportable] box. This system, as yet, does not provide a complete package, but the prospect of purchasing commercially produced equipment, does have attractions, both in funding and procurement. For RM Commando units operating in the field, the Kavo Supraclave [autoclave] is being trialled to see whether it will provide an answer to sterilisation problems.

1988 also saw the award of the Harvey-Fletcher Medal and Prize for the fourth time. This time the recipient was Surgeon Commander (D) A J (Alan) Woodman. Woodman was, at that time Commander Dental Training at *HMS Nelson*.

His department was the much scaled-down successor to the old Royal Naval Dental Training School, where he had previously served as the Deputy Officer-in-Charge and, for a brief period, as Officer-in-Charge. The new department was only 'scaled down' in terms of numbers of training staff. The training task, even without the dental hygienist training, was as big as ever and growing and Alan Woodman and his staff were immensely busy. In addition to the routine training tasks carried out, Woodman also held the post of Adviser in General Dental Practice with responsibility for co-ordination of the RNDS Vocational Training Scheme. Undaunted by the volume and complexity of these tasks, Alan Woodman ran an efficient training organisation which was continually fine-tuned to meet the changing demands of both vocational and ancillary dental training. The award of the Harvey-Fletcher Medal and Prize was made in recognition of these achievements.

The advent of Information Technology was beginning to have an impact throughout the Royal Navy, including the RNDS. One or two 'home grown' attempts at creating data bases and records within the Royal Navy Medical Services had met with mixed success.

In order to address the future use of such technology, the Surgeon Rear Admiral Support Medical Services was to set up a 'Small Systems Group' (SSG) to advise him on the way ahead. At a meeting of the RNDS Managers, it was reported that DNDS anticipated a "firm input" into this group [97].

Surgeon Commander (D) S (Stephen) Lambert Humble had made it his business to acquaint himself with the current and potential use of computer applications in dentistry in general and in the RNDS in particular. Such was his expertise in this field, at a time when few within the profession or the military had any significant experience with computers, that Lambert Humble was selected for loan to the SSG and, in early 1989 was to become the Adviser in IT to the Medical Director General (Naval).

Whilst the Branch managers were grappling with the thorny problems of budgets, manpower reviews and, indeed, IT, life at the 'coalface' continued apace. Despite shrinking numbers and unabated demands for their professional services, members of the RNDS still found time for adventurous opportunities which would have been unlikely to offer themselves, had they been working in a civilian environment. Such opportunities were not only available to the officers of the Branch.

In February 1988, Petty Officer Wren Dental Hygienist Paula Drouet was working in *HMS Tamar*, the RN shore establishment in Hong Kong – itself a much sought after opportunity, when she was offered the chance to join a Joint Services women's expedition to the Himalayas.

Joining a mixed party of WRAC, WRNS, and QARANC [*] personnel, and accompanied by two male adventurous training instructors, one from the RN PT Branch and one from the Army, the group left Hong Kong by air for Kathmandu, the objective of the expedition being to trek to the Base camp of Mount Annapurna, which, at 26,500 feet is one of the highest in the Himalayas. Once again the RNDS Newsletter was the vehicle for Paula Drouet's very readable account of what turned out to be a strenuous and, at times, hazardous trek[98]. An abridged version of her article is reproduced below.

---

[*] Queen Alexandra's Royal Army Nursing Corps.

High Flyers

The flight to Kathmandu with the Royal Nepal Airlines, took just over four hours and [we] were met at the airport by the manager of our trekking company and taken by coach to our hotel. The moment you left the airport building, the 'Kathmandu atmosphere' hit you – the heat, dust and noise, the general poverty and squalor and the children begging for "rupees" – a sight that was to become quite familiar by the end of our trip. It was really like stepping back in time. Things hadn't changed in [many hundreds of] years and you could still see old craftsmen at work – potters, weavers, brass-workers etc.

[After two days of sightseeing and sampling the pleasures of Kathmandu] – On Tuesday morning, our 'bus' left at 0630. This was to take us to Pokhara, a journey of eight hours, from where we were to start our trek. The bus itself was quite amazing, "rickety" wasn't the word! As for the state of the roads and the bridges we had to cross, I'll never know how we made it in one piece! The bus was loaded with so much gear, plus ourselves and all of the porters…. going round the hairpin bends at full speed, with sheer drops below, I've never been so scared in my life! However, we arrived in Pokhara and there met up with the rest of the porters.

Altogether there were 20 'staff' – three guides, three 'chefs' and 14 porters to carry all the equipment and our luggage – quite an entourage!

All the lads were very young, some only 15 and Dendy, the head guide, was only 24. They were all so cheerful and hard-working and the loads they had to carry were amazing. Everything was carried in large wicker baskets on their backs. I did feel guilty because we only had to carry 'daypacks'.

From Pokhara at 3,000 feet, we had a short trek to our first campsite at Hyenja and then, over the next few days, climbed gradually out of the valley and up to a village called Ghorapani, at 9,000 feet. From here you got a magnificent view of the mountain ranges.

That part of the trek was 'up and down' and mainly along rocky paths and steep steps cut into the mountain sides. The weather was really hot and the scenery beautiful. There [was plenty] to see along the way [and] we would pass through little farms and villages every couple of miles.

The methods of farming hadn't changed in centuries. Every spot of land was used in the form of terracing up the hillsides and oxen and ploughs were still used. There were also constant streams of donkeys carrying supplies up and down the main trails and whenever you heard the ringing of bells you had to stand clear!

We [got up] at around 0620 every morning, when the 'cook boys' would bring a bowl of hot water for a wash and, after breakfast, we would walk until midday and have an hour or so stop for lunch. Then we would arrive at the next campsite at about 4 o'clock. ≫→

Everything on the trek was well organised, especially the food. The cooks would create the most delicious dishes in enormous quantities, all cooked over an open fire. It was mainly a vegetarian menu, as fresh meat was hard to come by along the trails.

From Ghorapani we headed east and passed down and through a huge rhododendron forest. The trees were just coming into bloom and were really beautiful. We stayed overnight in Chomra down in the valley and at this point were at the start of the main Annapurna Trail. From Chomra, the trail deteriorated and was very rough and muddy. We were to climb steeply from now on, following the Modi Khola River all the way up the mountainside. That day we had a very long trek up to a little lodge at Dovan.

As we were climbing higher, the weather got a lot colder and at night it was freezing! The lodges were very basic, but cosy and the average price was about 20 pence a night.

The next day, Tuesday 23rd, was the most dramatic of the trek. Having left Dovan early in the morning, we climbed for a few hours to a spot called Hinku Cave, where there was a little visited lodge, built under a huge boulder of rock. Here we discovered there had been an avalanche a few days earlier, which covered the main track completely. All the girls waited at the cave, whilst Dendy, George and Ian [the RN and Army leaders] went to check out the situation, to see if it was possible to get across the avalanche. [Now] the snow started to fall and it was freezing! We waited a couple of hours, [until] they returned and said it was possible to continue. We very carefully made our way across the avalanche – the boulders of snow were enormous and it was very icy and slippery, but we got over OK and arrived at the next lodge at Deurali (11,500 feet) by late afternoon.

From here we were only two hour's trek from the Annapurna Base Camp Sanctuary at 13,000 feet, but the snow was falling heavily, so we decided to stay the night there and attempt the 'final assault' the next day.

The lodge at Deurali was literally like a stable. It had had half the roof blown off the month before and was patched up with bits of wood and branches. We had to huddle together with three or four layers of clothing on and in the sleeping bags, to try and keep warm, as there was no form of heating.

Later on, as it was getting darker, we heard an almighty cracking sound and rumbling like thunder, which was an avalanche higher up the mountain! Shortly after that we heard another one and I think we were all pretty scared, although no-one would admit it!

When we awoke the next morning, there was a good three feet of snow covering all signs of the trail and, with conditions as they were, the risk of further avalanches and without proper snow boots and clothing, Dendy decided it was too dangerous to go any further. We would have to abandon the attempt to reach the Base Camp and go back down the mountain as more snow was forecast. The next part of the trek had got to be the funniest, as it was just »▸

> impossible to keep your balance and we literally slid all the way back to where the snow finished! How the porters managed with the heavy loads on their backs, I'll never know. We had the longest day's trek that day, all the way back down to Chomra, [experiencing] from snow to sun [and] rain to hailstorms. By the time we reached the lodge, we were really exhausted! The owner of the lodge was an [elderly] …ex Ghurka captain. He cheered us up with buckets of hot water, our first wash for a few days and plenty of Ghurka Rum!
>
> It was a real disappointment not to make the Base Camp, as we'd got so close, but you can't fight the elements and we certainly experienced "Adventure Training" in the true sense!

Paula Drouet's account concludes with a description of the final trek back to Pokhara, their farewell to the guides, when they donated much of their clothing to the porters and the bus ride back to Kathmandu.

1989 also saw the passing of another doyen of the RNDS; Surgeon Rear Admiral (D) L B ('Ginger') Osborne [99]. Born in Cheshire in 1901 and trained in Guy's Hospital Dental School, Ginger Osborne joined the Royal Navy upon qualification in 1923 as a Surgeon Lieutenant (D). Early in his career, he was given the task of changing the ethos of the Branch from an emergency service to that of a provider of restorative and preventive care. His career took him around the world, serving from Scotland to the South Coast and to the Far East, and to sea in the battleships *HMS Nelson* and *HMS Rodney* during the early part of WWII.

As a distinguished sportsman, he had also officiated both within the RN Rugby organisation and the British Rugby Football Unions. In 1957, he accompanied HM the Queen at a match at Twickenham. Appointed Honorary Dental Surgeon to the King (KHDS) in 1951, this was changed to QHDS upon the Queen's succession.

In 1954, he was promoted to Surgeon Rear Admiral (D) and as Director of Naval Dental Services. Osborne retired from the RN in 1957, but continued working clinically within the Sussex Health Authority Schools Dental Service until he was 70. He died at the age of 89.

In August 1989, Surgeon Captain (D) S N (Stewart) Bussell was appointed to the tri-Service Directorate as Assistant Director Dental Services (Navy) – ADDS(N) and as Surgeon Rear Admiral (D) David Coppock's, Branch Deputy.

August 1989 also saw the retirement from the Service of another RNDS stalwart, Surgeon Captain (D) P C (Peter) Wrigley. Peter Wrigley's last appointment was that of Fleet Dental Surgeon at Fleet HQ in Northwood, Middlesex. The Summer 1989 issue of the RNDS Newsletter carries a report that, following a Branch cricket match, in which the Fleet Dental Surgeon's XI beat that of the Director, "a farewell party for Peter and Mary Wrigley was held in the Wardroom, *HMS Dolphin*. It was indicative of the affection in which both are held by many in our Branch, that some had travelled from as far as *HMS Neptune* [the Clyde Submarine Base] and North East England to be there. We wish them both health and happiness upon Peter's retirement. They will be missed" [100].

Another appointment of interest, in October 1989, was that of Surgeon Commander (D) G W (Geoff) Myers to the Joint Services Defence Course at Greenwich. This was a first for the RNDS and one which would stand both Myers and the Branch in good stead in the years to come.

In the previous chapter, it was recorded that two RNDS dental officers had been the first in the Branch successfully to sit the examinations for the Membership in General Dental Surgery of the Royal College of Surgeons of England. These opportunities, together with the availability of Master of Science degree courses and the advent of Dental Vocational Training, pointed towards an increasing and welcome emphasis on what is now called Continuing Professional Development (CPD). The importance of such clinical and professional advancement to the Branch – and the Profession in general – was recognised in the Editorial of the RNDS Newsletter, published in Summer 1989[101]. This is reproduced below.

Professional Development

Amongst the Branch news items published in this issue, it was a pleasure to record the success of four more Naval Dental Officers in gaining their Membership in General Dental Surgery. This brings the total number of MGDS diplomates within the Branch to 11 dental officers, approximately 14% of our total strength. There are yet others in the 'pipeline'.

This relatively high number perhaps belies the effort and cost of obtaining such qualifications. The pressures of study and clinical attainment required to meet the demands of the examination and the preparation of Log Diaries of treatment histories to the high standards required by the examiners, are considerable.

These pressures are endured over a period of some 15 to 18 months, during which time the candidate is also required to fulfil the expectations of his Senior Dental Surgeon in producing a target amount of clinical output.

SDS's have, in their turn, been both commendably amenable and supportive ➢

of their dental officers' endeavours, despite pressures upon them to produce satisfactory Clinical Profiles. If one accepts that such training is often undertaken at the expense of clinical productivity, one must ask the question, "Is it worth it?" and "Are the penalties acceptable?"

In the dim, but perhaps not so distant past, when your Editor qualified, nothing much had changed in the field of dental technology, materials or equipment for 50 years or more. There was, therefore, little requirement for continuing education for the general dental practitioner and relatively few attended courses of training after leaving dental school.

Since those halcyon (?) days, dental science and technology have now taken off at, to some, a most alarming rate. The undergraduate syllabus has had to absorb more and more basic science at the expense of clinical experience. Techniques change and equipment and materials become obsolete and are replaced almost as soon as the necessary new skills are acquired. It is now unthinkable that dentists, Service or otherwise, should not update themselves regularly on the changing requirements of their profession and it is to this end that the RNDS supports and encourages Vocational and all other forms of continuing dental education and training, accepting, whenever possible, the penalties.

It is not only the dental officers who seek to keep pace with the changing dental scene. As well as those who routinely undergo updates during normal advancement training, many Wren DSAs continue to come forward for Dental Hygienist and National Certificate courses.

The Armed Forces recruiting authorities are facing, with concern, the approach of the so-called 'Demographic Trough', the effect of which is already beginning to bite. In a vocational profession such as dentistry, we believe that it is of the utmost importance that potential recruiting problems should not lead to a lowering of professional standards. This would create a 'second class' dental service, capable only of meeting the most basic treatment needs of the man in the Fleet, rather than striving to maintain his dental health and thus, his operational readiness.

Long may there be Dental Branch personnel willing to accept the pressures and penalties of further training. Knowledge and the Pursuit of Excellence are obligatory if we are to continue to provide effective support to the operational task of the Royal Navy.

The same issue also reported the second award of the Alan Acton Davies Memorial Prize to Petty Officer Wren Dental Hygienist Debra Peake, in recognition of outstanding performance, both in providing a high standard of care in carrying out her clinical duties and as a departmental administrator[102].

Clinical advancement was not all that was required of RN Dental personnel. Dental officers were also expected to be able to meet operational challenges. To this end, the Combat Casualty Care Course (C4) had, as previously recorded, proved its worth during the Falklands Campaign. Now, in addition to dental officers, all New Entry Medical, Nursing and newly promoted Medical Services Officers were required to do this training. RNR Medical and Dental Officers and occasional officers from foreign navies had also boosted the numbers on this much acclaimed course.

Now, DNDS had decided that those dental officers who had so far missed out on this training, due to their seniority, should be included. Thus a number of 'older' colleagues were surprised to receive 'the call'!

One such was Surgeon Commander (D) P G (Peter) Edwards, Senior Dental Surgeon at the Royal Naval Air Station, Culdrose, whose amusing account in the Newsletter is reproduced below [103].

The Oldest Swinger …?

It was one of those rare, sunny autumn days at Culdrose. Small, fluffy, white clouds were chasing each other across a bright blue sky. I had finished treating my patient early and had ten minutes to spare before the next. My in-tray was empty and for once I sat in blissful peace, a cup of coffee beside me and gazed out of the window. The phone rang. It was always a pleasure to hear from my old friend [the Director of Dental Training and Research] and today he seemed in a particularly jocular mood.

"How would you like to go on the Combat Casualty Care Course?"

It took a minute or two before I realised he wasn't joking. Swiftly my mind formulated the myriad reasons why it would be quite impossible, when he laid the first bit of ground bait. The conversation went something like this:

"You don't have to do it, you know".

"Oh good!"

"Nobody will think any the less of you, if you'd rather not".

"Er, no".

"After all, at your age …"

"Well now, hang on a minute!"

"If it makes it any easier for you, we've already asked someone younger than you and he refused as well".

"Hold on, I haven't actually refused you know".

And then, like a skilful angler feeling his victim nibbling on the bait, he struck!

"It's physically demanding. On one course we had to withdraw someone.

He was younger than you too. You're right. It was a silly idea. Forget it".

"What do you mean? I never said I wouldn't … Of course I'll go!"

A chuckle from the other end of the phone told me that DDTR, who has known me for many years, knew me better than I had realised. I had been well and truly conned!

*

It was with some trepidation that I arrived on course on the Monday morning, to find, to my relief that I wasn't the only 'sucker'. There was one delightful RNR Surgeon Lieutenant Commander (D), who had thought that he had volunteered for a week's quiet first aid course in classrooms at Millbank and was looking forward to spending each evening with his wife, looking around the shops in London.

He first suspected that something was amiss when he received a [travel] warrant for Portsmouth and his suspicions deepened further, when he was told to bring a stout pair of walking boots! At least he was spared the months of horrid anticipation.

It is not my intention to give a blow by blow account of what we did on the course, surprise being an integral part, but I append some of the memories which have stuck and, I'm sure, will stick for a long time.

For example, I will never forget the night in the life raft. We were overcrowded to start with. Although there was just enough room around the circumference for the bottoms, the problem lay in where to stow the legs. One person moving meant everyone moving. And then, after an hour, it was discovered that water was pouring in through a hole.

We panicked not. "Quick! Cut the rope! Swim for the shore!" shrieked one of our number – calmly. But our duty CO, young Surgeon Lieutenant (D) (Tim) Elmer, assured us that all would be well and that we should sit it out until morning.

The fact that he was on the 'light' side of the raft and sitting high, rather than on the other side, where we were up to our waists in icy water, may have influenced him. But the night passed eventually, with continual bailing and with one member with his hand in the hole. I thought it singularly appropriate that he happened to be a Dutchman!

I noticed one interesting phenomenon, Sleep being impossible, we nevertheless organised a duty watch-keeper. It was fascinating to find that the only time any of us felt any drowsiness was when we had the watch. We would, each of us, sit there in extreme discomfort, trying desperately and unsuccessfully to sleep. Then it would be our turn to be on watch. Instantly, our eyelids would become heavy and we would have to fight constantly to stay awake. We would only snap into full wakefulness as we handed over our duty to the next man. ➤

Never was a cold, grey, wet dawn greeted so enthusiastically and, after swimming ashore and the longed-for and promised cup of coffee, failed to materialise, we were into the hard slog.

And hard it was! "Picking 'em up and putting 'em down." I was reminded of Kipling's "Boots". And, a stretcher, even an empty one, gets BLOODY heavy after a few hundred yards. And the only sustenance was cold water. One passed through the stage of feeling normally hungry and reached a point where one's body simply felt the need for fuel. I well recall saying, with complete honesty, that if I was faced with two rooms, one containing a large bed upon which lay a beautiful young lady and the other, a table with food, I would go for the latter. At which someone else said "I agree; and after eating, I would go back to the first room, throw the girl out and go to sleep!"

Before the course started, I had considerable anxiety over the prospect of killing rabbits. It was the one part of the syllabus about which I had serious personal doubts. As it turned out, my fears were groundless. After more than forty hours of discomfort, physical exertion and no food, those little, white, fluffy bunnies were no more or less than hopping meat, to be dispatched, cooked and eaten as quickly as possible. And nothing before or since has EVER tasted as good as that stew!

After a wonderfully refreshing sleep – and if you've never slept in a draughty tunnel on a bed of wet bracken and animal (I hope) excreta, don't knock it – it was time for more cross-country navigation and walking, walking, walking, ending with a most interesting river crossing exercise, about which I will say no more, not wishing to spoilt it for all you enthusiasts who are undoubtedly besieging DDTR for a place on the next course.

The final serial was in a local pub and here we relaxed for the first time since I know not when. Yet we behaved ourselves quite well, although our sensitivities had been somewhat blunted by our experience. For example, I had no compunction about removing my boots and socks, wringing out the latter and putting them back on while sitting at the table – all right, it was in the conservatory, but even so … . And after we had polished the last scrap from our plates, we gratefully accepted the odd lettuce leaf etc., which amused fellow diners, had left.

The dreaded weekend was over and the rest of the course seemed almost an anticlimax. I felt really sorry for the lecturers on the following Monday. With the best will in the world, we all kept nodding off from time to time. We hope they understood.

Although the weekend is the part that looms largest in one's mind, before, during and after the course, possibly the most valuable serials were the lectures and practical casualty handling exercises at the end of the first week. However, I found I learnt a great deal about myself during that physical module, not all of it bad and I am sure that the course would be very much the poorer without it.

Surgeon Lieutenant Commander (D) G (Gillian) Boswell had been increasingly recognised within the Branch and the Navy as a gifted athlete. In 1989, she reached the peak of her athletic achievements. In the RN Athletics Championships of that year she set new Championship records in both High Jump and Long Jump. In the High Jump, her record of 1.68 meters broke the previous record which had stood for 26 years. She also won the 100 metres Hurdles. In the Interservice Championships, two weeks later, she achieved two silver and one bronze medal.

In July 1989, she competed in the Interservice Heptathlon Championships, breaking another RN record on the first day – this time in the 100 metres Hurdles. Despite a disaster in the Javelin event, she went on to a personal best in the 800 metres, winning the Interservice Gold Medal for the overall event.

Boswell's performance won her a place at the Commonwealth Games Trials in September 1989. Sadly, she sustained a stress fracture during the trials and had to withdraw. This disappointment was offset when, in November 1989, her own athletics club, Atlanta Fareham awarded her the title of Athlete of the Year and she was ranked 40th in the UK for the Heptathlon[104].

The 1980s ended for the RNDS on a particularly sad note. Surgeon Rear Admiral (D) Philip Duly CB OBE died in the Royal Naval Hospital, Haslar after a short illness and after an all too short six years of retirement. We have met Philip Duly a number of times in the earlier pages of this volume of the RNDS History. It is worth here recording his achievements during his long and distinguished career in the RNDS[105].

Born in 1925, he trained in Dentistry at the London Hospital during World War II, qualifying in 1947. Duly joined the Royal Navy in 1948, transferring to the Permanent List in 1956. After service at the Royal Naval Air Stations at Lee-on-the-Solent and in Malta, he served at *HMS Dolphin* as the Staff Dental Surgeon to the Flag Officer Submarines and then in the carrier *HMS Hermes*, during which commission, he was promoted to Surgeon Commander (D). It was shortly after that appointment that he was appointed, in 1965, as Officer-in-Charge at the Royal Naval Dental Training School.

This, as we have ventured previously, was the 'turning point' of Philip Duly's career. Initially tasked with the training of Wren Dental Surgery Assistants, he commenced work on setting up the first training programme for Wren Dental Hygienists.

The School was quickly accredited for this training by the Central Examining Board for Dental Hygienists, (an offshoot of the General Dental Council), thus allowing Wren hygienists to practice their profession in civilian life, on completion of their Service careers. It also enabled the School to take on civilian students (paid for by the Department of Health and Social Security), to top up training capacity.

The first DH course started in 1967 and it was Duly's proud boast that during his time at the School, no DH student failed the National Qualifying exams.

In due course Philip Duly was appointed as, firstly, Deputy Chairman and then Chairman of the Central Examining Board. As if the work involved in launching and running the DH courses was not enough, Duly also found time to produce an update of the Handbook for Royal Navy Dental Surgery Assistants (B.R.888D).

On completion of his time at RNDTS and in recognition of his achievements there, Duly was awarded the OBE.

Leaving RNDTS in 1970, after five years in post, Philip Duly moved to London as Assistant to the Director and was promoted to Surgeon Captain (D).

In that rank he also undertook a number of staff and administrative posts, including Director of Dental Training and Research at the Institute of Naval Medicine, Command Dental Surgeon to Flag Officer Naval Air Command and to C-in-C Naval Home Command. During the latter appointment, he was appointed as an Honorary Dental Surgeon to the Queen

In March 1980, Philip Duly was promoted Surgeon Rear Admiral (D) and took over as Director Naval Dental Services. He became DNDS at a time when the first of many intensive studies into the viability and future of the Branch was taking place; a cause of concern to both himself and his successors. In 1982, he was further honoured with the award of Companion of the Order of the Bath (CB). Philip Duly retired from the Service in September 1983.

Philip Duly was a man of many qualities and talents. He was in his element when asked to mend anything from a grandfather clock to a car, but his great love was music. An accomplished organist, he was often to be seen (and heard) accompanying services in the various churches around his home town of Gosport. At the annual 'Blood Red' Dinner of the Medical and Dental Services at the Royal Naval College in Greenwich, it became a tradition that, after the dinner, diners would 'repair' to the magnificent Wren chapel to hear a short recital by Philip Duly.

So passed another illustrious member of the RNDS and so ended the momentous 1980s – momentous for the RNDS, for the Royal Navy and for the Nation. The Falklands Conflict had come and gone. Both the Royal Navy and its Medical and Dental Services had been tried and tested in the heat of war and had not been found wanting. Despite this, downwards pressure on manpower and resources was to continue into the 1990s, when the collapse of the Berlin Wall and the Warsaw Pact was to hand the politicians an even larger axe to swing in their endeavours to make ends meet in terms of the national budget. It was to seem that the lessons learned at the time of Operation Corporate*, when the Royal Navy was about to lose those very resources needed to contest Galtieiri's annexation of the Falkland Islands and South Georgia, were, yet again, to be ignored.

Whilst coping with the difficulties and anxieties at Directorate level, the RNDS, with its sister Services continued to keep abreast of, and sometimes to lead in developments within the Dental Profession. To do so relied on a continuing input of dedicated and talented young men and women of all ranks, prepared to advance themselves professionally and to face the challenges of preparing themselves to be able to work in an operational environment. Without these, the Branch would fail to provide the Fleet with the service it both deserved and needed.

*****

---

* Operation Corporate was the Service designator for the Falklands Conflict.

Chapter 7

"Change is here to Stay"
1990 – 1992

The final decade of the 20th Century dawned upon a Royal Naval Dental Services, still providing, in its 70th year, a comprehensive and much valued dental clinical service to the men and women of the Royal Navy, the Royal Marines and, most importantly to the ships' companies of the Fleet.

The successes of the RNDS came however, despite the continuing battles at Directorate level to maintain and protect the Branch's dwindling resources and manpower. In common with the sister military medical and dental services, the RNDS had been and was continuing to be, subjected to a series of government and MoD reviews, each of which inevitably lead to further shrinkage and re-organisation – always in the pursuit of 'Cost Efficiency'. Even year on year management processes were subjected to this 'squeeze' and when annual budgets were submitted in accordance with already agreed 'Long Term Costings', they were almost invariably subjected to further 'Efficiency Savings' of around 10%.

When one senior member of the tri-Service Medical Directorate complained about yet another review of the Medical and Dental Services, he was treated, by a senior civil servant, to the now immortal phrase: "Change is here to stay!"

It will be remembered that following rejection of an 'in house' manpower study which recommended status quo, by the Principal Personnel Officers in 1988, the Head of Management Services (Organisation, (Man S. Org), had been commissioned to carry out a comprehensive manpower review within the Defence Dental Services. The review had kicked off in late 1989 and was carried out by a team comprising two civil servants from Man S. Org, together with Air Vice Marshal John Jones, the now retired first Director of the Defence Dental Services and Professor G B Winter from the Eastman Dental Institute[106]. Both the latter could be perceived to be friendly towards the Defence Dental Services and to have a comprehensive understanding of the problems facing military dentistry in trying to achieve its aims.

The team visited Service dental clinics throughout the UK and in Germany during the first three months of 1990, interviewing clinic managers and clinical staff. In April 1990, their report landed on the desk of the Deputy Undersecretary of State (Personnel and Logistics) DUS(PL), at the Ministry of Defence[107].

Once again, this study was rejected at nearly all levels. Whilst more or less recommending the status quo, it had failed to give sound reasons for this. In a letter to DUS(PL), another senior civil servant, the Head of Medical Finance and Secretariat wrote: "In my view, they [the Man S. (ORG) team] have not carried out this task satisfactorily. The report carries 27 recommendations on a wide range of relatively minor matters, but covers the major issues superficially and perfunctorily."[108]

Thus, yet another scrutiny of the Dental Services was kicked into touch and the three dental branches braced themselves for yet more investigation.

It should be noted that at no time during this or any of the preceding studies, had it ever been suggested that the RNDS and its sister branches were not meeting the requirements of their operational masters. It was always and ever would be about money! It is perhaps appropriate here to quote the Editorial from the Spring issue of the RNDS Newsletter, which attempts to put these events in perspective[109].

Progress or Change?

In a letter to the senior managers of the three Defence Dental Services and dated November 1989, the Director of Defence Dental Services announced the setting up of a study team whose task is to progress and complete the review of the Defence Dental Services, which had commenced early in 1988.

As this issue of the Newsletter goes to press, the review is up and running and it would be nothing short of foolhardy to attempt to predict the outcome.

Whatever the final result there is little doubt that changes are in the pipeline yet again, be they small or of great consequence. We can almost hear your groans as you read this. "Not more change! When will they ever let us get on with the job and make progress, instead of reorganising us yet again?"

It is true that during the past two decades the Defence Medical and Dental Services have been subjected to almost continuous scrutiny to an extent that one is tempted to indulge in a degree of paranoia. This can be further fuelled by browsing through some of the past reports.

If you wake up screaming in the middle of the night, thinking about the possible permutations of "the Way Ahead" for our Branch, consider this:

A working party set up by the Secretary of State for Social Services under the chairmanship of Mr Laurie Pavitt M.P., published its report in April 1976, entitled "A Challenge for Change in the Dental Services". Under the heading "Dental Services for the Armed Forces", the report states:

"The system of recruitment and dental staff education in the Armed Forces is good and should be applied in the civilian sector. Shortcomings of the Service require attention. Firstly, there is under-utilisation of dental personnel and second, ➠

duplication of specialist services. In addition, they do not accept responsibility for all dependants at home and abroad and do not use enough ancillary personnel.

To overcome these problems, the Armed Forces Dental Services should be fully incorporated into the Community Dental Services and come under the control of the Area Dental Officer.

Overall planning of the Armed Forces Dental Services should be carried out by an Armed Dental Services Group [sic] consisting of one dentist from each of the Services and Area Dental Officers who have large Armed Forces bases in their areas. This Armed Services Group will be responsible for planning the services and arranging for overseas postings.

The salary scales and conditions of work for all dental personnel treating the Armed Forces, will be the same as those in the Community Dental Service.

Dental Services will be provided in a dental centre by a dental team, which includes dental auxiliaries, hygienists and preventive dental ancillaries."

You win a few ….. you lose a few! But the question remains: "What is it they want of us? Don't we give good value for money? Do they really want to get rid of us? Is this change or is this progress?"

Consulting various dictionaries and Roget's Thesaurus we discovered that "Change" can be defined as "to make or become different" or "to transform". "Progress" is "movement forward" or "to advance towards completion, maturity or perfection". It is to be hoped that the latest review will bring about progress rather than just change. Progress towards what? Maturity? Perfection?

Perhaps it would be timely at this point to remind ourselves what it is we are trying to achieve. The primary purpose of the Royal Naval Dental Services is: *"To promote and maintain a level of dental fitness which insures that the operational effectiveness and efficiency of the Royal Navy and Royal Marines are not impaired."*

Whatever changes are in the pipeline, the task of achieving the above purpose will remain as a worthwhile challenge for all of us in the Royal Naval Dental Services. It is, of course, a challenge which has been with us for some considerable time.

Unlike our sister Services, we have not (sadly) seen fit to celebrate our past Golden and Diamond Jubilees. With this issue of the Newsletter, we celebrate two notable anniversaries. Exactly 70 years ago, in January 1920, the Dental Branch of the Royal Navy was established by Order in Council. Exactly 10 years ago, in January 1980, our Director designate, Surgeon Captain (D) Brian Robinson published the first issue of this Newsletter. There have been occasions in the past when both the future of the Branch and the future of the Newsletter have been in doubt.

We are both still here and, we sincerely believe, we are both doing a good job.

Happy Birthday to you!

      and

           Happy Birthday to Us!

As mentioned in the above Editorial, early in the year, it had been announced that Surgeon Captain (D) Brian Robinson was to supersede Surgeon Rear Admiral (D) David Coppock as the Director of Naval Dental Services in the rank of Surgeon Commodore (D). Brian Robinson needs little introduction to the readers of this History. Since relatively junior rank he had been in the forefront of innovation and progress within the RNDS.

His achievements had included the design and introduction of not only the Branch Newsletter and the Combat Casualty Care Course, both of which had significantly enhanced the reputation of the RNDS, but also his untiring work in a series of senior appointments, to keep the Branch one step ahead of those who would diminish its capability or consign it to a subsidiary role within the overarching Medical Services. In pursuing these objectives he had always shown himself to be a master of 'lateral thinking' – a skill he would need even more during his tenure as DNDS.

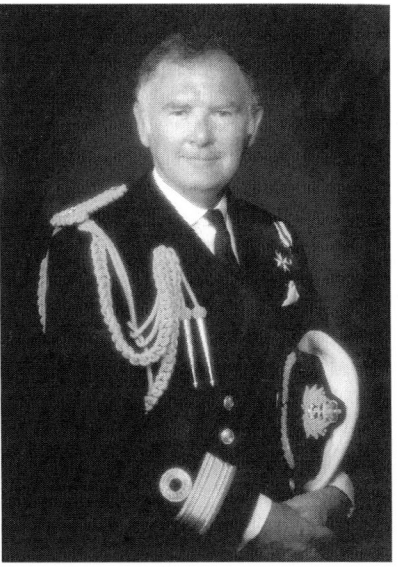

Surgeon Commodore (D) Brian Robinson OStJ QHDS

After qualifying from the dental school at King's College Newcastle in 1958, and on completion of two house appointments, Brian Robinson joined the Royal Navy and the RNDS in May 1960. Having married just before joining, 1962 found him and his wife and family at *HMS Phoenicia* in Malta.

Promoted Surgeon Lieutenant Commander (D) in 1964, he then spent three years at the new entry training establishment *HMS Raleigh* in Cornwall.

During his time at Raleigh he spent a short time at sea in *HMS Tenby* providing dental treatment to the ships of the 17th Frigate Squadron. His time in *Tenby* included a visit to West Africa and the Cape Verde Islands. After *Raleigh* and time ashore in Scotland and the West Country, in 1969 Robinson (now in the rank of Surgeon Commander (D)), joined *HMS Ark Royal* (the 'old' *Ark Royal*) as the Senior Dental Surgeon of the two dental officers borne in this 50,000 ton carrier. His account of the *Ark*'s collision with a Soviet destroyer in 1970 was included in Chapter 2 of this History.

Back ashore in 1971, Robinson spent two years as Senior Dental Surgeon in *HMS Daedalus*, the Royal Naval Air Station at Lee-on-the-Solent. In 1972, he embarked upon the one-year course for a Master of Science degree in Periodontology at the Eastman Dental Institute in London.

Upon graduation, in early 1973, he was appointed as Officer-in-Charge at the RN Dental Training School. Further clinical appointments followed this until, in 1980 he was promoted Surgeon Captain (D) and appointed as Director of Dental Training and Research at the Institute of Naval Medicine (INM). Here, as previously recounted, he took on the additional task of Head of the Training Division at the Institute and launched both the Combat Casualty Care Course and the RNDS Newsletter.

Leaving INM in 1983, further senior staff appointments followed: Deputy Director Naval Dental Services and Dental Adviser to Commandant General Royal Marines (1983); Command Dental Surgeon to C-in-C Naval Home Command and as Staff Dental Surgeon (Reserves (1987); Fleet Dental Surgeon to C-in-C Fleet and as Staff Dental Adviser to C-in-Cs Channel and Eastern Atlantic (both hats worn by C-in-C Fleet) and as Flotilla Dental Surgeon to Flag Officer Submarines (1989). He was the second recipient of the Harvey-Fletcher Medal and Prize in 1983 and in 1990 was appointed as Honorary Dental Surgeon to HM the Queen and as an Officer Brother to the Order of St John. His appointment as Director in 1990 was a popular one throughout the Branch.

Times were not only changing for the RNDS, other significant changes were afoot within the Royal Navy, which would themselves impact significantly upon the Branch. In February 1990, it was announced that women were to serve at sea[110].

Although promoted as obeisance to the feminist lobby, this decision was taken just as much as a solution to chronic manpower shortages in the Fleet.

As well as opening up sea-going appointments and drafts to wrens and female medical and dental officers, it would lead firstly to Women's Royal Naval Service personnel coming under the Naval Discipline Act* and, in due course to the abolition of the WRNS, with female personnel taking on equivalent naval rank and wearing naval rank insignia rather than the blue insignia and badges of the WRNS. Wrens already serving were to be given the option whether or not to serve at sea. Their decisions were to reach the appropriate authority by March 1990.

All joining after that date would automatically be included in sea rosters. Volunteers for sea service must be fit, would be trained to bear arms and should pass standard swimming tests.

Throughout these somewhat turbulent times, it was 'business as usual within the Directorate and during the previous two to three years, work had been progressed on an RNDS reference manual "Dentaims". Most of the work done in compiling this publication had been carried out by Surgeon

---

* Up to this time, unlike their sister Services, Wrens had not been subject to the NDA.

Commander (D) D C C (David) Alexander. Dentaims was intended as a 'handy guide' to Dental Branch administration for Senior Dental Surgeons and practice managers in the clinics. The editor of Dentaims was the Assistant Director, Surgeon Captain (D) Brian Robinson and his assistant editor, whose task was to keep the publication up to date, was Surgeon Commander (D) I L (Ian) Kelly.

The Managers' Meeting in March 1990 was informed that a submission had been made to the Medical Finance and Secretariat, for Dentaims to be awarded the status of 'BR' – a 'Book, Reference'[*], to be published as such in 1993[111]. Sadly, Dentaims was never to achieve such official status.

1990 had brought with it two potentially momentous world events, both of which were to impact upon the RNDS. One was the increasing belligerence of Sadam Hussein, the Tyrant of Iraq, towards his neighbour, Kuwait. The other and at the time, more significant of these, was the collapse of the Warsaw Pact and with it the Berlin Wall. This was to give the cash-strapped Government the undreamed of opportunity to 'take the Peace Dividend' and, with axes freshly honed, ministers turned once again towards the Armed Forces, launching yet another study – "Options for Change" – of which, more below.

Despite the trials of the senior staff officers in the Directorate, there was still some light relief to be found for those lower down the 'ladder'. Service personnel, including members of the RNDS had always had a front row seat, when it came observing in close up, such global events as the reunification of Germany. In April 1990, Surgeon Sub Lieutenant (D) Simon Wolstencroft, found himself on a dental student elective at the University of Munster[†]. Whilst there, he took the opportunity to visit the now undivided city of Berlin.[112] An abridged version of his account for the RNDS Newsletter is reproduced below:

Loose Chippings!

I wouldn't advise anyone to go to Berlin in a Mini Metro. They are too small and mine needed a new engine on return to the UK! Competing with BMWs on autobahns is not to be recommended. However, in West Berlin it was well worth the 5DM, just to get through the East German border control.

West Berlin is a thriving example of Western capitalism and all those thoughts evoked can be experienced in some form. A marked contrast is the despondent ➤

---

[*] All official Royal Navy administrative and operational written regulations and guides bore the prefix "BR" followed by an index number.

[†] Since the early 1970s, one productive recruitment path for the RNDS had been 'Dental Cadetships', whereby dental students were able to join the Royal Navy as Surgeon Sub Lieutenants (D), on an appropriate salary, with the costs of their training being borne by the MoD.

situation in the East side of the city.

To see West Berlin, one really needs to progress on foot and use public transport. I must have walked about four miles to the Brandenburg Gate, only to be disappointed to see it surrounded by scaffolding. According to one local, this was to protect the gate from 'eager beavers' chipping the Wall away, graffiti artists and also, in an attempt to restore the gate to its former glory.

From the gate I decided to walk along the wall towards Checkpoint Charlie. On the way I came across various characters selling fragments of the wall for about 3DM and others selling Warsaw pact accoutrements.

I walked on and soon came across a number of people happily chipping the wall away. I had been carrying with me a hammer and chisel [as one does!] and now was the time for some uninhibited destruction!

It was good fun, but surprisingly difficult to chip away any fragments. After some success and a few poses for the camera, I proceeded towards Checkpoint Charlie, passed through it, paid another 5DM and there I was on the other side!

My first impression was that of a building site, with cranes, lorries and men working. As I continued to walk, I noticed the monotony of the East German car industry. I don't think there has been any progress in car design since the war and they certainly don't show any imagination with regard to colour.

There didn't seem to be many people walking around and those we did see, seemed rather reserved, going about their business and paying little attention to tourists. East Berlin seemed to me to be an uneventful sort of place. Not somewhere I would have been in a hurry to get back to. Having said that, with the unification of Germany, it will be interesting to return at a later date and see the change in character which is bound to occur.

I left the East in the early evening and returned to the West. West Berlin is certainly a buzzing place at night. The German people that I met from the West were friendly and keen to speak English and I left Berlin with fond memories of a good time and a hope that the East side of the city will soon share some of the assets of the West.

In April 1990, a farewell 'ladies night' dinner was held at *HMS Collingwood* to honour the retiring Director, Surgeon Rear Admiral (D) David Coppock. After an excellent meal, he and the assembled company were treated to a well researched and slickly presented 'This Is Your Life' presentation of Admiral Coppock's career. As a keen salmon angler, he was presented with both an engraved silver salver and a mounted salmon fly, specially tied in the Branch colours of orange and gold and named "The Golden Dentist". It was explained to non-anglers in the audience that there was already a well known and successful fly named "The Silver Doctor"!

During his speech, Coppock, who had been widowed in 1985, surprised and delighted all present, by announcing that he had, the previous week, married his partner of several years – Sally Arnold. From that memorable occasion they both took with them the goodwill of all in the Branch.

May 1990 saw a less happy event in the untimely death of Mr Ken Pritchard who had been the Civilian Instructional Officer both at the RN Dental Training School and its successor – Commander Dental Training – since 1975. A former RN Sick Berth Attendant, for 15 years Ken had taught the practical aspects of the handling of dental materials to many generations of Wren Dental Surgery Assistants. Over time, his duties had expanded to include stores administration, the training library, Navy Days displays and clinical photography. A man of many parts who would be much missed[113].

Hong Kong and the Naval Base at *HMS Tamar* had featured strongly in the life and History of the Royal Navy during two centuries.

The RNDS had maintained a clinic within *Tamar* for many years, although in these times of 'rationalisation' responsibility for the clinic now fell under the command of the RADC unit in the colony.

Despite this there were still billets for an RN dental officer and a Leading Wren dental hygienist. Chairside and dental laboratory support were provided by locally entered Chinese personnel.

We last met Surgeon Lieutenant Commander (D) Lynford Thomas in Naples, anticipating the next major earth tremor. Now promoted Surgeon Commander (D), he found himself in the enviable appointment as Senior Dental Surgeon, *HMS Tamar*. Once again, he had produced an account of his impressions of life in 'the far flung' for the RNDS Newsletter. Seen through the eyes of a 'man from the valleys', it makes amusing reading[114].

Dai Pan

[Hong Kong] is, in fact more "foreign" than I expected. A century and a half of British influence seems only to have left a veneer over a remarkably unchanged Chinese culture.

I will give you a brief idea of some of the things that surprised me. The built up areas are desperately overcrowded, but there is a surprising amount of lush greenery remaining, due to the fact that half the land is designated "Country Park". The locals are highly superstitious and will congregate in large numbers for various festivals at different parts of the island. Temples and shrines abound. They are also gambling mad and vast sums of money change hands at horse racing meetings. ➤

The shopping is amazing and most places are open seven days a week until late evening. My wife lost her American Express card a few weeks ago, but I haven't reported it, because the thief's bills are less than hers!

The fish and meat markets are not for the squeamish and an AGR [anti gas respirator] is advisable in summer, as some of the innards etc. just get thrown into the drain. Frogs seem very popular and now is the snake season – even up-market hotels serve snake dishes!

Dogs are also sold for eating (on the quiet) and this is another winter dish. It is said that if something has four legs and is not a table, the Chinese will eat it!

Spitting is an art form and a good old clear out can be heard on most street corners. Hence the proliferation of "No Spitting" signs even in the most up-market places. The hotels are as plush as anywhere in the world and each new one tries to outdo the others. The Hong Kong Dental Association meets in the Hilton – a change from the St Mary's Postgraduate portacabin in Portsmouth!

The number of expensive cars on the road is quite staggering when one takes the size of Hong Kong and the New Territories into account – less than 20 miles North to South and East to West. Only the biggest-engined models will do for the rich locals and it is quite normal for me to be travelling in a convoy made up of only Mercedes, BMWs, Porsches etc. You can't miss me – I'm the one in the beat up Toyota. Because so many well-off people live in flats, the car is a much more important symbol of affluence here than it is at home.

There are a great many very wealthy people in Hong Kong and the basic rate of tax is 15%. Wealth is flaunted, but most of the population live in very cramped conditions with few of the facilities we would expect. There is a very limited welfare state and much of the social work carried out depends on the many charities in existence.

Dental Musings

The Services dental set-up in Hong Kong is administered by the Army and my clinic has an RADC sign above the door. It is a modern clinic overlooking the two *Tamar* swimming pools.

The staff are locals, apart from the Dental Hygienist, Jo Milford.

Jo is disgustingly healthy and sporting (apart from when she has strained this bit or pulled that bit of her anatomy!) She cycles and runs everywhere and has recently been chosen as a member of the Women's Hong Kong Triathlon Association team at the Commonwealth games in Auckland in January 1990!

Many aspects of the dentistry itself are different. Approximately 50% of my patients are locally employed servicemen. The caries rate out here has been lower than in the UK for longer and patients have generally had less conservation treatment and require less.

The perio [gum disease] picture is less rosy, with more widespread problems –

a factor of the often poor oral hygiene. Occlusal [tooth surface] wear is more of a problem and must be diet-related, although the locals do clean with far more gusto than the average "Foreign devil". There is a cultural taboo related to tooth loss (ageing and virility figure prominently in the equation) and it is difficult to persuade the locals to have an extraction, even when it is obviously necessary.

My main surprise was the high proportion (up to 30% or so) of locals with noticeable tooth staining problems. This is either a typical severe fluoride mottling or pronounced Tetracycline staining. Up to about 12 to 15 years ago, two parts per million of fluoride was added to the water supply and this [being 100% more than the recommended optimum] has caused the ruin of many a smile. Tetracycline is self-medicated willy-nilly during the chilly and moist winter months, for chest infections. Many drugs (e.g. antibiotics and the contraceptive pill) are freely sold without prescription.

I am told that approximately 50% of the local population have antibodies to the hepatitis B virus, which puts a new and powerful perspective on cross-contamination procedures!

Strangely enough, extraction forceps and all sorts of surgical equipment are readily available in normal Chinese chemist shops, as well as antler horn, pickled snakes, dried sea horses etc. What price alternative medicine?

The problems of the future of Hong Kong post 1997 (when the lease on the New Territories and, by inference, Hong Kong Island, is due to expire), naturally figure large on the local news and many people who have the means, are making plans to leave Hong Kong unless there is a fundamental change of regime in China.

There will be a 'brain drain' flood over the next few years with great problems in maintaining the infrastructure of government and of commerce. It all seems pretty gloomy, although there are constant exhortations to keep Hong Kong a viable commercial centre and thus indispensable to China.

The Royal Navy will keep a presence to the end, but *Tamar* will close in 1991/92 and be moved from its marvellous central location on Hong Kong Island to a small island – Stonecutters – in the harbour. There has been no decision yet on relocating the Sick Bay/Dental Centre, but it might very well stay on the Island where most of the facilities will be.

So here we are in our flat on the Peak – the most desirable area of Hong Kong. Our married quarter would have a rent of £6,000 or so per month on the open market and the views over the islands are wonderful.

The heat and humidity of summer were unbearable and the tropical storms spectacular, but winter is now here and the sunny skies and mild spring weather make me feel pretty smug. Apparently we will be living up in the clouds from January to March and every thing will go mouldy!

Hope your Christmas was white – mine will be blue overlooking the South China Sea – Eat your hearts out! ❧

Another note in the pages of the same issue of the RNDS Newsletter is worth mention here. Little has been said in these pages of the development of the RNDS 'sub-Branch' of Oral and Maxillo-Facial Surgery. Its story is covered separately in an Appendix to this History.

It is, however, worth recording here that, following a visit to the Royal Naval Hospital, Haslar, by the 'Visitors' of the Royal College of Surgeons, the Department of Oral Surgery at Haslar received, in early 1990, accreditation for training for the Fellowship in Dental Surgery (FDS) for the forthcoming five years[115].

Mention has been made, a number of times in this History, of the role of RNDS personnel serving with the Royal Marines. From some of the already described experiences, in the Falklands Conflict, in Northern Ireland and in the Arctic, it will be well apparent to readers that service with a Commando is a tough and physically demanding assignment.

Not only must a dental officer and his support staff be able to survive in combat conditions in any climate, but it is important that they are not seen as 'lesser mortals' by their Commando colleagues. To this end, the majority of RNDS personnel serving with Commando units will have undergone the extremely demanding All Arms Commando Course and, on passing the rigorous tests involved, are eligible proudly to wear the Green Beret.

In early 1990, Surgeon Commander (D) M (Malcolm) Hocking held the appointment of Staff Dental Adviser to the Major General Royal Marines (MGRM). In the Spring 1990 issue of the RNDS Newsletter, he describes the rigours of Commando training[116]. The following is an extract from his article:

Man or Superman?

Seven dental officers with appropriate numbers of auxiliary staff are spread through the Corps. Those with the Commandos deploy with their units to Norway, Northern Ireland and on exercise within the UK or elsewhere. As a rule they are accompanied by dental trained [and Commando trained] Medical Assistants, but as these are in very short supply, it is not unknown for Wren DSAs to substitute, although, so far, none have volunteered to attempt the All Arms Commando Course (AACC)!

This course is designed to introduce experienced Service personnel to the joys of life as a 'Bootie' and, if successfully completed, is a passport into the adventurous world of these elite forces.

While a modicum of physical strength and athleticism is helpful, mental determination is of overriding importance and is an area where the older candidate can often outshine the young 'superstar' on the course. Having completed a month's fitness and military skills training, the AACC proper starts. It lasts five weeks and completes with five tests in the final week. These are:

1. Nine Mile Speed March – To be completed as a squad in 90 minutes. This requires a fast marching pace interspersed with doubling, along roads and cross-country tracks. Dress: fighting order.

2. Endurance Course – Comprises a one mile cross-country course, with a series of water, mud and tunnel obstacles, to be negotiated, followed by a four and a half mile run back to camp, in syndicates of three. The whole course is to be completed within 72 minutes. At the end of the course there is a shoot, using the rifle carried throughout the course, where time can be gained or lost, depending on the score. Dress: fighting order.

3. Twelve Mile Load Carry – A march in full marching order, along roads and country tracks, to be completed within four hours.

4. Thirty Mile March – A march in fighting order which, in the winter, is 10 miles across Dartmoor and the rest on roads and, in the summer, the route is mainly across Dartmoor, to be completed within eight hours.

It is hardly surprising that not all dental officers appointed to the Royal Marines, successfully complete the course and, although failure does not necessarily disbar them from joining a Commando unit, success does put a glint in their eye which remains for many a long year!

As if the AACC was not sufficient, Arctic Warfare Training is another delightful requirement to be completed by those deployed to the Northern Flank of NATO in winter. As this largely consists of learning to ski, then resting in a nice warm sleeping bag in a snow hole for the remaining time, the pass rate for dental officers is rather better! Naturally there is a tendency for those acquainted with the Corps to capitalise on all the training and they return at regular intervals in their careers to resample such delights!

At the Institute of Naval Medicine, Surgeon Commander (D) D C C (David) Alexander was now well established as Head of Oral Research. In keeping with the ethos of the Institute his research projects were designed to support the operational capability of the Navy. They were not always only concerned with dentistry, but in early 1990, he launched the Caries Risk Assessment Study (CRAS). The purpose of this study was to determine whether the provision of additional information derived from a patient may assist the clinician in treatment planning decisions. He also reported on an investigation into 'The Occurrence of Dental Pain at Sea' and published a brief report on his investigation of the health problems of Royal Marines recruits during their stressful training period [117] [see above!].

The 'Peace Dividend' had, as already mentioned, given a cash-strapped Government the opportunity to wield once again, a freshly honed axe.

It would now of course, no longer be necessary to maintain the Armed Forces at Cold War strength and further swingeing cuts were in the pipeline. The new defence review was given the reassuring title of 'Options for Change' – but it held unpleasant manpower implications for all the Services; not just the medical and dental cadres.

Surgeon Commodore (D) Brian Robinson now found himself in the forefront of the fight to retain a Naval Dental Service, sufficiently viable to provide the required level of support to the Fleet. Sadly, the Ministry of Defence practiced an effective policy of 'Divide and Conquer' and it was not only the politicians and civil servants who had the knives out!

In a personal communication to the author of this History, Robinson has given a fascinating backward look at the background and the actions taken by him and his headquarters staff, to 'keep the show on the road' at that time. Ironically, as at the time of the Falklands Conflict, apparent salvation in the shape of a new operational threat, was just around the corner. But this time, the process of change would continue regardless. Surgeon Commodore (D) Brian Robinson now takes up the story[118]:

> ### *The End of the Cold War*
>
> In 1989, the Cold War, which had dominated Western Defence Policy for over 40 years, was drawing to its close. I was then the Fleet Dental Surgeon at Fleet Headquarters in Northwood. Down in the Ops Room I watched the Soviet naval assets slowly dropping off the plot as the months passed. By the autumn it was hard to spot anything outside their own territorial waters.
>
> The West had won this protracted battle of attrition and perhaps by some small miracle, in the process, the World had avoided a nuclear holocaust.
>
> As the USSR and the Warsaw Pact countries collapsed both economically and politically, America remained as the only superpower and we, as a small but largely loyal ally, basked in the reflected glory of this victory.
>
> The scenarios which had controlled defence strategies appeared no longer relevant and virtually all western governments with significant military forces sought to reduce their heavy defence spending.
>
> In very short order, British politicians declared that we could reap the benefits of the so called "Peace Dividend". To this end, the whole of the defence structure was placed under the microscope. The review was known as "OPTIONS FOR CHANGE".
>
> In rough terms, UK overall service manpower was reduced by some 18%. »→

In the case of the Royal Navy, this meant a reduction from 75,000 to 60,000 or a 20% drop. Additionally, the Reserve Forces and other warning and monitoring units were either to be drastically reduced, or cut over the next four years.

It was against this background that I became Director in May 1990.

The Directorate had become a very different place to that which I had experienced some seven years earlier, when I had been appointed Deputy Director to Surgeon Rear Admiral (D) Philip Duly. Then I had responsibility only for the Royal Navy Dental Services. By the time I returned, it was as Deputy Director Defence Dental Services (Personnel and Training) first and the Director Naval Dental Services a poor second.

At that time the new dental headquarters structure was not well conceived and internecine struggles were never far below the surface.

Our medical colleagues were also under tremendous financial pressures.

The 'Defence Medical Establishment' was endeavouring to maintain its estate of 24 military hospitals worldwide and whilst one or two might have to be sacrificed, the Headquarters staffs still believed in 1990, that the bulk of these units could and would be retained.

This was wishful thinking. From the purely naval viewpoint, it was my belief (and remains my belief) that my dental services were under threat of serious contraction both in manpower and rank grade and also in autonomy at that time, as the system tried to reduce costs.

Because the naval dental strength is a function of overall naval manpower, its size must shrink in line with Service reductions. This had been taking place for several years, as the Navy slowly contracted after the Second World War, but dental manpower reductions had largely been achieved by cutting the short service officer career lines. This was a painless way to meet the objective, but it did not help the structural balance of the Branch. At a time when harsh financial penalties were being applied to the Defence Budget, neither was it the most fiscally efficient.

A look at our Branch structure soon revealed that we were very vulnerable to attack. We had a dental officer/rank profile which, although not an inverted pyramid certainly had a large bulge in the middle and an increasingly small footprint. In other words we had far too many expensive full career commanders and not enough cheap, short career lieutenants to do the basic dentistry!

A further threat came with the new budgetary systems which were being rolled out in the Naval Commands. Establishments were being given significant financial control over their operation, which included manpower. At the time our uniformed dental service was not well costed or its peacetime worth evaluated. Against this background, some commanding officers had already questioned whether their dental services could be provided more cheaply from civilian sources.

My deputy and I started by looking at the officer rank profile. Our future model had to be aligned with the structure required by DNMP (Directorate of Naval Manpower Planning). Broadly speaking this controlled not only overall numbers but the levels in each rank and thus the rates of promotion.

Whichever way we worked the figures, it was apparent that we had far too many non specialist commanders. A new model was constructed to meet our needs and it was clear that some redundancies would be necessary to satisfy DNMP. Rather than pass on this unpalatable fact to the Branch by letter we held a series of road shows around the Commands to explain what and why this must be undertaken.

Redundancy costs money, and whilst DNMP accepted our model they also informed us that we would have to achieve savings of £2M plus, to pay for this and other penalties which they had managed to think up.

At this time we had no sound financial data to support the retention of uniformed personnel. Of course the capitation costs of manpower were clearly spelt out, as were the costs of equipment and consumable stores. What we did not know was the true cost to the Service of providing an equivalent service from civilian sources. It had always been our belief that we could bear comparison and even better the care, which might be provided by our local NHS colleagues, but we had little or no evidence to support our views.

With a degree of secrecy, for internal political reasons, we set about trying to gather information to support our case. Surgeon Commander (D) Geoff Myers was then the SDS [Senior Dental Surgeon] at Faslane, the nuclear submarine base on the Gareloch. He also possessed an astute financial brain. He undertook a detailed costing on the provision of equivalent dental services from both service and civilian sources. Factors such as patient time away from duty, availability of appointments to operationally constrained personnel and travelling costs were factored in and these produced a very favourable bias towards the retention of a uniformed service. Of course, a nuclear submarine base in Scotland was an ideal choice for our first comparison. If we had failed here, then our prospects elsewhere would have looked bleak. However as we gained more information and costing experience, the results showed that we could bear a favourable cost comparison with a civilian alternative. We were of course, helped by the fact that the NHS dental services were already under severe strain and that in almost all areas the sudden dumping of several thousand service men and women on an overstretched system could not be handled. To be fair most Commanding Officers were aware of this and it is true to say that the service we provided was greatly appreciated in most cases.

As is always the case in such matters, I was invited to present a paper to the Second Sea Lord's Management Board. As the Paper developed several other issues emerged. It became clear (to me at least) that the most effective way to deliver dental services in the Navy was to have budgetary control of resources.

The MDG(N) already had significant budgetary power over secondary medical services with his two subordinate Surgeon Rear Admirals controlling the budgets for hospitals and operational medical services. At the same time, the Director RAF Dental Services was in the process of being given some limited budgetary control over his Service.

I therefore stuck my neck out and asked for this power and in return suggested that greater savings could be made without any significant decline in standards. To achieve this, dental manpower would be used more efficiently by the use of mobile dental teams based in the large base port clinics supplementing a core dental support team in the establishment as required. Strangely this latter concept was suggested to me by a 'black stripe' captain employed in MoD on management services.

The paper was duly presented to Second Sea Lord's Board but was shot down in committee by the Medical Director General (SRA Lammiman) this, despite the fact that he had received a copy of the paper for over a week before the meeting and my office was only a few doors down the corridor from his. I believe that he was being manipulated by others in his management team.

It was clear that the Medical Directorate did not wish the dental services to have financial autonomy.

I suppose I already knew what the outcome would be before the meeting, but I think that my proposal might just have gained Second Sea Lord's approval if the MDG(N) had backed me, but this I always guessed was highly unlikely. Of course everything else was accepted as the structure represented significant savings.

The other major factor which dictated the outcome was the fact in the 'big Navy', budgetary control of manpower was delegated to establishments through the Top Level Budget Holders such as C-in-C Naval Home Command. To take the establishment dental officer out of the ship system would have set a dangerous precedent and this I recognised.

If nothing else was achieved, I believe that this paper pre-empted a strike on the Branch from one or more areas. This was confirmed later by several comments which came from within the MoD via several sources.

The redundancy plan proceeded and our call for voluntary redundancies was oversubscribed. It was quite a generous package that the Service offered and, in fact, we later had quite a lot of bother from one individual who wanted to leave but was refused, because he did not fit our criteria. He did eventually resign from the Service, but not with quite the financial perks he had hoped for! Dental teams were introduced and proved to be quite a successful innovation. Of course, it meant that certain dentists had to work a bit harder, but the Clinical Profile Monitoring System, which was up and running, helped Commands to decide where the high loads were occurring and vice versa! In all truth, we could no longer afford to provide a spare 'staff officer' for Captains in lightly loaded establishments. Those days had gone. ⇒

> The concept of the dental services having budgetary control over their assets did eventually come to pass some years later with the establishment of the Defence Dental Agency. I believe that this is a good concept but as always, even when successful, such systems are forever being tampered with as various factions wrestle for control of power.
>
> The moral of the story is that the dental services will never be allowed to proceed independently of the larger medical organisation. My successors have recognised this fact and now work on the principle of "if you can't beat them join them". This though, is as much due to the fact that, for many senior dental officers, it offers the only route to higher promotion.

Another change for the dental profession as a whole was announced by the General Dental Council in early 1990, which required all personnel involved in prescribing, taking or developing radiographs to have undergone 'Core of Knowledge Certification' courses. Although dental radiography was well covered in Commander Dental Training's syllabi for both Dental Surgery Assistants and Dental Hygienists, this now had to be addressed on a separate course and the subject was discontinued from mainstream training. Courses were set up at the Royal Naval Hospitals at Haslar (Gosport) and Stonehouse (Plymouth), as well as at *HMS Cochrane* at Rosyth in Scotland. Without due certification, it was now illegal for dental personnel to participate in these procedures[119].

For some time, DNDS and his predecessor, Surgeon Rear Admiral (D) David Coppock had been seeking places for dental officers on senior staff courses, with a view to raising the profile of the Branch within the 'Big Navy'. As a result, Surgeon Commander (D) Geoff Myers had undergone the Joint Services Defence Course (JSDC) at Greenwich and Surgeon Commander (D) John Hargraves had attended the RN Staff Course, also at Greenwich. These, the first of such selections had resulted in Myers being appointed as Fleet Dental Surgeon and Deputy Fleet Medical Officer at the Fleet Headquarters at Northwood, relieving Robinson as he stepped up to become DNDS.

Hargraves, to the delight of the Branch senior staff, was appointed into a medical staff billet as Chief Staff Officer to the Surgeon Rear Admiral (Operational Medical Services).

Thus it was both officers were in prime positions to influence operational policy, during further momentous events shortly to take place.

Readers of this History will remember, from a previous chapter, the Civilian Dental Stores Officer at Naval Home Command, Mr Ron Coote. All in the RNDS were saddened to learn of his sudden and unexpected death in March 1990. It was previously described how his personal knowledge not only of the complex range of dental stores, but also of the needs and preferences of individual dental officers, enabled him to provide a highly efficient supply service as well as much appreciated advice to the less experienced officers. Until the late 1970s, RN dental clinics had been required to account for, periodically, every single item of equipment, including all hand instruments. Many a young dental officer, upon failing to find a particular excavator or scaling instrument, had been known to telephone Ron for help, to be met with the assurance that he would provide a replacement from his 'lay-apart store'! This happy liaison with RNDS staff led, during the Falklands Conflict, to Ron setting up his highly efficient stores replacement service to those in the field and at sea, circumventing the cumbersome and bureaucratic 'official channels' which led, more often than not to wrong or unwanted items being supplied. The sadness felt throughout the Branch at Ron's passing, is best summed up by the obituary published in the RNDS Newsletter at that time: [120]

Ron Coote BEM

As we go to press it is with great sorrow that we have to report the death of yet another staunch friend and supporter of the Dental Branch. Ron Coote died suddenly on March 15th 1990, less than two years after his retirement as Command Dental Stores Assistant to CINCNAVHOME. The affection and esteem in which he was held by all in the Royal Naval Dental Services was demonstrated by the number of dental officers and staff who attended his retirement party and who contributed to his leaving gifts in June 1988.

The same affection, coupled with sadness at his untimely passing, was shown by the very high turnout of members of the Dental Branch, past and present, who attended Ron's cremation service at Portchester on 23rd March 1990.

We believe that it would be appropriate here to reproduce part of the appreciation published in the Autumn 1988 Newsletter on the occasion of Ron's retirement. The sentiments expressed therein have not changed:

"The Royal Navy is by nature, a young man's Service and therefore, most of us are not around for too long. Every now and again someone 'breaks the mould' and serves for so long that he becomes an Institution! Such a person is Ron Coote.

Ron has given his dedicated and expert service to the RNDS for so long, that apart from very recent new entries, there are no currently serving dental officers or Wrens who do not know him or know of him.

The great majority of us have also been helped out of difficult spots by him on many past occasions when we have had 'problems with stores'. Ron's Alladin's Cave, whence he could produce replacements for any missing item, was legendary in the Branch.

> Alas! All good things come to an end. After two careers in the RNDS, his first taking him to CPO Sick Berth Attendant (D) and the award of the BEM, while his second as Civilian Stores Officer extended his service a further twenty years to Command Dental Stores Assistant. Ron Coote retired on 6th June 1988….."
>
> We will miss you Ron! … ❧

As recounted in his piece on "The End of the Cold War", above, the Director, Brian Robinson and his senior staff were only too aware that, at a time of rapidly shrinking manpower, their medical colleagues were casting covetous eyes upon the strength and structure of the Dental Branch. Although autonomous in its operation, with the advent of cascading budgets, DNDS was not only answerable to the Medical Director General (Naval), but depended for his budget, on a slice from the same cake as that passed down to MDG(N) by the Second Sea Lord.

Alarm bells began to ring in the Dental Directorate when, at the annual dinner of the RN Medical Club *, the MDG(N), Surgeon Vice Admiral Sir Godfrey Milton-Thompson proclaimed in his 'State of the Union' address: "The Dental Services continue to maintain their high quality service to the Navy and this is appreciated by the Fleet. Nevertheless, the Dental Services are small and getting smaller. I have no doubt that they must consider coming closer to the doctors. Do we really need a separate command structure? Why should we not have a common promotion list? Why should dental officers not be considered for any Surgeon Rear Admiral's appointment – or even as MDG(N)?"[121] A genuine offer or a baited trap? The Directorate view, with little hesitation was that it was the latter!

After much preparation and some concern, April 1991 saw the full implementation of devolved cost management within the Armed Forces – the New Management Strategy (NMS). The new buzzword at all levels of management was "accountability" and the NMS structure introduced a cascading system of fiscal and management authority, bringing into general use the system whereby the whole defence budget was divided among 'Top Level Budget Holders', each of whose budgets were sub-divided at various levels, right down to individual units.

The implications of this meant that, as well as a case being made at Directorate level for 'a fair slice of the cake', senior dental surgeons in

---

* The Annual Dinner of the RNMC was known in both the Medical and Dental Branches as the "Blood Red Dinner", in recognition of the coloured 'distinction cloths' worn between the gold rank stripes on the uniforms of both Branches.

establishment clinics would have to compete with other departments for enough money with which to fulfil their objectives. Inevitably, mistakes were made at first and it was not unheard of that a clinic might run out of some essential stores item, such as amalgam! Senior dental surgeons soon learned to fight their corner at establishment budget meetings.

April 1991 also saw the appointment of Surgeon Captain (D) E J (Ted) Grant as Deputy Director to work with Surgeon Commodore (D) Brian Robinson, wearing the tri-Service 'hat' of Assistant Director Dental Services (Naval) – ADDS(N). Grant's appointment was made at short notice to relieve Surgeon Captain (D) S N Bussell, who had elected for early retirement for personal reasons. Ted Grant had been preparing to move to the headquarters of C-in-C Naval Home Command, as Command Dental Surgeon. This appointment was filled, also at short notice by Surgeon Captain (D) R S (Dick) Hambly.

Grant's departure from the Institute of Naval Medicine marked the end of the long-standing post of Director of Dental Training and Research, which had existed in one form or another since 1952. All Branch training matters were now devolved to other authorities within the Branch. Postgraduate Dental Training would be controlled and supervised by the Adviser in General Dental Practice (Surgeon Commander (D) A J (Alan) Woodman). Dental officers undergoing MSc training outwith the Branch would have a point of contact and control with the Assistant Director Naval Dental Services.

Dental Cadets would be supervised by the Adviser in General Dental Practice and Commander Dental Training (Surgeon Commander (D) S (Stephen) Lambert Humble) would run or oversee 'in house' dental courses, book and slide libraries, dental training films and would edit *Dentaims* [122]. Research would continue, for the time being at the Institute of Naval Medicine, in the hands of the Head of Oral Research, now Surgeon Commander (D) C R (Colin) Priestland. The second 'hat' of Head of Training at the Institute was handed to an officer of the Instructor Branch, who had held the post as Grant's deputy. Sadly, Brian Robinson's and the Branch's 'baby', the Combat Casualty Care Course was almost immediately downgraded and the challenging New Forest module discontinued.

The partial demise of the 'C4' course was untimely. Following his aggressive stance over a period of some months, on 2 August 1990, Saddam Hussein invaded Kuwait.

*****

Chapter 8

Sand, Sea and Saddam
1990 -1991

Iraq's invasion of Kuwait was, of course, not unexpected and preparations had been in hand for some months. With regard to medical and dental support, one of the last actions of the Director of Dental Training and Research was to arrange update casualty care and resuscitation training for ten RN dental officers. Some of these attended the Army's Advanced Trauma Life Support training courses, to enable them to give combat casualty care support to the Army medical organisation ashore, should they be required.

Elsewhere, much thought had been given to the provision of a 'hospital ship' to be deployed to the Gulf in support of operations both ashore and afloat. The ships which had been so hastily, but efficiently converted to this role at the beginning of the Falklands Conflict in the early 1980s, were no longer available. The Falklands experience had shown the value of seaborne secondary medical care facilities, which could enter zones of conflict and which could, on occasion, be deployed in other roles.

Under the Geneva Conventions, ships with such flexibility of purpose could not be afforded the protection given to a hospital ship. They were therefore designated, Primary Casualty Receiving Ships (PCRS). It was known that the US Navy would deploy two large hospital ships to the Gulf in the event of conflict, so it had been decided that the British contribution would take the form of a PCRS. A search for a suitable 'platform' for this had come up with *RFA Argus*. *Argus* was a former 'Ro-Ro' ferry which, by virtue of its large upper deck, had been converted to the role of a helicopter training ship. Its conversion to PCRS is best described by an article from the RNDS Newsletter[123].

> ### *The 'Instant' Hospital – Just Add Water!*
>
> In a time when the minds of most Service managers are concentrated frequently upon the often nugatory process of keeping operations and objectives within continually increasing and severe financial constraints, it is worth recording here what can be achieved when the financial fetters are removed.
>
> In late September [1990], MoD (Navy) announced the requirement for a fully equipped and staffed PCRS to be deployed 'with utmost despatch' to the Gulf. During the next very few weeks, some impressive teamwork, involving a number ≫

of authorities, including Surgeon Rear Admiral (Operational Medical Services), Fleet Medical and DGSS in Bath, sought and identified a suitable ship and converted it to the medical role. This was *RFA Argus*.

Argus is a helicopter training and support ship of 22,266 tons, originally converted from a Ro-Ro container ship. She is 574.5 feet in length and has a large flight deck of almost 'carrier' proportions. The former Ro-Ro deck has been converted to a hangar deck with three watertight bulkheads. The hangar is served by two aircraft lifts. The main superstructure, including the bridge and crew accommodation is forward of the flight deck and a small 'island', which includes the funnel and a radar mast, occupies part of the starboard side of the flight deck.

Between the 8th October 1990 and 29th October 1990, the date on which she sailed (a period of exactly three weeks), the teams involved, co-ordinated by our medical colleagues Surgeon Commanders Paxton Dewar and Rick Jolly, achieved the near impossible.

It was decided that the forward compartment of the hangar would be used for the hospital conversion, this being served by the forward aircraft lift.

During the ensuing three weeks, a one-hundred bed hospital was constructed within the hangar, using two tiers of 'duplex' Portacabins in a roughly 'L' shaped configuration, allowing room for casualties to be transported from the upper deck, by lift to the hangar area, immediately outside the hospital entrances, on both levels.

The facilities constructed included: two operating theatres, with two operating tables within each; recovery rooms and full supporting services; a 24-bed Intensive Care Ward and other wards, the latter being mostly in the upper tier. A scissor lift was installed to carry patients from the OT, triage and intensive care areas on the lower deck to the low-dependency wards above. Storage facilities were planned and all mains services were built in and connected. The whole complex is served by double-door, air-lock entrances and has been constructed to maintain suitable positive pressure for collective protection purposes in the event of chemical threat.

Argus, in addition to her normal RFA officers and crew, is manned by an approximately 100-strong Medical Group of doctors, dentists, medical assistants and nursing staff, representing all the relevant clinical and medical support specialties.

The medical capability of the ship is further supported by an Air Group of four, CASEVAC-equipped Sea King helicopters, with aircrew and support personnel, totalling approximately 100 and a 40-strong Royal Marine Band, borne in their war role as medical ancillaries.

The Medical Officer-in-Charge is Surgeon Commander Dewar and the Dental

Branch contingent are:

Surgeon Captain (D) George Rudge – Oral Surgeon, Triage Officer and Medical Group Executive Officer.

Surgeon Lieutenant Commander (D) Charlie Killick – Dental Officer and Resuscitation Officer.

Leading Wren DSA Rita Burnside and MA (D) Alex Speight.

The *Argus* sailed from Devonport on 29th October and after a small 'glitch' concerning her main propulsion, which necessitated a quick, albeit short, return to port, she is now on station.

The achievement of getting this ship converted, equipped and manned in so short a time is tremendous by any standards and is a feather in the caps of all concerned, from the planners to the contractors and the staff themselves. It shows what can be done when 'the chips are down'!

We are confident that, if required to do so, the 'Argonauts' will meet any challenge which presents, but we hope and pray that they will not be required to exercise their considerable medical skills.

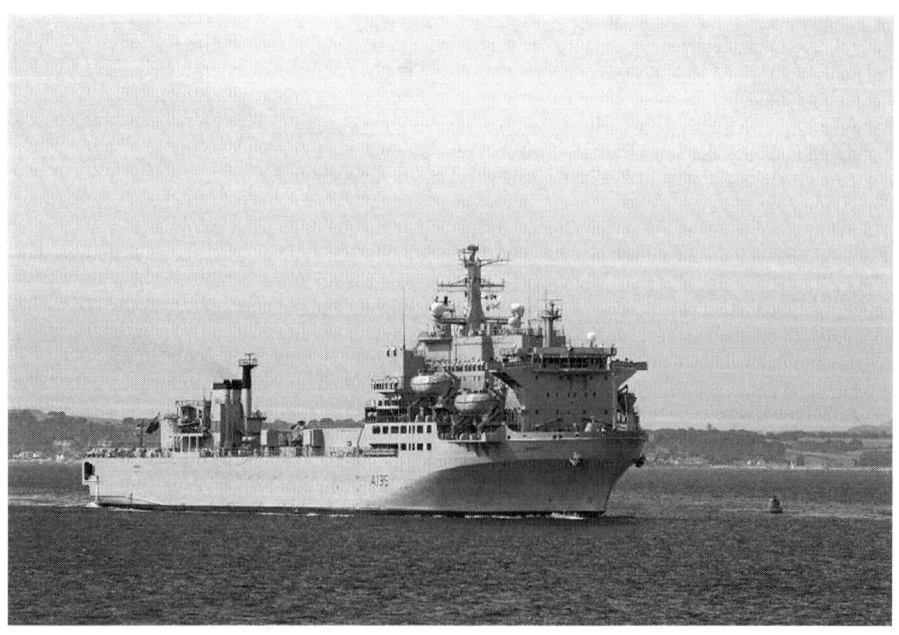

RFA Argus leaving Plymouth – October 1990

For the Royal Navy in general and the RN Medical and Dental Services in particular, the Gulf War – 'Operation Granby' as it was designated by the Ministry of Defence – was to provide a very different set of experiences to those encountered during the Falklands Conflict.

During and since the Iran/Iraq War, the RN had established a permanent presence in the Gulf in the form of the 'Armilla Patrol'. This took the form of one destroyer or frigate, which usually carried a dental team with portable equipment which could be set up in the sick bay.

The team, a dental officer and a dentally trained MA (Medical Assistant) could and often did, deploy to other ships in the area as circumstances required. Most RN ships were equipped with a 'lie flat' operating table which could double up as a dental chair and some were fitted with an appropriate compressed air supply, although the 'Frigate Portable Dental Unit' usually included a small compressor, with which to drive the dental handpieces, mouth sprays etc.

Apart from those in *RFA Argus*, the Naval dental personnel present in the Gulf immediately before and during hostilities were Surgeon Lieutenant (D) N P (Nigel) Mallon, supported by Leading Medical Assistant (LMA) Wallace. These two, were later relieved by Surgeon Lieutenant (D) D V (Dominic) Flanagan, supported by Leading Wren DSA Karen Calderbank.

Despite having been called forward for update casualty care training, none of the previously mentioned ten RN dental officers were deployed during the conflict.

Surgeon Commander (D) C R (Chris) Sanderson, at that time undergoing Oral Surgery training, was deployed with a Naval Medical contingent to 32 Field Hospital RAMC, established in Saudi Arabia, ready to receive the anticipated casualties from the pending conflict. 32 Field Hospital was the most forward UK hospital in the war zone and once Coalition forces had launched their offensive, was established in Wadi al Batin on the Kuwait/Iraq border. It was to treat 1250 patients and perform 105 surgical operations during the war [124].

These, together with the team in *RFA Argus* made up the RNDS front line contribution to Operation Granby.

Although many female medical personnel had been deployed in hospital ships and ashore, during previous operations and wars, Leading Wren Rita Burnside had the distinction of being the first ever Wren to find herself at sea in a conflict zone.

Before, during and after the Gulf war, Surgeon Commander (D) Geoff Myers held the appointment of Fleet Dental Surgeon and Deputy Fleet Medical Officer. He played a highly significant and effective role in the planning and day to day management of the RN Medical and Dental contribution to the operation.

As previously encountered in these pages, several in the above 'cast of characters' have committed their experiences to the printed word in the

RNDS Newsletter. Let them, therefore, tell their own stories.

As first on the scene, let us begin with an account of his experiences by Surgeon Lieutenant (D) Nigel Mallon who, not only writes well, but was a most talented cartoonist, illustrating his account with a highly amusing 'strip cartoon entitled "Top Gum". The following is a slightly abbreviated version of his article[125].

Have Drill – Will Travel!

When I was told that I would be joining the 'Group X-Ray' Armilla patrol, my initial expectations were of cocktail parties, trips to the Seychelles, the Far East and Christmas in Mombasa - in fact, I had arranged 17 port visits with *HMS London's* Operations Officer. 2nd August 1990 and Saddam Hussein's invasion changed all that!

I had never been to sea before, let alone war! The first time I heard the general alarm was in the DRIU [Damage Repair Instructional Unit] at *HMS Phoenix* during my Pre-Joining Training.

The second time was in *HMS Brazen* in the Red Sea as the Royal Marines fast roped from a Lynx helicopter to board an Iraqi tanker, trying to break UN sanctions. We had visions of this "act of piracy" – as quoted by Iraq – as the initiating factor of World War III!

On 26th September 1990, I joined *HMS London* in Cyprus. After a short period at sea with the Portable Dental Unit, I found myself established in *RFA Diligence* – A forward repair ship based in Jebel Ali, south of Dubai. From the well equipped dental surgery on board, I could treat all the RN and RFA ships as they came for their maintenance periods. A casualty service was also provided for the Allied Navies.

With the invaluable chairside assistance of LMA [Leading Medical Assistant] Wallace, we worked hard to treat as many patients as possible, so as to reduce the amount of potential 'pain cases' which could emerge later. In the first month we had seen over 500 patients and by January 1991, we had seen our 1000th. Clinically, I had expected a high degree of stress-related problems – I was surprised that this was not the case. Despite the high volume of work done in the initial months, pain cases did not dwindle completely. It would seem that the more the supply of dental care provided, the larger the patient demand became.

Dubai is a multi-cultural city – a bit like the Hong Kong of the Middle East. This is where the waiting started: the 'phoney war' period, leading up to January, was difficult. We had rushed down, having seen street maps of Kuwait in Northwood [Fleet HQ] and were expecting a swift start to the war ….. now we were waiting. ➢

Due to accommodation problems in *RFA Diligence*, I had ended up in a Dubai hotel – on subsistence, with a car ….. waiting! I was all for letting sanctions take their full effect!

By this stage, I had moved from Cyprus to *HMS London* to *HMS Brazen* to *RFA Diligence* to *RFA Fort Grange* for exercise, then back to *Diligence*, then to a hotel. This moving around made it difficult to establish any sense of camaraderie or identity. I was pleased to get a chance to settle down in one place. I had made good local friends and took the opportunity to see some of the Emirates, go camping in the desert and take up scuba diving. At weekends, expats would take us 'Wadi bashing' – Wadis are dried up river beds. They would charge in their four-wheel drive Jeeps and Landcruisers, over terrain of scrub desert, sand or mountains. After frequent beer stops, it would usually end in a BBQ. Life in fact soon proved to be rather expensive, as I acted as host for numerous runs ashore! My dilemma now was whether to use every waking moment to train to be a potential anaesthetist/oral surgeon/doctor, for a war that may never happen, or make use of every opportunity the UAE offered. I ended up staying awake all night, doing both!

Prior to the arrival of *RFA Argus*, Naval Party 1036 – Surgical Reactive Team, based in *RFA Fort Grange*, provided medical support. In Exercise Copper Bottom, I and two of the dental team were vital in administration, medical treatment and triage, especially in the large holding areas.

The arrival of *RFA Argus* in theatre, with Surgeon Captain (D) Rudge and Surgeon Lieutenant Commander (D) Killick, allowed me to lose my dubious title of Senior Officer Dental (Middle East) – SODME. This left me with the more envious position of *Diligence* Dental Officer – DILDO. The dental staff (dragged kicking and screaming) joined *Argus* on 11th January 1991, to lead the First Aid Reaction Team (FART) to damaged ships. Suddenly life had stepped up a few gears and a heavy sense of realism appeared. We studied the Advanced Trauma Life Saving system – an American triage and casualty handling programme, as used extensively in US accident and emergency departments. The thought of being winched down on to the burning deck of an RN ship was chilling.

I gave up general dental duties, allowing Surgeon Lieutenant Commander (D) Killick to take over. Part of my day was spent using computers to update 'Souls on Board' lists, as part of the medical casualty reporting cell. It was conceivable that, on returning from a damaged ship, the dental team would have to do the casualty signal on the patients we had seen.

17th January 1991 – Our rude early morning call at 0415 was unforgettable.

In 11 minutes a sleeping ship was dressed for action, secure and ready. It was strange, but there were smiling faces – the waiting had ended, we were going to get on with it – but in the pit of your stomach you knew you were at war and that there would be casualties. ➤

> Personally, I felt quite at peace and had a God-given calm to accept whatever might come my way. I guess, statistically, you always feel that things will happen to the next man. As a Christian, I was interested to see if people would be more interested in God, when faced with the possibility of death. I had heard of this happening in the Army, but perhaps their tensions and fears were greater with the prospect of an impending land battle.
>
> However, I was not aware of any increased interest. Maybe we were more confident in our resources and safety at sea, as compared with those on land. Sources of tension for us were the mine threat, possible air attack and boredom.
>
> Morale in *Argus* was low due to the issue of *roulement*. When would we return? 'Group Yankee' had arrived, but were seen as reinforcement, rather than replacement. Commodore Craig (Senior Naval Officer Middle East) eventually announced release of part of 'X-ray Group'. Within eight hours I was in *HMS Brazen* heading for the Straits of Hormuz. The elation on board was incredible, but we could not allow ourselves to believe it until we were home safely in the UK.
>
> The return through the Med. was an opportunity to unwind, with good runs ashore in Sardinia and Barcelona. There was a sense of fraudulence to be dealt with. What had we actually done? As the doctor in Brazen put it: "*Veni, Vidi – Video*" – "We came, we saw, we watched videos!" [In fact], The Royal Navy had completed 42% of the operational sea duties, despite having a fleet one eighth of the size of that of the US Navy. Effective deterrence, air cover, mine hunting and a host of other duties had been performed at a very high professional level. [After] I returned, there was much enquiry into the war role of the dentist. To say that you are a 'flexible asset' does not add up to much on paper, when governments are still determined on Service cuts. The dental staff had provided dental care, medical cover, and had supported the reporting cell and 'FART' in *Argus*. It was a rich experience, in which I am glad to have played a part.

Despite the self-deprecating remarks and doubts about the role played by himself and his team in Operation Granby, Mallon had played an invaluable part in the preparation for a conflict which, potentially, could have produced many Allied casualties, both ashore and afloat.

Apart from his somewhat 'roving commission' once the war had started, he provided a huge amount of dental support to all personnel congregating in the Gulf in preparation for the conflict. This will always be the primary role of the RN dental officer. His or her ability to fill other functions are just a valuable bonus.

Now let us hear from Leading Wren (DSA) Rita Burnside – the first ever member of the Women's Royal Naval Service (WRNS) to serve at sea in a theatre of conflict. She too has provided an insight into her experiences during Operation Granby, for the Branch Newsletter [126].

Reflections of an Argonaut

I was asked by Surgeon Captain (D) Rudge if I would like to go on a cruise to the Mediterranean and beyond. As the weather was pretty bad at home, I agreed with only the slightest hesitation. My husband, Paul, was willing to let me go and immediately took out a huge insurance on me!

At this stage I don't think I realised what I was letting myself in for. The following week, things were a bit clearer. I was to join *RFA Argus* a Primary Casualty Receiving Ship (PCRS), which was in Devonport, undergoing a few changes at the time.

For the next few days things were rather hectic. I went to *HMS Raleigh* to learn about fire fighting, which I think must have been one of the worst experiences of my life!

I spent most of my time on my back, with the hose attacking me, dressed in a fireproof suit, which was so big, I barely touched the sides. Then I explored the DRIU, which I rather enjoyed. Finally we tested out the swimming pool in our 'Once Only Suits' and I jumped from the high board and swam to our life raft at the other end of the pool.

On board the *Argus* with me, were 27 QARNNS [Queen Alexandra's Royal Naval Nursing Service] junior rates and 13 senior rates and officers, so there were about 40 females in all.

Getting kitted out in sea-going uniform was amusing, nothing seemed to fit and my kit bag was huge.

Eventually the day came when we were due to join the ship. It was massive, but unfortunately our mess and the lads' accommodation weren't. All the female junior rates were put in a 27-woman mess.

Once we had sorted out our belongings and squeezed as much as we could into the tiny wardrobe provided for each of us, it was time to explore the ship. As I have said, it was a big ship and full of boxes of stores. The hospital complex, at that stage, was full of workmen and completely empty of equipment.

By the Saturday, the medical team was complete. We were allowed home that night and were to set sail on the Sunday morning. I was quite sad to leave home and it finally sank in what was going on and how dodgy the political climate was looking. My family and friends were very worried about it all.

The next day came too quickly and, after a tearful goodbye, I boarded the ship, ready to sail. We sailed out to an ammunitioning buoy on the Sunday and set sail on the Monday – only to return on the Tuesday with rudder problems! I was lucky not to suffer from sea-sickness, but some of the girls were quite bad. Anyway, we finally set sail the next day after another night at home and, this time, we were really on our way.

We had to be on station by November 15th, with the hospital ready to receive ⇒

casualties. I was working with Surgeon Lieutenant Commander (D) Killick in the sickbay hospital.

We had a portable dental unit, which luckily I had used in Norway. The PDU was squeezed between the beds and it was rather cramped.

After a little readjustment to the bedding arrangements, we managed to gain a larger working area. Our days [on passage] were filled with stores lifts, cleaning, lectures and seeing dental patients. The reaction to females being on board was mixed, but because of more worrying events, it was less of a problem than expected.

En route, we stopped at Suez and a group of us went to visit the pyramids, which I really enjoyed – especially jumping back on board the fast moving ship from a boat that was on fire! We had to board *Argus* while she was moving, as ships are not allowed to stop in the Canal, so our boat had to go at full speed for quite a time, which had exciting effects on the engine cooling – hence the fire.

The hospital complex was, by now, looking more like it was intended. The medical staff had really worked non-stop to put it together. We had lectures and exercises to prepare us for the possibility of war. My war casualty role was patient documentation. When we eventually arrived at Jebel Ali, we were allowed ashore. After being confined to the ship and wearing 8's [working uniform] continuously, it was a lovely feeling.

We had to abide by the strict dress customs; so no shorts or tee-shirts were allowed. Christmas was spent in Sharjah, where we were entertained by Surgeon Lieutenant Commander (D) Mallon, in his five star hotel! New Year was spent at sea and after returning to port to restock and refuel, we set sail again with the rest of the fleet, on 4th January to await events.

We didn't have long to wait. On 15th January, the war started. We were woken by the action stations alarm going off at 0430. Our mess was at panic stations at that time – 27 girls jumping out of bed at once were a sight to see! Somehow, everyone managed to be at their action stations, complete with IPE [Individual Protection Equipment – anti-gas respirator and anti-flash hood and gloves], within eight minutes. In practice, it had been 12 minutes! From that day on, wherever I went, so did my IPE – even to the loo!

Morale amongst the girls was quite good. We still managed to apple-pie each other's beds and tease each other. Being the only Wren amongst so many QARNNS, I was the butt of many of these jokes. Fortunately I was able to retaliate quite well, especially after my IPE bag was drawn all over with "I wish I was tall enough to be a QARRN" and other similar quotes. Lieutenant Commander Mallon came in quite handy; he drew a cartoon strip called the QARRNWEILLERS, which depicted two nurses as dogs wanting to be Wrens. We carried it on after he left the ship and it was appreciated by the crew.

We were still seeing dental patients every day and a new duty was mine watching. ⇒

> We were near the top of the Persian Gulf and there was a strong threat. Life on board was very boring. We just seemed to be waiting for the land war to start.
>
> A 'brief' we attended, brought it home to me just how badly the troops could be injured, if things went wrong. Once the land war had started, it was clear that things would be over fairly quickly. We did receive three casualties from the American ships which were mined and they were very well looked after by the nursing staff.
>
> We stayed at sea continuously for 60 days before we started our journey back to the Southern Gulf. The day before we entered Jebel Ali, we had a celebration on board, which equalled New Year's Eve. The following day, the 11th March, my birthday, we flew home to our families and a nice hot bath! Fortunately, *Argus* never received the number of casualties expected and the surgeons' and nurses' skills were only needed for minor accidents and injuries. For that, I will always be thankful. ❧

Later in the year, Leading Wren DSA Rita Burnside was awarded the Alan Acton Davies Memorial Prize for her impressive contribution to life and work in *RFA Argus* during Operation Granby. Her citation read: "Throughout the Operation, often in difficult and arduous circumstances, she performed her duties, (both dental and as a medical auxiliary), in a cheerful, efficient and exemplary manner, which drew both admiration and commendation from those who worked with her, in the best traditions of the RNDS and the Royal Navy."

Surgeon Commander (D) Geoff Myers, the Fleet Dental Surgeon, who in his secondary role as deputy to the Fleet Medical Officer, had played a very significant role in the planning, deployment, support and control of all RN medical and dental operational assets before and during the Gulf War, was honoured with the award of the OBE in recognition of his outstanding contribution.

It is now well known that for political reasons, following the capitulation of the Iraqi forces, no attempt was made by the Coalition to 'follow up' and Saddam Hussein remained free to lick his wounds and then to turn his attention to those whom he saw as worthy of his particular style of retribution.

The dust of the Gulf War had not yet settled when the Kurds in Northern Iraq, thinking Saddam to be finished, rose up against the Iraqi leader, who then proceeded ruthlessly to suppress this rebellion*.

---

* It was against these same people that in March 1988, Saddam's henchman, who later became known as "Chemical Ali", deployed chemical weapons. At Halabja, it was reported that this attack resulted in up to 5,000 fatalities and up to 10,000 non-fatal casualties.

Following this reprisal, well over half a million Kurdish refugees fled their villages into the mountains of the Iraq/Turkish border, amidst appalling weather conditions. Stranded and helpless in the mountains, living in makeshift camps, without infrastructure or sanitation the people in the camps were soon overwhelmed by disease and privation. Many hundreds died, before, in response to global outrage, a huge, multinational relief operation was launched. The British contribution to this was named "Operation Haven" of which the principal force was that of 3 Commando Brigade, Royal Marines[127].

A significant part of this operation was to provide medical support to the refugees and these included the dental teams deployed with 40 and 45 Commandos and the Medical Squadron of the Commando Logistics Regiment. These included Surgeon Lieutenant (D) C D J (Chris) Redman (40 Commando), Surgeon Lieutenant (D) C (Crawford) Elrick (45 Commando) and Surgeon Lieutenant (D) R (Richard) Colbeck (Medical Squadron – Commando Logistic Regiment). The latter was accompanied by Petty Officer Wren DH Mary Norris, Leading Wren DSA Charlotte Freeman and Wren DSA Liz Edwards. The two commando dental officers were supported by commando (and dentally) trained Medical Assistants.

A number of personal accounts of 'Op. Haven' exist, therefore, as previously in this History, we will let some of those involved tell their own stories.

Firstly, an extract from a letter sent back to DNDS by Chris Redman[128].

Dispatches from Kurdistan

In the last 24 hours we have moved south and have taken over from 45 Commando who are shortly to be going home. The job we did further north is now complete and I think everyone is surprised just how quickly some sort of order has been resumed.

For the first two weeks I spent my time with Charlie Company as a 'medic'. I must admit to doing very little, but it was good experience, spending some time in the field with a fighting company. I went out on a number of patrols with the guys and also managed to get up to the large refugee camp above us on the Turkish/Iraq border. This particular camp held about 70,000 Kurds and I've never really seen anything quite like it. I was actually amazed as to how cheerful and healthy the majority of the refugees appeared to be, considering the foul conditions in which they were living. However, I also stuck my head into one of the tents in the German field hospital up there and you quickly saw the flip side of the coin. A forest of drips maintaining dozens of dehydrated and undernourished infants – they were losing about four a day. I hear that there is now nobody there. ≫→

Having spent my time with "C" Coy, I returned to the RAF setup, which was co-located with Support Company at a place called Kanai Masi. For three weeks this area was a hive of activity and seemed to be very much a showpiece for the relief effort. Many distinguished visitors came to see for themselves what we were doing there, including Tom King [the Secretary of State for Defence], most of the US generals (about one a day!) and our own Commandant General.

Kanai Masi was ideally placed for a way-station for the Kurds who had come down from the mountains and were waiting for Dahuk to be 'liberated'.

We provided about 50,000 Kurds (when we were at our busiest) with food, water and medical support, as well as laying on large convoys of trucks to help them continue their journeys back to the villages from which they had fled.

The medical setup was like a large field hospital which had medical teams from Holland, Canada, UK and the US. At the height of it all, about 850 Kurds were being seen in the complex, each day.

I set up a dental tent in the compound for emergency cases and, being the only dentist there, had all dental cases sent to me.

It never ceases to surprise me how inadequately trained many doctors seem to be, when it comes to primary pain relief of dental origin. Anyway, once set up with a Kurdish interpreter, we opened up shop and were snowed under with patients every day for about a week and a half. Generally their mouths were in appalling condition, with gross caries [decay] widespread and very advanced cases of periodontal [gum] disease. We had a couple of children with externally draining sinuses [from dental abscesses] and a number of cases with multiple abscesses. [There was] very little evidence of any dental treatment, so I can only assume that there were no dentists. The three most difficult cases I dealt with were small children in acute pain. Fortunately, I had a 'tame' civilian doctor who was extremely handy with the Midazolam, so we did quite a few sedation extractions. In the space of 10 days, I did 168 extractions!

The Kurds were really pathetically grateful for everything we did for them, but it was extremely interesting and very rewarding. MA [Medical Assistant] Speight was with me for most of the time, but also got involved with the medical side of things too – helping out in the dressing tents. Charlotte Freeman and Liz Edwards came up from the Medical Squadron for a few days, to help out, as did PO [Petty Officer] Mary Norris.

It is extremely hot at the moment, over 100 degrees on most days. Although we are living in the field, conditions are not bad and we have such luxuries as showers, some fresh rations plus NAAFI goods, etc. One of the worst things is the insect situation – there are hordes of them and they all bite or sting!

We had some more excitement one afternoon at Kanai Masi, which I forgot to mention. Four US guys who were clearing a ridge just behind the location, tripped a booby-trapped mine. When we got to them, they were quite severely peppered with shrapnel, covered in blood and quite shocked. We dripped

> a couple, gave one morphine and within 35 minutes, they were on their way to hospital without loss of life or limb. We have since seen three of the blokes, who were fine – the fourth was sent back to Germany to have his eye dealt with.
>
> Well, that's about all the news I have. I personally think that the security [role] we have taken over will be less interesting than what we have been doing. Still, you are right when you say that I wouldn't have believed it, if you had said I would be in Northern Iraq this time last year! It hasn't been a bad past 18 months really – 10 foreign countries, courtesy of Her Majesty, with a couple of free suntans thrown in!

In Summer 1992, the Journal of the Royal Navy Medical Service devoted its issue to the experiences of medics and dental teams during the Iraq War and Operation Haven. Among these are two graphic and moving accounts by RNDS personnel, both of which are worth reproducing here. The first is by Petty Officer Wren Dental Hygienist Mary Norris, who was awarded the British Empire Medal for her outstanding work during Op. Haven [129].

> ### *A Mission of Mercy*
>
> Almost a year has passed since I received the invitation to join Med. Squadron [of the Logistics Regiment, Royal Marines] en route for Northern Iraq – for the purpose of Operation Safe Haven 1991. Though a while ago now, the memories of the plight of the Kurdish people are still vivid in my mind, as I am sure they are with many other servicemen and women who were also involved. No-one could have prepared us for the sights we were to be confronted with, during the two months we were there.
>
> Our first two weeks were spent in Turkey, visiting Zakho refugee camp and hospital. Each day a team, consisting of two medical officers, two or three DSAs [WRNS Dental Surgery Assistants] or MA(Q)s [female RN Medical Assistants] and several general duty Marines, were assigned to the camp to treat a constant stream of refugees being transported from the mountains to safety. Each family, on arrival, was given a tent, allocated blankets, clothing and food and given a full check up at the medical screening tent by Service personnel. It became evident, quite quickly, that almost every child under the age of five years, was suffering from severe dehydration and malnutrition, not to mention numerous cases of scabies, head lice, infected wounds and even rickets. Each patient was seen by a medical officer and treatment was given there, in situ. All severe cases were forwarded on to Zakho hospital nearby. A special intensive feeding tent was set up at the camp itself after only a few days, as the hospital was soon inundated with very sick children. This basic tent proved to be a life saver to many of the very small babies and children brought to us.
>
> Zakho hospital [became] our second undertaking. The hospital itself was already in the hands of the Canadian and American forces, with French paediatricians

and doctors working all hours to cope with the flood of refugees.

It was in a very poor state of repair and we joined with other service people in clearing up the corridors and wards. Here we saw rooms full of beds occupied by dozens of children. There was a shortage of blankets, no sheets and very little medicine or supplies. Improvisation was definitely called for. After a little instruction, the Royal Marines added another string to their bow in providing nappies for the patients. It is surprising what you can come up with, using rolls of gauze and cotton wool!

The weeks spent in the two areas of Zakho camp and hospital, saw many emotions shared between Kurdish people and British forces together. I will never forget my first night duty at the hospital, when a small child lost his battle for life after many attempts to revive him. Knowledge of first aid and Combat Casualty Care certainly was useful, but a little inadequate when requiring instructions on how to lay out a body.

This was to be the first of many such deaths over the coming weeks. In many cases we had arrived there a little too late. Many tears were shed by all, of course, but there were also tears of joy as new babies were being born amidst the severe conditions. Seeing new life certainly brought hope to all of us there.

After Turkey came Northern Iraq. Here our first task was to clear up a rather dilapidated building, once a school, and produce a treatment centre. As the Marines set to work rebuilding walls, clearing fallen masonry and repairing the roof, the girls cleaned and scrubbed walls and floors and even painted walls white, to create a clean working environment. Rooms were designated for wards, casualty and even an operating theatre and dark room. We had stretchers, beds and bedding and electricity.

The patients attended in truck loads and soon we were up and running, treating young and old with a wide variety of ailments. We also received many casualties from accidents involving mines and other such exploding devices. The entire area was scattered with weapons such as these and small children and Kurdish males, attempting to rebuild their lives, became victims.

The arrival of the surgical support team from [the Royal Naval Hospital Haslar], came just in time, as a severe accident involving six young Kurdish boys, turned our centre into a full working hospital.

In addition to these Kurdish patients, we nursed American and Canadian servicemen and women and civilian aid workers alike. And, as the weeks went by, more and more of our own personnel began contracting stomach disorders – a hazard of our living conditions out there. Food came in the form of ration packs for five weeks, until fresh food was obtained via the US Army. Home was a tent and a sleeping bag, often shared with many strange visitors. It was David Attenborough's paradise out there, I can tell you – snakes, locusts, scorpions and frogs! »+

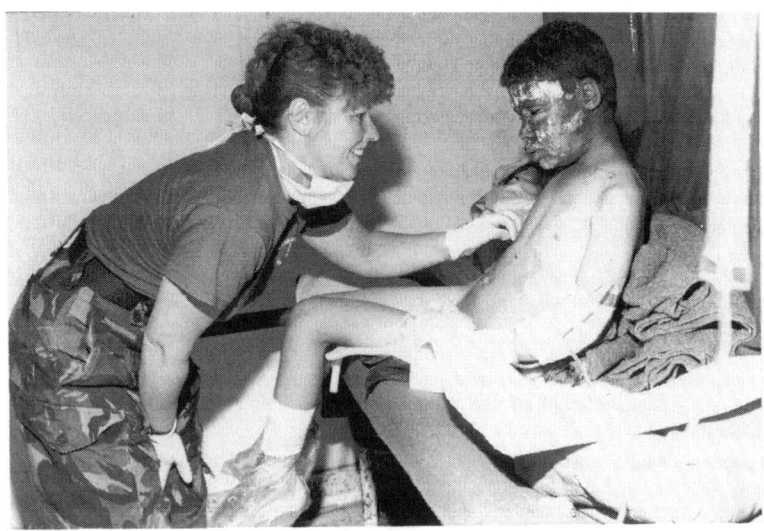

PO Wren DH Mary Norris with a young Kurd land mine victim

I think that by the end of our stay, we had overcome our phobias of creepy-crawlies, one way or another. Our washing facilities consisted of a bowl and stream water. Later a length of piping and a plastic bottle became the makeshift shower for daily ablutions.

The toilet facilities had to be seen to be believed. Another length of pipe, pushed into the ground and a blue plastic funnel for one function and a bucket with a black plastic bin liner, for the other.

Sounds OK – well it was until you had to empty it! Enough said! The Marines who built the walls of corrugated iron for privacy, added a nice touch in the way of fresh flowers in a jar, at the opening ceremony!

Throughout each day we ran a watch system, some working away at outstations nearby (smaller refugee camps), others at smaller hospitals in nearby towns and the remainder in our hospital named Sirsenk – "Haven amongst Holocaust".

The work, albeit sometimes arduous and long, was certainly beneficial to thousands of Kurdish refugees. We gained their trust gradually, by healing the sick, trying to learn their language and understanding their customs – the latter being the most difficult.

The ways of these people, combined with their religious beliefs, took a while to understand and we often failed in convincing them that the treatment we were prescribing was correct.

I have often been asked, "Has it affected you being there?"

The answer has to be yes. Actually living alongside and seeing so many seemingly innocent people, wandering, homeless and helpless, looking for lost members of their families, is a sight firmly imprinted on my mind. »➔

> Hopefully our small contribution to the campaign has restored some dignity to these people and left them with a positive look towards the future. I was certainly proud to be a member of the Armed Forces during Operation Safe Haven and learnt the value of comradeship and trust. That is what it is all about.

The other RNDS contributor to the same issue of the RN Medical Journal was Leading Wren Dental Surgery Assistant Charlotte Freeman. Her account covers the same ground as Mary Norris, but it is worth seeing the same events through different eyes.[130]

Haven or Hell?

We left the UK in a Hercules from RAF Lynham on 30 April 1991. I was now an 'attached rank' to the Medical Squadron, Commando Logistics Regiment, Royal Marines. We were all quiet and very subdued; our minds were filled with apprehension of what we might have to endure and sadness at the thought of leaving loved ones behind.

One of the worst things was not knowing for how long we were being deployed. We were told it would be as long as six months, but nobody could give us a definite time span. Although I had served in the WRNS for seven years, most of which had been with the Royal Marines, I had never experienced field conditions. My memories of life in a tent were good – most mod cons, hot showers on hand. I was in for a big shock in more ways than one – no plug socket for hair dryers!

After a long and tedious flight, we eventually arrived in Turkey. We were then split into our flight groups for the journey to Silopi by American Chinook helicopter.

Medical Squadron were setting up their complex on the border of Iraq and Turkey, with the mountains of Syria facing us. Tired, dirty and feeling bedraggled, we staggered over the rough terrain which was to be our home for however long we were needed.

The following morning, after spending an uncomfortable night on a rollmat, we were taken to a refugee camp situated at a town called Zakho, just inside the Iraq border. The camp was large enough to hold 25,000 Kurdish refugees in tents that had been provided by the UN.

The camp comprised of living accommodation for the Kurds and four tents used by the medics for initial screening, minor treatments and intensive feeding.

Transport had been provided by both 40 and 45 Commando RM, to assist the Kurds in the journey down from the mountains. Those who were too ill to withstand the journey by road were airlifted by Sea King helicopters to a landing strip close to the main screening area, as they would require immediate medical attention. Screening was carried out by a team of doctors and medics from Medical Squadron, one of whom was a qualified paediatrician. Routine checks were then carried out on the children, paying particular attention to the eyes, ears, head and the torso, for scabies.

We found that the majority of the under-fives had severe diarrhoea and vomiting, resulting in dehydration. This was measured by pinching loose skin on their stomachs.

Babies who had more than half an inch of loose skin, were transferred to Zakho hospital for rehydration. The ones with less than half an inch of loose skin were sent to the intensive feeding tent, where a mixture of vitamins and Dioralyte was administered orally. The last thing we had to do at the refugee camp was to inoculate as many Kurdish children as the time allowed.

Zakho hospital, which was run by 18 Canadian medics during the day time and by the Medical Squadron at night, was not the ideal hospital we are accustomed to in the UK.

It was very filthy and run down; medical equipment and stores were in very short supply, because they had been stolen and sold on the black market when the hospital had been attacked.

The ailments we had to treat, ranged from typhoid, cholera and tuberculosis to leukaemia, leprosy and severe malnutrition. Our night shift were very hectic on the paediatric wards, rehydrating small babies, using intravenous drips into their jugular veins. Problems arose when the mothers tried either to remove the drip, or increase the flow, hence killing the baby by flooding its lungs.

During our time at Zakho, there were many tears of sadness, when we were unable to save some of the children's lives, as they did not have the strength to breathe by themselves. Although we attempted mouth to mouth resuscitation for several hours, it was all to no avail. We were also hindered by the fact that there was no oxygen in the hospital.

One busy night I and another DSA, who were the only medical cover on watch, were guided down to the labour room by one of the Kurdish mothers. In this room was her friend going through the last stages of labour and who was obviously in a lot of pain.

We knew that she was relying on us to deliver her baby. Neither of us had faced this situation before and, although we had read about it in the text books, this was reality and there was no room for mistakes. After a few tense moments, our natural instincts took over and we delivered a healthy 7lb baby boy, which was to be the first of several that evening.

Three weeks later we were given our orders to move forward to set up a new location and complex, deeper within Iraq, after the area had been made safe by other RM units. Our new camp was to be a place called Sirsenk, which was about 20 kilometres from Dahuk. We handed over Zakho hospital into the capable hands of Dutch medics and proceeded on our way south.

On arrival at Sirsenk, we faced a rundown building, which we transformed into a small hospital, consisting of minor and major treatment rooms, a dental surgery, a ward and a fully equipped theatre, which saw a lot of action! Firstly, we had to clean and repair the building, before we could even erect our tents. It was about 2300 by the time we had whitewashed the walls and the building resembled a hospital. I was employed in the ward and also the dental surgery. We were split into three watches so that we would have a different task each day.

The majority of our patients were suffering injuries from mines, which were scattered just about everywhere; many amputations had to be carried out on lower limbs, [often on] children who had been injured while out playing. One of the most horrific sights was of a young boy of about eight years who had been accidentally run over by a four-ton lorry; despite all our efforts, he died.

I also went to assist 40 Commando RM at Kani Masi, which was a small village at the base of the mountains. At this camp, there were several [other] organisations working alongside us, [such as] the Overseas Development Agency, Médecins sans Frontières and Canadian and Dutch contingents.

The set up was similar to that at Zakho refugee camp, with two additional cholera tents. The doctor from 40 Commando RM, along with a team of medics, saved numerous children and women in these tents. Just like Zakho, there was an intensive feeding tent, where I worked alongside RGNs, who showed me how to put nasogastric tubes into children. They found that this was a more satisfactory method than using IV drips.

I was able to do some dentistry in between the night shifts in the cholera tents. [In such poor conditions, the Kurds were not able to practice much in the way of hygiene] and their oral hygiene left a lot to be desired. We only treated Kurds with toothache, which was mainly [associated with] abscesses. The only treatment for this was extraction, as antibiotics would probably be sold on the black market, rather than taken.

It was a few weeks after the Defence Secretary, Mr Tom King, had visited Sirsenk that we heard the news that we were going home – four months earlier than expected. I never thought I would ever have an experience like Operation Haven while I was serving in the WRNS and, although conditions were bad, it was very rewarding in being able to adapt, improvise and overcome the various problems that were posed to us. It was an experience that I will never forget.

Two young women amongst many, who, although their basic training was in dental support, found both the skills and resilience to deal with the enormous and daunting problems thrown up by such a vast humanitarian crisis.

Such is the variety of experience to be expected by those who serve in the Armed Forces, regardless of profession or trade.

*****

Chapter 9

Options for Change
1991 – 1993

As the dust settled following the challenges of the Gulf War and its aftermath, Surgeon Commodore (D) Brian Robinson and his senior managers were to be found grappling with the implementation of his "Options for Change" restructuring of the Branch. In order to achieve the significant savings required from the RNDS, Robinson's 'Mobile Dental Teams' concept had been launched. Manning priority was given to these and to the manning of the Fleet and the Royal Marines. Elsewhere, the 'Core Dental Teams' within dental departments in the establishments, found themselves very tightly stretched. They could, however, be supplemented by the mobile teams, when these were available.

It will be remembered, from a previous chapter in this History, that the Royal Naval Reserve (RNR) Dental Branch, was a small, but highly regarded cadre of civilian dentists and dental support staff, who gave much of their spare and vacation time to work in uniform in support of the RNDS. As such, not only did they bring to the Branch additional expertise, particularly within the specialty of Oral and Maxillofacial Surgery, but they acted as an invaluable 'force multiplier' to cover absences of RNDS personnel due to leave, courses or sickness.

Thus it was that the unplanned and unexpected announcement that the Reserve Dental Branch was to be disestablished was met with disbelief and dismay amongst both the RNR dental officers and their regular RN colleagues. The Directorate was inundated with calls from long-serving and loyal RNR dentists, wishing to know why they were to be thrown on the scrap heap! It was embarrassing for Robinson, Grant and the senior staff, that they had no answer to these calls for explanation.

The order had come from the Commodore Reserves on the staff of the Commander-in-Chief Naval Home Command (CINCNAVHOME). Further enquiries revealed that a staff officer in CINCNAVHOME, whose organisation, in common with the Armed Forces as a whole, was being pressed for more and more savings, had 'taken' the Reserve dentists as a 'Savings Measure'. This was done without any reference to the RNDS and little research to evaluate the costs and benefits of such a measure! By the time DNDS became aware of the order, it was *fait accompli*.

One very disgruntled RNR dental officer wrote to his MP, the Rt. Hon. Paddy Ashdown, leader of the Liberal Democratic Party, asking him to find out why such a measure had been taken and what would be the benefits to the Exchequer? Ashdown passed on this request to the Secretary of State for Defence, the Rt. Hon Tom King.

Not surprisingly, King passed the letter to his 'minions' for reply and in due course it arrived on the desk of the Deputy Director Naval Dental Services, Surgeon Captain (D) Ted Grant, amongst whose Terms of Reference was the task of dealing with Parliamentary Questions on the RNDS.

One of the important tasks of the RNR dental officers had been the dental examination of all other RNR personnel, in order to determine that their dental fitness levels were such that they could be deployed at short notice if necessary and to advise them to seek treatment if required.

The Government had recently introduced charges for dental examinations within the National Health Service, where all RNR personnel would now have to go for their 'fit to fight' certification.

Grant's research showed that this would produce costs significantly higher than the savings achieved by the abolition of the RNR Dental Branch. These facts and figures were included in his draft reply for Tom King to Paddy Ashdown. When handed to a senior civil servant for onward transmission, the man blanched, saying, "We can't give this to the Minister. He won't like it at all!" Grant explained that his brief had not been to "Please the Minister", but to give an explanation of the measure, including an analysis of the projected costs and benefits perceived. The letter which was finally received by Paddy Ashdown had very little in common with Grant's draft.

On 14 June 1991, many RNDS members met at the Institute of Naval Medicine for yet another Wood Lecture and Clinical Day The programme included presentations by RNDS officers on a number of clinical subjects as well as a 'washup' on Operation Granby (the UK's contribution to the Gulf War) by Surgeon Captain (D) George Rudge. The Fifth Wood Lecture was given by Professor Aubrey Sheiham, a sometimes controversial public dental health expert who had upset the civilian dental 'establishment' on several occasions, once by pronouncing that dental examinations should be carried out less frequently because dental treatment itself was a principal cause of dental disease! His presentation was well received by the audience. This was followed by the 'Directors Dinner' in the Wardroom at *HMS Dolphin*, where the principal speaker was Vice Admiral John Coward DSO, the Flag officer Submarines, who proposed the toast to the Branch. At the dinner, Surgeon Commodore (D) Brian Robinson announced the latest award of the Harvey-Fletcher Medal and Prize. The Award went to Surgeon Commander (D)

D C C Alexander, the Head of Oral Research at INM, for his outstanding research into the epidemiology of dental disease in the Royal Navy.

The fight under 'Options for Change' for a viable future for the Medical and Dental Branches continued and at a meeting of the RNDS senior managers, held on 12 July 1991, DNDS announced that the situation with regard to the future of the Naval Medical Services remained 'fluid'. He told managers that the "main battle" was being fought over the future of the military hospitals and secondary care. He was able to temper this gloom with the good news of Surgeon Commander (D) Geoff Myers' award of the OBE for his outstanding contribution at Fleet Headquarters in the medical support to Operation Granby (the Gulf War). In the same vein, he also announced the selection for promotion to Surgeon Captain (D) of Surgeon Commander (D) John Hargraves[131].

The inevitable consequence of the 'Wrens at Sea' policy was the gradual subsumation of the WRNS into the Royal Navy. As time passed, the WRNS blue rank, category and cap badges would be replaced by the RN gold badges, the title of Wren would be dropped and Wren Officer ranks would realign with the naval ranks of their male colleagues. Wrens were now subject to the Naval Discipline Act and were expected to 'bear arms'!

This latter fact brought with it more training and more duties, as illustrated in an amusing short article by Wren DSA Sara Stone in the RNDS Newsletter[132].

Women at Arms!

Oh my God! DSAs with guns! Whatever next? *HMS Drake* Divisions were looming and, as per tradition, a guard of honour was required. Unfortunately, *HMS Drake* had insufficient male ratings to make up the guard. The First Lieutenant sent round the bearer of bad tidings, in the form of a very persuasive CPOGI [Chief Petty Officer Gunnery Instructor], to each department for names to make up an all FEMALE guard.

The deciding factor as to who were to be the 'lucky' ones, was the size of our feet! Basically those who had the feet which fitted the parade boots were selected! Four of the twelve Wrens chosen came from the Dental Department. The fortunate few were: Leading Wren Helen Rust, Leading Wren Nicki Moore, Wren Ann Taylor and myself.

Prior to Divisions on 26 October 1991, we had 'Drill'. We had muscles like the Field Gunners! (No! – we are not running for the Devonport Field gun Crew either!) Despite not being too keen at the start of training, on reflection it was quite good fun and apart from minor aches and pains, it has to be said that we were proud to be the first, all women's guard at *HMS Drake*. We recommend that all dental staff should try this sometime – the muscles developed from holding a gun for hours on end can come in handy in the surgery!

Despite the usual embattled routine at the Directorate, as the above article demonstrates, at the 'coal face' all was not 'doom and gloom'. In the same issue of the Branch Newsletter, there were two reports from dental officers, each of whom had taken part in separate trekking and climbing expeditions in the Himalayas and an account by a dental cadet, Surgeon Sub-Lieutenant (D) N (Nick) Turnbull of an Easter elective attachment to *HMS Tamar* in Hong Kong.[133] The adventurers in Nepal were Surgeon Lieutenant Commanders (D) S (Sarah) Howe and G (Gio) Sidoli[134]. Sarah Howe's fascinating account is reproduced below[135].

Highs and Lows

Late in October 1991, a team of twelve intrepid walkers set off for Kathmandu on Expedition Pisang 91. I was lucky enough to be included as team dentist. Our main objective was to climb Pisang Peak (19,983 feet) and to encircle the Annapurna range of mountains.

We travelled on Biman Bangladesh Airways – the cheapest, but also the most disorganised. The flights did not connect, so we ended up in Dhaka for a day, unexpectedly. We were able to travel around the city in a convoy of rickshaws – something which made the delay worthwhile.

We finally arrived in Kathmandu and spent three days exploring while our trek agent sorted out the tiresome details, such as provisions and trek permits.

The city was bustling and busy. Petty Officer Wren PT [Physical Trainer] Val Hodgkinson and I, soon discovered the delights of shopping in Nepal, buying mounds of clothing and jewellery. This was not the sort of behaviour expected of great mountaineers, so we told our team leader, Chief Petty Officer Bob Fordham that we were searching for Surgeon Lieutenant Commander (D) Gio Sidoli, believed to be in the area. We never did find him, but little pools of blood on the road, led us to the local dentist instead. Dark and hung with strange instruments, it was similar to a torture chamber.

Eventually, running short of money and with most of the team suffering from the local food poisoning (called Kathmandu Dog), we set off by bus for Pokhara. The journey took 13 hours on virtually non-existent roads. After our first night under canvas, we met our porters and Sherpas, who numbered more than 30. They were led by Sherpa Shera, the Sirdar, or boss. The porters carried the majority of our equipment and the Sherpas were responsible for all the cooking and selection of a good campsite. All we had to do was walk – a treat compared to previous British expeditions.

After all the planning, we were finally off. For the first five days we walked through lush, green countryside on a good path. There was little level ground. We were either toiling steeply uphill, or rushing steeply down again. To keep the porters happy, we only covered ten miles, daily, so there was plenty of time for gazing at snowy mountains or shopping at roadside stalls. It sounds idyllic, but there were perils. At the first campsite it rained heavily and we were besieged by leeches.

Later there were river crossings in freezing water and terrifying scrambles over rickety bridges. There seemed to be ferocious water buffalo and relentless mule trains round every corner. We kept our morale up by eating fruit and nut chocolate and drinking endless bottles of Coke at tea houses. In my position as dentist, I could only be ashamed of our diet. Shera improved things by serving up excellent meals. But as the trek progressed, we all got fed up with Dhal Bhaat, a rice, lentil and vegetable concoction.

Soon the terrain became harder and more barren as we climbed towards the Thorung La Pass (17,700 feet). There was little vegetation and no villages for a considerable distance. As the altitude increased, we made less and less progress. To while away the time, I decided to learn to speak Nepali. Two of the Sherpas, Habon and Big Karma (a giant by Nepalese standards at five feet, eight tall), taught me some traditional folk songs and some words that they thought would be useful.

It was only later that I tried them out on Shera, that I realised that they were rather rude! All the porters started calling me "Thulu Didi Dutsak". I was flattered to have a nickname until Shari explained that it meant "Older Big Sister with the Fat Bottom"! I gave up Nepali soon after, turning my thoughts to dentistry. I felt I ought to earn my "Team dentist" title. In the town of Jomsom, I managed to get my wish. The porters were more terrified of me than the average English patient. To gain their trust, I had to examine most of my team mates. This took place in a dusty hotel courtyard in gale-force winds. Once one porter relented, they all wanted a check up. They all had excellent teeth.

By now a crowd had gathered. One elderly man came forward, pointing to a mobile upper molar. Using elaborate miming techniques and Shera as interpreter, I offered to extract it. The patient thanked me in perfect English and asked if he could have an injection! My audience, which included most of the team, were delighted. Shera, though, was horrified. An extreme dental phobic, he developed convenient memory loss, when asked the whereabouts of the dental valise, in future.

From Jomsom onwards, life became less enjoyable. Crossing the pass was a nightmare. We camped at 15,000 feet and set off very early to ascend the last 2,700 feet to the summit. We were soon overtaken by the porters, still wearing T-shirts and flip-flops, despite the extreme cold.

The British contingent was not so hardy. All were suffering from varying degrees of Acute Mountain Sickness (AMS) – headache, nausea and dizziness being the commonest symptoms.

By the time I reached the top of the pass, I could only walk five steps before a five-minute rest. For a while, I thought I was going to die, but survived long enough to win the dubious distinction of being the only team member to be sick at altitude!

This renewed my resolve and I made it over the top. It was worth it for the tremendous views (I think!). For the next three days we were all rather exhausted and bad tempered, so the production of yet another bowl of Dhal Bhaat almost caused a riot, but Shari calmed things down with her timely production of cheddar cheese and flapjacks.

I had my first row with my tent companion, Leading Radio Operator Angela Ellerington, over something very trivial. Her red hair made the porters believe she was a witch, so for several hours I was terrified she would put a spell on me. We were all rather irrational on account of 'altitude lassitude'.

For the next three days we made better and more cheerful progress downhill to Pisang Village. It was a tiny, primitive place, where we were to leave most of our equipment, while we attempted to climb Pisang Peak. We stayed in the Yak Hotel – the fifth establishment of that name we had seen. It had no windows, a large hole in the roof and open fires with no chimneys. Sleeping there was like being smoked alive, but a luxury after camping.

Pisang Peak rose huge and menacing behind the village. The weather, which up until now had been fine, turned snowy. After a long day slogging up the foothills, we reached Base Camp at 15,000 feet. We had expected to be alone on the peak, but found three other groups in residence. The most bizarre and unfriendly were twelve identically dressed Germans, complete with female yodeller! They all walked in line, taking identical steps.

We spent a horrible night in a blizzard, awaking to heavy snowfall.

The cold had caused chest problems and AMS had returned. Less than half the group were able to proceed much further and even the fittest had to abandon their attempt due to avalanche danger and extreme cold. Because of the snow and concern that we would not get back to Kathmandu, we turned back immediately.

This was the worst part of the whole trek, as we were cold, filthy and demoralised. The porters, needless to say, seemed unaffected by the snow and flip-flops became snow shoes.

Shera explained that we had failed the climb because somebody had cooked fresh meat and offended the gods. We were obviously cheered by this as it lessened our guilt feelings. Our vegetarian Dhal Bhaat tasted almost like real food that night.

It was downhill all the way to Kathmandu. There was a blissful stop at thermal springs for the first bath in two weeks, though certain male purists remained dirty and without friends. Our final night under canvas was in a village called ⇒

> Bhuli-Bhuli. The porters sang and danced for us. As the evening progressed they became amorous and uncontrollable. The cause was *rakshe,* a fiendish local drink with the taste and consistency of wallpaper paste. Luckily for the team, there was also rum at eighty pence for a large bottle.
>
> The next day we arrived at Besisahar to catch a truck to civilisation. All of the porters, Sherpas and team, plus the equipment, crammed into the back for a very uncomfortable ride. All too soon, we arrived in the city for a bit more shopping and another dose of 'Dog'!
>
> My trip to Nepal was the most interesting and physically exacting thing I have ever done. The people were lovely and the scenery, spectacular. The only bad thing about the whole experience was the Dhal Bhaat. I would love to visit again in future.

The experiences of Surgeon Lieutenant Commander (D) Gio Sidoli on the *Fearless* expedition were similar. They too were eventually turned back by a combination of AMS and unseasonably heavy snowfall, having reached an altitude of 15,800 feet. On the return trek to Kathmandu, the *Fearless* team were able to indulge in some exciting white-water rafting, a pastime which afforded Sidoli the opportunity to brush up on his suturing technique!

The final closure of the RNR Dental Branch came on 31 January 1992. This sad occasion was marked by a dinner held in the Wardroom of the aircraft carrier *HMS Invincible*, at which the Director, Surgeon Commodore (D) Brian Robinson gave a speech of thanks to all the reservists who had served the Navy and the RNDS so well during the past 77 years, since 1915. At midnight the Branch ceased to exist, an ensign was symbolically hauled down to the accompaniment of Royal Marine buglers. The ensign was presented, in a suitably inscribed case, to the President of the dinner, the currently serving Senior Dental Officer, Reserves, Surgeon Commander (D) D M (David) Higgs RNR. Past and present members of the RNR Dental branch were each presented with engraved glasses as a memento of the occasion[136].

The majority of problems with which the Directorate had to grapple were, inevitably, linked to savings measures.

Since the demise in the mid-1980s, of the cadre of civilian dental technicians, employed within the RNDS, these had been replaced by uniformed RAF dental technicians. This arrangement had been beneficial to both the RNDS and the RAF Dental Branch, not only providing an expertise still much needed within the RN Branch, but also enabling the RAF to maintain its perceived requirement of uniformed personnel with a 'war role'.

During the early part of 1992, the RAF Dental Branch, also under great pressure to achieve savings, required the return of four of its technicians, leaving the RNDS dental technical support fragmented and less able to meet its targets. At a meeting of the branch senior managers, it had been discussed that the remaining technicians should all be moved to the Command Dental Laboratory at *HMS Drake* in order to provide a better organised central facility. The Advisor in Dental Laboratory Facilities, Surgeon Captain (D) R S (Dick) Hambly, was instructed to carry out a study to determine the best way ahead for the dental laboratory services in the future[137].

Within this History, it has been written on a number of occasions that the trials and tribulations experienced at Directorate level, did not affect morale or the sense of purpose at the 'coalface'. To a large extent this remained true throughout the difficulties experienced during the 1990s. However, it was inevitable that some of these uncertainties would percolate beyond the 'corridors of power'.

The RNDS Newsletter had been up and running for over twelve years, during which time it had been an excellent vehicle for disseminating news and views and for sharing experiences at all levels. A two-way traffic, which enabled those 'at the top' to keep the Branch informed, but also to 'hear' what was going on around the Branch.

The Newsletter had, it seems, for the time being, fallen upon hard times. The reader of this History, will be aware that the author has relied upon a great deal of excellent input from this source, covering the years since its launch by the then Surgeon Captain (D) Brian Robinson. The Editorial, written by Surgeon Commander (D) J V (John) Holland for the second issue of 1992, is an impassioned plea for 'copy' and gives a flavour of the 'mindset' of the RNDS at that difficult time[138]. An extract is reproduced below.

Hard Times

I feel most people enjoy reading the articles [in the Newsletter], written in a variety of styles about a variety of subjects. In the past twelve years, we have enjoyed many serious, clinical, travel and just plain amusing articles from a wide range of contributors. The principle has been to inform in an interesting and readable way. Now, I appreciate that morale may not be what we would wish, with redundancies and cut-backs heaped one upon the other; time served to promotion is getting longer and the chances of serving abroad, ever more remote, but dwelling on what has been, is a worthless pursuit. The Navy of the Nineties will bear little resemblance to that of the Sixties, when I joined, but that does not make it any less worthwhile, either as a career or as a broadening experience, before entering NHS general practice. There is still much to write ≫▸

> about and share with one's fellows: changes in equipment, stores, materials, clinic refurbishments, DSAs at sea and abroad, working alongside sailors who think the 'little woman' should stay at home, preferably doing his darning! Come on! It's all happening out there. Tell us about it, we want to know. The Newsletter is also a good way of giving some feedback to "Them in Charge".

Little has been written in this History of the work of the specialists and consultants within the RNDS. A separate account of the History and progress of those RNDS officers with higher qualifications in Oral and Maxillofacial Surgery and in Orthodontics has been prepared in parallel with this History and is presented as 'Appendix 1' to this, the main text. Nonetheless, it is fitting to include here a brief insight into the 'Specialist World', written for the Newsletter by its Editor, Surgeon Commander (D) John Holland, himself an Oral and Maxillofacial Surgeon[139].

> ### *A Surgical Diversion*
>
> Those who have not visited Haslar lately will not know of the external changes to our defences. The hospital has, like other establishments been ringed by a high wire fence topped by rolls of razor-wire, in the popular concentration camp style. It is believed that this is to keep evil-doers out, but perversely, it has been placed behind the high walls, built originally to keep the patients in; so, we are not absolutely certain of its intended purpose.
>
> Funnily enough this preoccupation with keeping people out is not new. At one period of the nineteenth century, the number of patients trying to escape was surpassed by the number trying to climb in over the walls, when the local population decided that the treatment available inside was probably superior to that outside. Nursing staff, who not many years before, were punished for helping patients out, were now being punished for helping them in! This popularity, we like to believe, is still the case, but the fact that the hospital is now in an area of increasing population and happily takes civilians to improve training opportunities, may have something to do with it.
>
> To preserve security and improve traffic control, only staff vehicles may enter the hospital through the altered main gate; all others are diverted to a much enlarged car park outside the secure area. Those, now on foot, who have not been put off, have to pass under the beady eye of MoD Police as they walk into the hospital grounds.
>
> Some of those not put off were attending the Tri-Service Oral Surgery and Orthodontics Symposium, held this year in Haslar. This has been held annually, although last year it was postponed because of the Gulf War. It is held over two days in June and is an opportunity for specialists under training and their training

posts to be assessed. The meeting also gives them a chance to give presentations to a relatively sympathetic audience, although the standard of papers is now high and most would be well received by the most critical audience.

Each year, a guest of high professional stature is invited to give a lecture on a subject of their own choosing. This year, Professor Kursheed Moos from the West of Scotland Oral and Plastic Surgery Centre in Canniesburn, Glasgow, gave a presentation on "Severe Trauma of the Naso-Ethmoidal and Orbital Regions". All Naval Oral Surgeons have spent time at Canniesburn, which is noted for the high incidence of traumatic injuries it treats. On my first day, I was confronted by 17 fractures (it was 2nd January!) and they continue to see 60 or so facial injuries a month. Professor Moos is therefore, well qualified to speak on this subject and, as expected, he gave a very full and interesting talk on what is, thankfully, a rare injury. Members of other specialties on the hospital staff were also invited, as were the Oral Surgery Department at Queen Alexandra Hospital, Cosham. The conference room was satisfyingly packed for this special occasion.

Of course, a meeting such as this is also a chance for old friends to meet, old memories to be revived and new experiences shared. Thus the social programme was almost as full as the clinical, with the symposium dinner held on board *HMS Warrior 1860* and visits before this, either to *HMS Alliance* [A preserved WW II submarine] or *HMS Victory*, followed by drinks in the Old Naval Academy. As is customary, the three Service Dental Directors also attended the dinner with our guests and local civilian consultants to the Royal Navy. This was generally considered to be a successful meeting and well worth the effort it undoubtedly took.

The changes in the National Health Service have gradually caught up with Haslar and we are now required to give returns of our waiting lists and justify their length. On top of this are returns for hospital costings, which now take up much of the dental staff's time and patience. With the Portsmouth hospitals gaining "Trust Status" in the next financial year, the pressures are bound to increase. For instance, in the past, we have been happy to treat [Service] dependants from the South of England, who have been unable to reach the top of an NHS waiting list, because of moving house so frequently.

While we are still happy to see them, now paper work has to be raised to get their local health authority to pay a nominal sum towards the treatment, which adds considerably to the administration of these patients.

Staff changes have been considerable over the past year. PO Wren Suzanne Owen is now Clinic manager and responsible for coping with the ever increasing quantity of paper that crosses her desk. She updates the admissions board, arranges the operating lists and oversees all the varied activities of the department. Leading Wren Sue Beckett runs the Staff Dental Clinic, where ➤

> Surgeon Captain (D) Geoff Sharpe is busy five sessions a week.
>
> Wren Kay Crump has progressed from the Orthodontics side to Oral Surgery. Her place in Orthodontics has been taken by Wren Netty Read. A comprehensive knowledge of the many small brackets, wires and elastics is necessary, so replacements can be ordered and the treatment runs smoothly. Surgeon Captain (D) (Timothy) Hall and Lieutenant Colonel Phil Sims RADC, who does three sessions a week, do the tricky bits. Sergeant Steve Graham is our RAF dental technician [a specialist support post retained at Haslar], making up a true tri-Service team. All the DSAs are expected to take a turn in the operating theatre, assisting the surgeon and as scrub nurse, which makes the job very different from a normal dental clinic.
>
> We do two operating sessions a week. On morning sessions we also do day-cases, using the day-case ward as well as our own, enabling us to keep on top of the work. New referrals are 55% up on last year, so a rapid throughput is essential to prevent waiting lists building up.
>
> On top of this, there is the continual search for the patients' hospital notes, which seem to have a life of their own in the nether regions of the hospital! All hospital patients have notes made up, which contain out-patient and in-patient sections, the whole being known as the "bed ticket".
>
> These are stored in Central Medical Records, when not in active use. However, frequently they are mis-filed or have disappeared into 'Typing' or other parts of the administration scattered around Haslar. The search for individual notes can be tiring and frustrating, requiring a high degree of low cunning and the detecting abilities of Sherlock Holmes.
>
> Last, but not least, we should mention Surgeon Lieutenant Commander (D) Steve Liggins, who passed his medical finals in June and is the first medically qualified member of the Dental Branch in living memory. He is going through his exhausting year as a pre-registration house man, before returning to his career in Oral Surgery.

It had recently been ordained that all new candidates for careers in Oral and Maxillofacial Surgery, should have both medical and dental qualifications. Together with Fellowships in both Surgery and Dental Surgery, the training pathway for Oral Surgery, now extended beyond twelve years! Although some periods of training were spent in Service hospitals, during much of this period, trainees were not available for Service deployment. Since Service oral surgeons had an important war role, the dental branches were obliged to 'bite the bullet' on the cost and manpower implications of this new requirement. Surgeon Lieutenant Commander (D) Steve Liggins was the first in the RNDS to follow this training pathway.

At a meeting of Branch senior managers on 20 March 1992, DNDS announced that, as a further savings measure, it was likely that a decision would soon be made to move all single-Service staffs 'from the centre' (i.e. out of London). He had recently submitted a draft paper for '2-star' circulation, setting out his proposals for meeting the savings required under 'Options for Change'. The final draft would be presented to the Second Sea Lord's Board of Management in June.

At the same meeting, it was explained that a site for the new 'out of town' headquarters had been identified in the Portsmouth Naval Base. The new HQ was scheduled for completion by the end of 1993 and for occupation by March 1994.

The Director, Surgeon Commodore (D) Brian Robinson, then explained to those present at the meeting, his vision for the future of the RNDS and what changes he foresaw, in order to meet the new budgetary constraints.

He had been told that savings of 14% to 16% were required from the Branch. It was his belief that this could be achieved mainly by restructuring. If pressed, however, up to 20% savings in cash terms might be possible, but this could only be met by some degree of financial control from the Directorate. In order to achieve this, he had embarked upon the 'useful' exercise of costing all Branch activities.

He outlined his concept of the 'Single Business Unit' (i.e. a Dental Branch which would hold its own budget and be responsible for its own expenditure). He believed that in terms of savings achievability, this was the preferred option. However, he explained, this idea ran contrary to the principles of the New Management Strategy and had therefore been vetoed.

This was a Navy decision alone and the RAF Dental Branch had received approval to go down that road and had been given full budgetary control over their activities. Within the Navy, commanding officers would retain responsibility and control of their dental facilities. However, DNDS intended to retain flexibility of response within the Branch by the deliberate under-resourcing of Establishment Dental Teams, which could be supplemented as required by the deployment of personnel in mobile Area Dental Teams.

Robinson then went on to explain why and how the Branch would be restructured in order to achieve the required savings. He explained that the RNDS was at present top heavy with senior (and expensive) dental officers. In order to rebuild the rank 'pyramid' with fewer senior and more junior officers, either there would have to be a block on promotions to Surgeon Commander over, probably, the next ten years or there would have to be a programme of redundancies. The latter was the probable and much more desirable solution.

These manpower savings would achieve a 15.5% reduction in the number of dental officers, which would equate to approximately 20% in cash terms. As a result of these reductions, the officer strength of the RNDS would reduce to 74.

Finally, Robinson explained, in order for the restructuring to work, whilst still maintaining a viable and vibrant Branch, recruiting of new dental officers would need to be vigorous. A new recruiting video 'Dentists with a Difference', had now been released and selected dental officers would be invited to give presentations in their old dental schools. Morale within the civilian dental profession was currently low and recruiting should be buoyant[140].

The use of computers, word processing and spreadsheets was now a fact of life within both the Directorate and many of the dental clinic administrative offices throughout the Royal Navy. Now the computer had arrived in the dental surgery. In mid-1992, the new dental charting and records system was introduced into the clinics at *HM Ships Nelson, Drake, Raleigh* and at the Commando Training Centre Royal Marines.

Training was provided to clinic staffs in the use of the new system and a one-day Module of training in Word Processing was added to the courses for Leading Wren DSA and Petty Officer Wren DSA, run by the Commander Dental Training[141].

Although manpower reductions had yet really to bite, within those busy dental clinics which provided direct support to the Fleet, worrying trends were being seen.

In preparation for the mid-year meeting of RNDS senior managers, the Fleet Dental Surgeon (FDS), Surgeon Commander (D) Geoff Myers and the Staff Dental Surgeon to Flag Officer Plymouth, Surgeon Commander (D) John Hargraves, both reported declining levels of dental fitness among personnel at sea.

The latter was of the opinion that more dental effort should be applied to identifying and treating those who needed one appointment only, rather than those who required complex, multi-appointment treatments.

The FDS wrote: "Dental health continues to decline. Currently just hovering above 70%. Submarines remain the most worrying area, although there may be some evidence that the bottom of the trough has been reached. Devonport is levelling out, but Portsmouth, although still acceptable, appears to be starting to deteriorate. Rosyth is the only area that has shown improvement.[142]"

In the meantime and after some minor adjustments, Brian Robinson's 'Post Options' plan for the restructuring of the RNDS had been accepted by the Second Sea Lord (2SL), who announced his decision in a 'Loose Minute' to members of the Navy Board[143].

In order to explain the outcome of Robinson's efforts and its relation to problems which would arise in the immediate future, it is worth reproducing the Second Sea Lord's minute here:

> ### *Review of the Royal Naval Dental Services*
>
> 1. The Director Naval Dental Services has recently completed a fundamental review of his Branch in the light of post-OPTIONS requirement and the planned integration of my department and [that of] the Commander in Chief Naval Home Command. His paper has undergone a thorough 2* [Rear Admiral level] scrutiny and I have accepted the recommendations of his review which meets the war and operational peacetime needs of the Navy with a realistic structure.
>
> 2. In summary, I have agreed the following changes:
>
>   a. Director Naval Dental Services will transfer his department from London to the new headquarters within the Portsmouth Naval Base, when integration occurs, to form a Dental Division as part of a new MDG(N) [Medical Director General (Navy)] organisation. Responsibility for all [RN] dental activity in the UK, with the exception of the operational aspects, will be transferred to the 2SL/CINCNAVHOME TLB [Top Level Budget] area.
>
>   b. A new concept is introduced for resourcing the dental manpower requirement to meet the objectives of increasing efficiency and manning flexibility. In future, multi-manned clinics will be complemented with dental staff, comprising a core Establishment Dental Team (EDT) who will be under the line authority of the Commanding Officer. The size of this core EDT will be set by DNDS. This will generally be <u>below</u> that indicated by the approved Dentist/Patient Ratio. Dependent upon any shortfall between tasking and the performance of the EDT, as measured by Command determined targets, additional manpower will be made available on a priority basis.
>
>   c. To meet this demand, the Command will establish and control, Area Dental Teams (ADT), which will be made available to establishments within geographic areas on the advice of the Command Dental Surgeon. When not deployed, ADTs will be held within the Base Port dental clinics and occupied primarily treating ships alongside. ADTs may also provide some of the manpower for Fleet DD/FF [Destroyers and Frigates] task group deployments subject to agreed MOUs [Memoranda of Understanding].
>
>   d. A redundancy program affecting some eight to ten Surgeon Commanders (D) will be phased over two tranches. There will, however, be no requirement for rating redundancies. ➤

> e. The resultant Branch structure will encompass a significantly smaller full career officer cadre. Some minor adjustments to career factors will be inevitable, but it is not envisaged that there will be significant degradation to career prospects.
>
> 3. The effect of the proposals is to achieve manpower savings (both uniformed and civilian), which equate to 14.7% (16.75% in cash terms). Together with a programme of de-enrichment and other savings measures, DDS(N)'s plan would yield savings of at least £6.8M over the LTC [Long Term Costings period]. This figure could rise even further if Treasury funding is forthcoming for the redundancy package.
>
> 4. It is intended that these proposals will be implemented with effect from 1 April 1994, to coincide with the move of MDG(N)'s department to the new headquarters within the Portsmouth Naval Base.
>
> 5. The above changes will be promulgated in due course by DCI [Defence Council Instruction]. In the shorter term DDS(N) will inform Dental Staff by letter.
>
> 6. The result will be a viable Dental Branch which will provide the best option for support to the RN as a whole, whilst remaining in step with the post-Options force structure.

Although drafted by Robinson himself, the minute was initialled by Admiral Sir Michael Layard, the Second Sea Lord and was addressed to all members of the Navy Board, which included the First Sea Lord, the Second Permanent Under Secretary at the MoD, the Commanders-in-Chief Fleet and Naval Home Command, the Controller of the Navy, the Chief of Fleet Support and the Assistant Chief of Naval Staff.

Thus it was that Robinson's plan for the future of the RNDS received approval in all the necessary 'High Places'. So, could he and his deputy, Surgeon Captain (D) Ted Grant now relax and get on with the job of providing a high standard of dentistry to the Royal Navy? Sadly, the answer was "No!" As ever, there were others lying in ambush along the path which led to this ultimate goal.

The Medical Director General (Naval), Surgeon Rear Admiral David Lammiman was also obliged to meet the requirements for savings dictated by 'Options for Change'.

The Dental Branch, although autonomous professionally, was still in terms of organisation and funding part of the Naval Medical Organisation and was therefore vulnerable to savings measures also being sought by MDG(N). In conversation with a senior member of the Medical Directorate, Grant had been given sight of a proposed new organisational diagram for the Medical Branch structure, once it had moved to the new Portsmouth Headquarters. This showed the Director's post on the same level as departmental heads in the rank of Surgeon Captain, with his Deputy relegated to 'Desk Officer' level as a Surgeon Commander (D).

Apart from the loss of status of the Branch within the Royal Navy as a whole and the inevitable collapse of morale among his career officers, Robinson believed strongly, that given the work-load carried within the present Directorate, which was not likely to diminish, the proposed organisation would be unworkable. The driver for the plan for the new HQ was the integration of the tasks and staffs of Second Sea Lord and the C-in-C Naval Home Command and MDG(N)'s proposed structure had been provisionally approved by the C-in-C's Chief of Staff (COS). Thus, at a meeting with MDG(N), Robinson sought his permission to meet with the Chief of Staff to put his case for maintaining the senior Branch structure at the present level. Lammiman agreed to this and on 17 December 1992, Robinson was able to put his case to the Chief of Staff.

Always a powerful advocate for the RNDS, Robinson had prepared his argument carefully and arrived in Portsmouth for the meeting armed with meticulously organised notes[144].

The meeting was a long one and Robinson started by informing COS that MDG(N) had agreed to his own 'wiring diagram' for the Headquarters Dental Organisation, if he could persuade COS to endorse it.

He told COS that he believed that he had not been presented with all the relevant information required for him to make this decision and then reviewed the history of his own efforts at restructuring the RNDS, pointing out that his proposals had been approved by the Second Sea Lord and the members of the Navy Board. Explaining that he was now encountering "not a little difficulty" in implementing his proposals, he highlighted the fact that, although he did not seek to change the position which had existed between the Naval Medical and Dental organisations within the Navy, Medicine and Dentistry are separate and autonomous professions. Nowhere, outside the Armed Forces, was there an hierarchical relationship between the professions, but they co-existed with parallel structures each with its own statutory governing body and professional associations.

Robinson then continued by explaining that there was little overlap in the daily activities of the two Branches, with the Medical Services being largely involved in the provision of secondary (hospital) care and the RNDS with primary care. He pointed out that "by and large", doctors and dentists could not carry out each others' tasks and that the inter-relationship could not be equated with that which existed between medicine and nursing, which was a true ancillary service.

Turning to his proposals for reorganisation, Robinson stated that he believed that he had taken his administrative organisation to an "irreducible minimum" and explained that after 1994, his Deputy, who was already heavily tasked, would assume the equivalent tasks held by four separate senior medical officers as well as being in charge of Dental Postgraduate Education. He pointed out that the tasking flowing to both the Director and his Deputy from the tri-Service Directorate, continued to expand, whilst at the same time there remained a need to direct and evolve new policies within the RNDS to enable it to meet the growing demands of the Fleet.

To put this in context, he explained that he would have three dental officers on his staff to carry out the functions of 23 similarly tasked medical and ancillary officers.

Robinson then turned to the tasks carried by his Deputy, whose position and rank within the organisation were now under threat. Listing his recent activities, he told COS that Grant had, since April, in his capacity as 'Appointer' made 70 new officer appointments. He had also written 270 letters concerned with recruiting. These activities represented 20% of his time.

Additionally, he had been concerned with Redundancy Boards and the specification and contracts for surgery protective clothing.

Together with DNDS, he had been involved in the restructuring of the Branch. He had chaired several committees, essential to the running of the Branch and had researched and identified a new Primary Dental Care Centre in London. He had been involved with the production of a new recruiting video; he had reviewed over 150 requests for approval of overseas dental treatments and also had to deal with many enquiries from retired dental officers.

Robinson said that he felt very strongly that such commitments could not be undertaken by a Surgeon Commander ((D).

After some discussion of the various points he had raised, Robinson took his leave feeling that his presentation had been well received.

A week or so later, he received the C-in-C's approval to retain the senior Branch management structure, when the move to Portsmouth took place.

The autumn of 1992 saw the announcement that Surgeon Captain T J C (Timothy) Hall OBE QHDS had been selected to succeed Robinson as the Director Naval Dental Services, in the rank of Surgeon Commodore (D), in April 1993.

At the annual 'Blood Red Dinner' of the RN Medical Club, held in the

Painted Hall of the RN College at Greenwich, the MDG(N), Surgeon Rear Admiral Lammiman announced, during his 'State of the Union' address that "The Director Naval Dental Services will follow 2SL [Second Sea Lord] to Portsmouth. With the exception of the operational elements, all naval dental activity in the UK will be transferred to the new Medical Directorate in the Portsmouth Naval Base. The smaller Navy will require redundancy of some senior dental officers, but it will not include any dental ratings. The new recommendations for the Dental Branch structure have been accepted and they will be implemented from 1 April 1994."

He continued: "Surgeon Commodore (D) Brian Robinson is due to be relieved on 8 April 1993 and I would like to take this opportunity of thanking him for all his hard work and wish him and Judy a very happy retirement.[145]" And, as a footnote, the MDG added; "None of these dinners would be complete without a mention of the Royal Naval Reserve. Sadly, after 77 years of continuous service, the [RNR] Dental Branch was disbanded on 31 March this year".

The beginning of the year 1993 seemed to be a quiet period at the Directorate, but this was deceptive. Like the proverbial swan, 'all serene above the surface, but paddling like fury beneath', the Director and his Deputy were busy with the implementation of the now agreed new structure for the 'Post Options' Dental Branch'. The actions which needed to be taken included the offer of and selection for a number of redundancies among the Branch senior ranks and some vigorous planning of new appointments by the Appointer. The objective of this activity was to have everything in place in time for Robinson's handover to Surgeon Commodore (D) Timothy Hall, in April. The Deputy Director, Surgeon Captain (D) Ted Grant, would continue in post as the 'link man' during and after the supersession.

April came and Brian Robinson started his well deserved retirement. It was marked by a splendid farewell dinner, attended by over 110 dental officers, past and present, and their wives on Friday 5 March 1993, in the Wardroom Mess at *HMS Nelson*. Fittingly this was the same mess that Brian Robinson had joined as a Surgeon Lieutenant (D), 33 years previously.

In an appreciation in the RNDS Newsletter, the Editor, Surgeon Commander (D) John Holland noted that he had fought "many battles with many people; all in the interests of the Branch and the continuing good dental health of the Navy, which has always been paramount in his actions. However, it was due to him that the new structure of the Branch has been accepted at the highest levels and will be implemented in its entirety"[146]. Holland went on to comment: "It is extraordinary that, after so much innovation and work for the Branch, he is the first Director to retire in the rank of Surgeon Captain

(D) since Surgeon Captain (D) Wood in 1950, forty three years ago"*.

Surgeon Commodore (D) T J C (Timothy) Hall OBE OStJ QHDS Royal Navy took up the baton as Director Naval Dental Services and as Deputy Director Defence Dental Services (Personnel and Training) on 9 April 1993. Born in 1937, his secondary education was at Bishops Stortford College from which he gained entry to Guy's Hospital Dental School in 1955. Qualifying in 1959, he joined the Royal Navy after a house appointment at Sunderland General Hospital, in September 1960.

After New Entry appointments and some brief shore appointments, Hall's first sea appointment was a 'loan' period to *HMS Venus,* a ship of the Dartmouth Training Squadron for a brief cruise to a number of Scandinavian ports.

He then joined *HMS Jufair,* the Royal Navy Base in Bahrain, as Staff Dental Surgeon to the Flag Officer Middle East, spending time in each of the ships of the Persian Gulf Frigate Squadron.

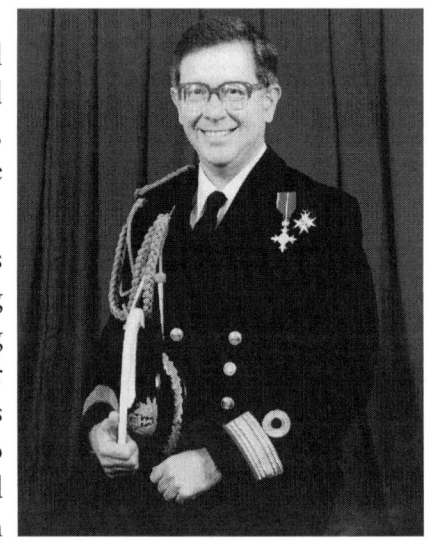

Surgeon Commodore (D)
T J C Hall OBE OStJ QHDS

Returning to the UK, Hall was appointed to *HMS Sultan* the engineering training establishment in Gosport. Having then made the decision to pursue a career in Oral Surgery, his next appointment was to the Royal Naval Hospital Haslar, also in Gosport. It was here that he met and eventually married his wife Gillian, then a Nursing Sister in the Queen Alexandra's Royal Naval Nursing Service. Here also, he studied for his Fellowship in Dental Surgery of the Royal College of Surgeons of England and was awarded his FDS in 1964. In 1965 he was promoted to Surgeon Lieutenant Commander (D) and was appointed to the Royal Naval Hospital Gibraltar, as a Specialist, arriving in Gibraltar as a newly married man.

In 1969 he returned to Guy's Hospital to train for and obtain the Diploma in Orthodontics, thus adding another string to his 'Specialist' bow.

---

* At that time the rank of Commodore in the Royal Navy, although equivalent to 'One Star' rank in the other Services, was considered a 'non-substantive' or temporary rank, which went with certain senior appointments. Thus, officers leaving or retiring from such an appointment would revert to the rank of Captain, unless promoted into another appointment. This 'anomaly' has since been changed and RN officers now appointed Commodore, retire in or retain that rank.

Following his step on to the Specialist ladder, Hall's appointments then became a rotation between the RN Hospitals at Haslar, Plymouth and Gibraltar, returning to the latter as Senior Dental Surgeon and with the Acting Rank of Surgeon Commander (D) in November 1971. He was confirmed in the rank in June 1972. Climbing the ladder towards Consultant grade, Hall also underwent short Oral Surgery training periods at Odstock Hospital in Salisbury and at Canniesburn Hospital Glasgow. In 1978, Timothy Hall was appointed as an Officer of the Order of the British Empire (OBE) for "services to oral surgery".

In November 1975, Hall was graded Consultant and although continuing mainly in hospital practice, as often happened at that time, he returned to general dental practice for two years, when he was appointed as the Flotilla Dental Surgeon to the Flag Officer Submarines at *HMS Dolphin*, the submarine base at Gosport in 1981.

Promoted to Surgeon Captain (D) in December 1982, Hall then found himself going through a number of senior staff and administrative appointments.

From 1983 to 1985, he was Director of Dental Training and Research and Head of the Training Division at the Institute of Naval Medicine. From there he was appointed as the Command Dental Surgeon to C-in-C Naval Home Command and in 1987 he was appointed to the Ministry of Defence as Assistant Director Naval Dental Services, Deputy to Surgeon Rear Admiral (D) David Coppock. In 1989, Hall returned to RNH Haslar as Consultant Adviser in Dental Surgery (Navy) and as Adviser to the Medical Director General (Naval) in Oral Surgery and Orthodontics.

When appointed as DNDS in April 1993, Surgeon Commodore (D) Timothy Hall was the first 'hospital dentist' to head the Branch since Surgeon Rear Admiral (D) W I N Forrest.

The new Director of Naval Dental Services, (DDS(N), in tri-Service parlance), held his first meeting of the Naval Dental Services Board of Management (previously known as the Command and Staff Dental Advisers) on 8 July 1993. The meeting was held at the First Avenue House, Defence Medical Services Directorate in High Holborn, London[147].

It was attended by the Command Dental Surgeon CINCNAVHOME, the Staff Dental Adviser to Flag Officer Plymouth, the Staff Dental Adviser to 3 Commando Brigade, the Adviser in Dental Laboratory Facilities, the Fleet Dental Surgeon, the Commander Dental Training/Adviser in General Dental Practice, the Staff Dental Adviser to the Flag Officer Scotland and Northern Ireland and the Head of Oral Research. The Consultant Adviser in

Oral and Maxillofacial Surgery and the Dental Adviser, Gibraltar were unable to attend. Hall's deputy (Grant) acted as Secretary to the Board.

Hall opened the meeting by stating his intention of continuing these meetings, which he regarded as invaluable to the management of the Dental Branch. Before going on to the general business of Branch administration, he announced that the move to the new HQ in the Portsmouth Naval Base was on schedule and would take place on or around 14 February 1994. He predicted that the move would represent a significant change in the way that the RNDS did its business. He believed that this would be of benefit by keeping the Directorate more in touch with the daily business of the Branch, but that tri-Service business might suffer due to less easy lines of communication.

Hall described the concept of the 'Dental Division' within MDG(N)'s Headquarters structure, the concept which would realise the high level agreements achieved by his predecessor. The Director also referred to the fact that he had been informed that, following the first tranche of Branch redundancies, the Director of Naval Manpower Planning had decreed that there could be no further RNDS redundancies. With the prospect of a significantly smaller Branch, this announcement had caused some disquiet.

Until the new structure had been agreed, there had been a block on promotions to Surgeon Commander (D) and it was asked whether the moratorium on further redundancies would lead to further delay in promotions. The Assistant Director (ADDS(N)) replied that it was hoped that promotions would recommence, as planned, in June 1994.

Although women were by now well established in sea-going billets, (ADDS(N)) (Grant) reported difficulties with medical colleagues in the establishment of sea billets for dental Wrens. The Fleet Medical Officer took the view that he would only accept Medical Assistants with dental training at sea, explaining that "it had always been required" that dental staff at sea could double up as medical watchkeepers. Grant had countered that dental staff in ships were borne for dental duties and not as a solution to the medical manpower problem. Medical Assistants in dental posts, although they received appropriate dental training, lacked much of the skill and experience of a fully trained DSA. He had suggested that Wren DSAs in sea-going drafts could be given, and indeed often were already given, advanced first aid training, widening their role in times of conflict or emergency.

After discussion at the meeting, Grant undertook to take the matter up with MDG(N)'s staff. This was, in due course, done and at Grant's request, MDG(N) wrote to the drafting authority at *HMS Centurion*, to confirm that he had not excluded dental Wrens from sea billets and that he saw no obstacle to all dental Wrens being eligible for sea service.

Meanwhile – back at the 'coalface'; whilst dental officers and staffs continued to busy themselves striving to keep the Royal Navy and the Royal Marines 'fit to fight', there were still those who found time for 'fun in the sun' and adventure. As readers of this History are, by now, aware, there seems to have been a tendency amongst dental officers and ratings, not only to scale teeth, but to scale the heights, whenever such opportunities presented themselves.

We have already shared in the experiences of several who undertook strenuous treks in the Himalayas. Now we go to Africa and an account of an attempt on Mount Kilimanjaro by Surgeon Lieutenant (D) B (Barbie) Jamieson. Her story is once again gleaned from the RNDS Newsletter[148].

How High the Honeymoon?

When your husband has a group of crazy friends, you end up doing crazy things. So when two of our friends decided that the idea of climbing Mount Kilimanjaro, at 19,340 feet Africa's highest mountain, sounded a good idea for a honeymoon, eight of us ended up packing our rucksacks!

You fly to Mombasa and immediately are taken half way to the mountain and stay at the Taita Hills Hilton Hotel – definitely to Hilton standards, an oasis in the middle of apparently nowhere. But there civilisation ends for the next week…..

After travelling along dirt roads, which cover everyone and everything in red dust, and the entertaining crossing of the Kenya/Tanzania border, you stay the next night at a small hotel in Moshi, where a rep. briefs you on the next five days.

For instance, you hear that the water purifying tablets brought from the UK are ineffective against some of the 'nasties' you are likely to come across – though the rep. does provide some effective iodine tablets. He tells you that you need to drink between three and five litres a day, to help fend off altitude sickness. He tells you which routes to ask the guides to take and about the person who was killed when lightning struck their climbing pole!

So, the next morning, we were driven to Kilimanjaro Park Gates, at approximately 6,000 feet. We were already well above the height of Ben Nevis and as a Pompey resident, working at *HMS Sultan*, my normal highest altitude is when I cross the Hilsea railway bridge! The key to altitude climbing is to do it very slowly, which anyone who knew me at Dartmouth will know suited me. In fact, it soon becomes impossible to do anything else. The first day is the easiest – taking six hours to climb through the rain forest at 9,000 feet to the first overnight at Mandara. It is already becoming apparent why no-one is allowed to attempt the climb without a team of porters and guides, who are so acclimatised that they run ahead of you and even serve lunch on the way and they have tea awaiting your arrival at the overnight camps. »+

The huts are wooden and house eight simple bunks. Although very primitive, the 'loos' and washing facilities become more interesting the higher you go.

The accommodation and the assistance given you by the team of porters, guides and cooks make it reasonably comfortable – except for the loos. If I say that one of the first things affected by altitude are your guts ….. I'll leave it to your imagination!

The next day was, for me, the absolute killer. Another 3,300 feet through moorland type terrain. Occasionally we would have to go down the side of a ravine, in order to climb wearily up the other side. Although a change on the calf muscles, this became demoralising. In total, Day Two was about 19 km. and about seven hours. I was beginning to have severe problems getting enough air into my lungs. In fact the only muscles really giving me grief were my intercostal muscles and diaphragm.

However, at Horombo Hut, Gilly was in a worse state than I, as she was affected by altitude sickness at the end of the second day. We were all taking Diamox, which helps to lessen the effects of altitude by decreasing cerebral and pulmonary oedema, but as it is a diuretic and we were all dutifully drinking our four litres of iodine water ….. So, Day Three dawned and leaving Gilly, her Diamox and her guts in the capable hands of her porter "Happy", the rest of us set off on to the saddle region between the two volcanic peaks. This is a sort of arctic desert and involved another 3,300 foot climb, past the Last Water Point. The porters carry what was needed, up from there to Kibo Hut at 15,520 feet. By now it is starting to get very cold and any incline at all, means going at a snail's pace.

We arrived at about 3.30 p.m., had tea at 5p.m., took our Diamox and Imodium and then got our heads down as best we could. I spent the next six hours wondering when would be the best time to make an expedition into the freezing cold for a wee! If I went then, I might have to go again later. If I waited till we got up (at about midnight), then I might have to rush to get ready (impossible at that altitude and not in my nature anyway).

Such dilemmas! – But even thinking becomes difficult after a while.

At just gone 1 a.m., we set off up the steep scree slope on the route to the summit. The idea of going at that time is:

i) So that the scree is still frozen and therefore easier to climb.

ii) So you can get to the rim of the crater before sunrise (it takes about six hours).

iii) So you can get to the highest point (another 11/12 hours) and back to Kibo for lunchtime, so that …..

iv) You can get back to Horombo for tea!

They make it <u>so</u> easy!! The unofficial reason for going during the night is so you can't see how bad the climb looks! ⇒

> After about an hour, though it felt like much less, I realised I was having trouble maintaining the pace at which we were going. I felt that if I went any slower, I would hold the others up and I wouldn't be able to get down to Horombo that day. As I've said, any physical effort at this altitude is torture – It is really difficult to make logical decisions - so I gave up. Almost immediately I began to regret it, but it was an irreversible decision. If I could press the rewind button ….
>
> However, I had climbed to 16,000 feet, four times the height of Ben Nevis and 5,000 feet higher than I had ever been before – but I didn't make it to the top, like Hugo and Rob, my husband.
>
> Having got down to Horombo, Day Five was spent going back to Mandara and then on to the Park Gates to meet the minibus which took us back to the border and then back to Mombasa. After all that Down, seven hours in a cramped minibus was not what our calves, hips or guts needed, but the week at the Whitesands Hotel in Mombasa was! ?❦

June 1993 saw the death of one of the RNDS' most illustrious officers. Surgeon Rear Admiral (D) William (Bill) Holgate CB OBE FDSRCS(Eng) had joined the Royal Navy in 1928, after winning the London and Haslar Gold Medal for gaining the highest marks in the then competitive entry examination.

Serving part of World War II in Malta and in Colombo, Ceylon, he returned to the UK in 1944 and in 1948, by then as a Surgeon Commander (D), he was appointed as Senior Dental Surgeon in *HMS Terror*, the base establishment in Singapore. Following his second return to the UK, he then pursued a surgical career in the naval hospitals, gaining his Fellowship in Dental Surgery along the way. In 1957, as a Surgeon Captain (D), he was appointed to the RN Medical School, Alverstoke (now the Institute of Naval Medicine) as Director of Dental Studies and Research. There, Holgate gained something of a reputation as an inventor and innovator. Amongst other things, he and his very able dental technician produced a series of models, demonstrating various dental procedures, which became a regular exhibit at national dental exhibitions and conferences.

He also devised and produced custom-made mouthpieces for divers, which proved far more satisfactory than the 'one size fits all' version. He also became a member of the Medical Research Council unit at Harwell, looking at the Strontium 90 content of extracted wisdom teeth, as a way of analysing the effects of fallout from the nuclear weapons tests in the Pacific, during the 1950s and 1960s*.

---

* When the office of the Director of Dental Training & Research at the Institute of Naval Medicine was closed in early 1991, a lead-lined, wooden box was discovered at the back of a cupboard, containing some of Holgate's original samples. The discovery caused a vigorous but brief reaction from the 'Health & Safety Police' and the samples (which were not highly radioactive), were safely destroyed by the nuclear accident response team at INM. For further details of this project, see Appendix 1 to this History.

Promoted to Surgeon Rear Admiral (D) and appointed as DNDS in 1960, he caused something of a stir by resigning the post in 1961, upon being offered the job of Chief Dental Officer for England at the Ministry of Health. He held that high office for ten years before retiring to the Isle of Wight. There in October 1987, tragedy struck in the form of the still-remembered, hurricane-force storm which, as well as causing significant damage along the South Coast and further inland, blew the roof off the house in which he lived with his wife of 54 years. Following this event, she succumbed to heart failure and died the following day. Holgate, subsequently remarried in 1989 and died in his 87th year[149].

We have heard before of the 'Armilla Patrol'. This was the RN guardship in the Arabian Gulf, usually a frigate or destroyer, which had been established as a permanent RN presence in the Gulf during and since the Iran – Iraq War of the 1980s. Its function, originally, was to provide assistance to any merchant shipping which might become inadvertently involved in the conflict and, since the War, together with ships from other nations, to police the 'peace'. As also mentioned previously, the Armilla deployment offered a wonderful opportunity for 'sea time' for a succession of young dental officers, equipped with 'Frigate Portable' dental equipment.

The turn of Surgeon Lieutenant (D) M F (Mike) Thomas, came in early 1993 and his account in the RNDS Newsletter gives a good flavour of the variety of work (and play) to be experienced on such a deployment[150].

Join the Navy – See the World!

My time had come! After two years working with the Fleet Air Arm at *HMS Heron* and *HMS Osprey,* I was to become part of the 'real' Navy as the Staff Dental Officer to Commander Armilla Task Group 5.

After the preliminary calls to the Fleet Dental Surgeon at Northwood and to *HMS Nelson*, to become acquainted with the Portable Dental Unit, I joined *HMS Coventry* on 9 January in Devonport.

My first dose of Stugeron [motion sickness medication] proved to be unnecessary, however, as the ship's sailing orders had been changed 24 hours earlier!

Therefore, after a week of storing ship, we sailed to become part of the first 'Operation Grapple' task group and headed for the Adriatic. After seven days of intensive workup, we [Thomas and his assistant LMA (D) I R Martin] transferred across to *HMS Brilliant* to begin our tour of the Adriatic.

HMS Brilliant saw the new portable dental unit put to good use, as the ship's POMA [Petty Officer Medical Assistant] managed to find more and more patients to treat (were there really only 280 on board?). After a rapid depletion ⇒

of stores, I transferred [again] to join Surgeon Commander (D) [Steve] Taylor on board *HMS Ark Royal*. Five days later, I was back 'home' in *HMS Coventry* and we left the Adriatic to begin heading towards the sun!

I was fortunate to be landed at Port Said with about 50 of the ship's company, for 24 hours in Cairo. This is what the Navy is all about – "Join the Navy, see the World!". It cannot be a bad job, being paid, whilst looking around one of the Seven Wonders of the World. It had been over a month since we left "Good Ol' Blighty" and the atmosphere in the ship improved as we began the planned part of the deployment. The Sick bay became a hive of activity as the Medical Officer, POMA and ourselves all competed for the chair, the operating table and the spare area of deck left in the corner ......

Jebel Ali is a huge port just inside the Arabian Gulf and is a frequent port of call for the Royal Navy. It was hot, even in February. A 45 minute bus-ride away was Dubai, a thriving mixture of cultures and people, with the first lesson in bartering! It was on the second day in port that we discovered the '10 dib-dob' curry, a treat not to be missed!

From Jebel Ali, we began our patrols and the first of many exercises which saw us working with the French, U.S., Kuwaiti, Saudi Arabian and Russian navies. I transferred across to *USS Hewitt* for two days, as part of the exchange between all the ships and had a taste of America (maple syrup pancakes for breakfast!).

After a short visit to Bahrain, which saw the first victory of the ship's cricket team and my being awarded the Geoff Boycott award for slow batting, we arrived in Muscat, Oman, just outside the approaches of the Gulf. Oman provided the first real taste of Arabia, as many of the old forts and mosques are preserved and the local culture is more readily apparent than in many of the Gulf States. The sea was warm, the sun was bright, the tan was coming along nicely and the Wadi-bashing was tremendous. Wadi-bashing involves cross-country driving, in this case up into the mountains and then an incredible scramble/swim/leap down a gorge, which took the breath away, as the splendour of the landscape was revealed. On my return to Oman, later in the deployment, we were taken to see one of the deepest gorges in the world. At over 1800 metres, it was deeper than the Grand Canyon, an almost unbelievable sight.

From Oman, *HMS Coventry* took us up to Kuwait, where we saw the ravages from the Gulf War. The expatriates had many sad tales to tell, but here and throughout all of the Gulf States, were perfect hosts, arranging all sorts of visits and activities for the whole ship's company. In Abu Dhabi, a visit to see Jasper Carrot performing had been arranged.

In between all the port visits, the [dental] fitness rate was creeping up, as the last few of the ship's company found their way to the sickbay. When we left *HMS Coventry* at the beginning of May, we had reached a fitness level of 99.6%, with just one 'not seen' document held onboard for someone yet to join. How frustrating! ≫→

> Due to the ship's programmes, we were to remain on station in the Gulf from February until July. Whilst waiting for an opportunity to transfer to *HMS Southampton*, the relief ship for *HMS Coventry*, we were accommodated onboard *RFA Brambleleaf.* Luxury!!
>
> The ten days onboard the RFA provided a welcome break, with a chance to unwind, have a bath, sleep in a real bed and prepare for our next ship. necessary, however, as the ship's sailing orders had been changed 24 hours earlier!
>
> The sickbay of *HMS Southampton* presented considerably more difficulties than *HMS Coventry*, in terms of space and layout, when it came to setting up the dental unit. However, the new portable dental unit proved to be very adaptable and is an excellent piece of equipment.
>
> With *HMS Southampton*, we visited some old favourites, such as Dubai (six visits in all) and some new ports of call, including Damman in Saudi Arabia. The Saudi government follow a very strict Muslim code and are intolerant of other religions being practised in their country. It was therefore a moving and wonderful experience to be able to meet with some Christians from the expatriate community and to share in their fellowship and worship in their homes.
>
> From Damman, we returned to Kuwait, Bahrain, Dubai, Muscat and Abu Dhabi until, all too soon, it was time for the handover to *HMS Cornwall* and leaving the Gulf. By now, most of the dental stores had been consumed, to be replaced by vases, coffee pots, brass camels, rugs and T-shirts. We left the ship in Cyprus to fly home at the end of July.
>
> During the deployment, there were over 1200 dental attendances and I placed just under 500 restorations. Sending dental teams to sea can certainly be justified! The Armilla Patrol is an excellent appointment which I found very enjoyable. This was what I joined up for! There are many challenges working in a completely different environment to a shore clinic. I can certainly recommend the Armilla Patrol as a superb opportunity to get to sea and to visit an interesting and exciting part of the world. … When can I go to sea again please? ❧

Vocational Training for new dental graduates had now become mandatory and the Services' pilot vocational training schemes had translated, almost seamlessly, into a recognised element of any newly graduated new entry dental officer's first year in each of the Armed Services dental branches. Clearly, this had implications for the appointing of new officers.

Traditionally, many young dental officers had been moved frequently during their first year or so, in order to give them experience of the varied aspects of Service life. Now, each new entry officer in the RNDS, on completion of his 'General Service Training' at the Britannia Royal Naval College in Dartmouth, would be assigned to a shore establishment dental practice. The Senior Dental Surgeon of each designated 'training practice' was himself, an accredited trainer within the national scheme. Each graduate would spend his first year in supervised practice with a proportionate amount of release time for courses and weekly group discussions and demonstrations.

The RNDS Vocational Training Scheme was administered by the Adviser in General Dental Practice, Surgeon Commander (D) S (Stephen) Lambert Humble. He had negotiated a scheme which 'cross-pollinated' with the local civilian training scheme, whereby, RNDS trainees would attend group sessions and courses with their civilian colleagues and the latter would also attend Navy-run training sessions in Commander Dental Training's department in *HMS Nelson*. This arrangement had the added benefit of providing those who left the RN after a Short Career Commission, with evidence of training within the National Health Service – sometimes a source of anxiety to trainees within the sister branches, whose VT schemes were entirely 'in house'. It also acted as fertile recruiting ground!

At Directorate level, DDS(N), Surgeon Commodore (D) Timothy Hall, sat as the tri-Service observer on the newly launched National Committee for Dental Vocational Training, thus ensuring that each single-Service scheme was in compliance with national requirements.

At a meeting of this committee, he raised the problem of those dental officers, pre-the vocational training scheme, who left the Services for civilian practice in mid dental career without the VT certification now required for employment within the National Health Service. After discussion at several sessions of the Committee, it was decided that exemption would be granted to any dentist who could demonstrate evidence of practice in Primary Dental Care in the Armed Forces, within the previous four years.

Preparations for the move of the Directorate to the new HQ building in the Portsmouth Naval Base were by now well under way. Some vigorous negotiation had resulted in the allocation of a very satisfactory suite of offices for DNDS, ADNDS and their supporting staff. The offices were immediately adjacent to those of the Medical Director General and his staff and, as well as housing the offices of the Commander-in-Chief/Second Sea Lord, all other personnel departments would be housed under the same roof, much facilitating the tasks of manpower management and recruiting.

The new Headquarters was to be named Victory Building.

The move had been set for April 1994, but by the end of 1993 it had become a possibility that this could be brought forward. Chief Wren (DH) Jacquie Watts had already been allocated as the Branch 'advance guard' in the building and local interviews were being held for the post of PA to DNDS.

Readers of this History and especially this chapter, may have come to the conclusion that dental officers in the Royal Navy spend more time climbing mountains around the globe, than at sea! This is not so. However, in keeping with demonstrating that RNDS personnel make a habit of achieving great heights, even within a rapidly shrinking Branch, not to mention the leavening effect of personal accounts of 'derring do' within these pages, here is the article, written by Surgeon Lieutenant (D) T B (Tim) Elmer, about a climb on Mount Kinabalu in Borneo. It is captured once again, from the RNDS Newsletter[151].

It will be remembered that the dental cadre within the Armed Forces of the Sultanate of Brunei, was provided by dental officers from the Royal Army Dental Corps and that the RNDS had been afforded two dental officer billets attached to the Sultan's Flotilla, the sea-going element of the Royal Brunei Armed Forces. The RNDS incumbents at that time were Surgeon Lieutenant Commander (D) A (Alan) Maxwell and Tim Elmer.

What goes Up …

Mount Kinabalu is the highest mountain in South East Asia, at 13,455 feet. It is the focal point of the Kinabalu National Park in Sarawak, Borneo, only a short jaunt from Brunei. As a result, Surgeon Lieutenant Commander (D) Maxwell and myself, comprising the entire RNDS contingent out here, decided we'd climb it.

Getting there from Brunei is easy. It's a 20 minute flight from there to Kota Kinabalu airport and then about two hours by car to the Park itself. We flew out and spent the first night in a hotel, drinking too much and watching the "Madonna Tour Video". The next morning saw us bright and early at the Park Headquarters to pick up our guide. Although the climb is very well marked, it is compulsory to have a guide. And so, we began to ascend the "Summit Trail".

As I've mentioned, the path is very well defined and a great deal of it has been made into steps, utilising the thousands of tree roots crossing the path or *de novo*. We had heard from others that the climb was relatively easy: "Just like climbing the stairs at home", they said. Utter tosh! - Unless your idea of easy is climbing the stairs for six miles. For botanical and zoological buffs, the height of Mount Kinabalu creates a unique environment, with unique fauna and flora to match.

The climb starts in Montane Oak Forest, more than 40 different species of oak tree, and, as you ascend, you pass through "cloud forest"- (6,400 to 7,300 feet). This is so called as it spends most of its time wreathed in cloud.

The trees here are gnarled and twisted, their branches loaded down with mosses, epiphytic ferns and orchids. Towards 9,500 feet the trees become shorter and ➤

more stunted, eventually being replaced by scrub and then mosses and sparse grass. The tree line is reached at 11,000 feet and above this there are just vast expanses of bare granite. It is at this height that you reach the rest house where you stay overnight. It would be possible to climb straight on to the summit and back in one day, but that's for masochists only. It took us four and a half hours to reach the rest house and by that time I was knackered and feeling the lesser effects of oxygen starvation – a bit of a headache and the urge to take huge lungfuls of air and to hold it in.

The rest house itself was a well constructed affair, two stories with about 30 rooms, a communal dining area and a decent galley. All their stores are carried up the mountain, using manpower only.

We were often passed by youths carrying woven rattan rucksacks, containing all sorts of things, from cases of beer to huge Calor Gas bottles. It turned out that the pay for carrying up a full gas bottle and taking down an empty was 40 Malaysian dollars – about a tenner.

The rooms were very basic with four bunks to each room. Maxwell and I ended up sharing with two continentals, Klaus and Jurgens. At about three o'clock in the afternoon, things took a distinct turn for the worse. We bumped into two officers from 10 Gurkha Regiment, Hong Kong, with 20 Gurkhas in tow. All of a sudden it was 11 o'clock at night, we were legless and stuffing ourselves with "bart". "Bart", is Gurkha goat curry (I didn't ask where they had found the goat) with "cili padi" as a side dish. For the uninitiated, "cili padi" are tiny red or green chilli peppers, which you eat whole, dipped in coarse ground salt. Pure dynamite! I haven't moved so fast since I took a swig of Dr Futtock's patent purgative!

We lumbered back to our billet and grabbed a couple of hours sleep. Our guide had advised us that we needed to be up at 2am, to continue the climb and attain the summit in time to see the sunrise. He had obviously not considered the potential of two cili padi powered dentists!

Above the rest house the ascent was mostly across smooth granite, with very little scree.

In places this was seriously steep and there are a series of ropes strung out from the summit, for several thousand feet, to give you some purchase whilst hauling yourself up. This was pretty tiring and close to the summit, I thought I was going to die. The lack of oxygen (honest!) was making my head spin and this was not helped by Maxwell lurching along ahead of me, coughing, retching and murmuring "Oh God! Oh God!"

However, worse was yet to come. We actually reached the summit at 4am, having fair hurtled up the mountain. Sunrise is not until about 6.15am and it was cold - very cold! Mind numbingly cold, with no shelter except gaps between the granite boulders on the leeward side of the summit. Even with all the extra ➤

> clothing I'd taken, I was still frozen. To give you an idea of what a low ebb I'd reached, I even considered asking Maxwell if I could sit closer to him, than is considered socially acceptable, in order to augment my meagre body heat. But then I thought, "Damn it, no! I'd rather get frostbite and die than cuddle Maxwell!" So I shivered in solitude.
>
> On the plus side, at nearly 14,000 feet above cloud and haze, the equatorial night sky was breathtaking. There was a full moon, which set like the sun, changing colour as it dipped towards the horizon. The sunrise, when it did arrive, was magnificent.
>
> So, to the descent. I can think of no adequate training that can prepare your thighs for walking downstairs for six miles. As we approached the bottom, I heard Maxwell laughing. "Why on earth are you walking like that?" I stopped. My legs, completely jellified, continued to do a Michael Jackson in the absence of any music. Enough was enough. We piled into a minibus, stopped at the Park HQ long enough to get our 'Been there, done that' certificates and headed for home.

On 8 December 1993, Surgeon Commodore (D) Timothy Hall held the final Board of Management meeting of 1993. It was also the last such meeting to be held in the Defence Medical and Dental Services HQ at First Avenue House in High Holborn.

It was now known that the move to the new Second Sea Lord/C-in-C Naval Home Command HQ in Victory Building in the Portsmouth Naval base, would take place early in the new year and much of the meeting was taken up with the planning of the move in such a way as to avoid any disruption to the operational tasks and day to day running of the RNDS. However, in his opening remarks, Hall announced the launch of yet another 'Study' which would affect the Defence Medical Services as well as many other aspects of the Armed Services. The study was borne of the 1993 Budget.

Despite the savings realised by 'Options for Change', the Government, still unable to make ends meet, was looking for ever more drastic 'efficiency savings'. The latest Armed Forces study was to be (ingenuously) entitled "Front Line First". The title implied that savings would be taken from the support elements of the Services, including medical and dental. Its authors seemed oblivious to the fact that medical and dental staff in the Armed Forces had an important front line task to play. The Front Line First study was led by the Minister for the Armed Forces, who had been tasked with finding savings of £1.2 billion over three years – a huge sum at that time. Hall warned that the RNDS and its sister services would soon be confronted by a team of 'mould breakers'. Elmer and Maxwell, from the summit of Mount Kinabalu, had witnessed a magnificent dawn of many hues. As the year turned, the RNDS would experience a dawn of a very different hue.

The year ended on a pleasing note, when, on 17 December 1993, the Director, Timothy Hall was invited to present the prizes at the Annual Prize-Giving of the Faculty of Medicine and Dentistry at the University of Birmingham.

*****

Chapter 10

A Purple Dawn?
1994 – 1995

February 1994 found the Dental Directorate team in their splendid new offices in Victory Building, the new Second Sea Lord/Naval Home Command Headquarters in the Portsmouth Naval Base. On moving day, there was snow on the ground!

The team comprised the Director, Surgeon Commodore (D) Timothy Hall, the Deputy Director, Surgeon Captain (D) Ted Grant, Surgeon Commander (D) Geoff Myers, who bore the title: Staff Dental Officer (Organisation) and Chief Wren Dental Hygienist Jacquie Watts, who ran the 'Admin' desk. Additionally, a civilian PA had been assigned as support to the Director.

Compared with First Avenue House, the office suite was modern, airy and reasonably spacious. It also had the huge advantage of not being in London! In fact, for the three officers, it was a less than a half hour journey from home to the office.

Not everything, however, was that easy. As they moved into their new offices, each member of the team found their desks equipped with a brand new "CHOTS" terminal. CHOTS (Corporate HQ Office Technology System), was a newly introduced MoD secure, wide area IT network, which would enable the dissemination of orders and command documents up to the level SECRET, as well as providing the means of communicating by email, between personnel in the same and different departments. Despite having attended 'CHOTS Familiarisation Days' and training courses, the team and their colleagues elsewhere in the new HQ, found the system anything but 'user friendly'!

The Directorate team were not given much time to enjoy their new surroundings. The 'Front Line First' study had now become the Defence Costs Study (DCS). That part of the study dealing with the future of the Defence Medical and Dental Services was "DCS 15".

DCS 15 would be coloured by two current preoccupations of the Government. The first being a belief that services within Government departments could be delivered more efficiently by 'Agencies'. An Agency was defined as a 'stand alone' unit, which would hold its own budget and which would be run by a 'Chief Executive'. The latter might or might not be a uniformed Service officer. The second preoccupation was with the continuing search for rationalisation within the Armed Forces.

At Directorate level and within the context of an Agency, the lines and differences between the three Services and their *modus operandi* would become more and more blurred, leading to a fear amongst all three Branchs' managers of the launch of a 'Purple' Service.

'Purple'? In the late 1960s, the Canadian Armed Forces had commenced an ultimately unsuccessful experiment in 'ultra-rationalisation'. The three Canadian Armed Services had been amalgamated, with common (army) ranks and a common (rifle green) uniform, referred to colloquially (and only half in jest) as the 'Purple Uniform'. This move by the Canadian Government had led, amongst other things, to the immediate resignation of all but one of the admirals of the former Royal Canadian Navy.

Although the overarching designation "Canadian Armed Forces" was retained, the original rank structure for each Service was reinstated in 1970 and the uniforms distinctive to each of the Armed Services were reintroduced in 1987.

Due to the disruption occasioned by the recent move to Victory Building, DNDS had decided to postpone the Spring meeting of his Board of Management to 9 June 1994, the day before the Wood Lecture. This was duly held in the Victory Building conference room where the Director was able to announce the recent selection of Surgeon Captain (D) Ted Grant to be his successor, in the rank of Surgeon Commodore (D). Grant would supersede him on 26 November 1994.

The meeting covered a wide range of problems dealing with budgets, stores and (lack of) manpower, as well as the apparent 'creeping civilianisation' of an increasing number of dental officer and support staff billets. The Adviser in General Dental Practice, Surgeon Commander (D) Stephen Lambert Humble, reported on progress since Dental Vocational Training for new graduates had become mandatory. The chief of the scheme in England and Wales, Mr David Rule, had recently visited Gibraltar

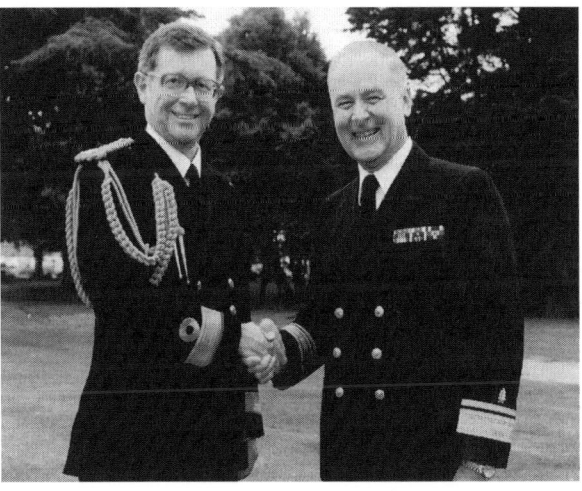

DNDS, Surgeon Commodore (D) T J C Hall greeting Rear Admiral Ron Morse DC USN, Chief of the US Navy Dental Corps – 9 June 1994

to observe RNDS vocational trainees undergoing a module in paedodontics at the families' clinic there. He had declared himself impressed, indicating that even in this area of dental practice, less frequently encountered by RNDS personnel, the Branch was well up to speed[152].

The meeting was followed by a lunch at *HMS Nelson*, in honour of the visiting Chief of the US Navy Dental Corps, Rear Admiral Ron Morse DC USN.

The following day, 10 June 1994, saw yet another Wood Memorial Lecture and Clinical Meeting[153]. The lectures and presentations were held at the Institute of Naval Medicine. The meeting was also well supported by a dental trades show. In addition to over 200 past and serving RNDS personnel of all ranks, the event was also attended by Rear Admiral Morse and his accompanying staff.

Before the eponymous lecture, there were presentations by several distinguished speakers. First Professor Martin Addy from the Bristol Dental School spoke on "Risk Assessment and Preventive Dentistry". After a sherry reception amongst the trade stands and a good lunch, the afternoon session kicked off with the presentation by DNDS of the Alan Acton Davies Memorial Medal and Prize to Leading Wren Dental Hygienist Caroline Hill, for her outstanding contribution to the dental health of the Royal Navy. This was followed by an "Historical Review of Dental Care in the Royal Navy", delivered by Professor M N (Tony) Naylor. He acknowledged that much of his material had been gleaned from the research of Surgeon Commander (D) Nick Daws.

A good day was then rounded off by the Wood Lecture. This was delivered in impressive style by Mr Derek Henderson, an oral surgeon of international renown, who was an Honorary Consultant to the Royal Navy and who had been responsible for part of the training of most of the then serving RNDS oral surgeons. He spoke on the development of orthognathic surgery. The day ended with the conviviality of the Director's Dinner, held in the Wardroom at *HMS Dolphin*. Guests included the Second Sea Lord and the Medical Director General (Naval).

Despite all the mayhem of pending re-organisation, the Directorate continued to seek and to preserve opportunities for RNDS personnel to serve abroad and at sea. An exchange agreement had existed for some time between the Royal Army Dental Corps and the RNDS.

The same issue of the RNDS Newsletter in which a report of the above Wood Lecture day appeared, carried an interesting account by Surgeon Lieutenant (D) J (Julie) Fenwick of such an exchange appointment and of life in post-Cold War Berlin[154]. An abridged account is shown below:

For You Ze Wall is Over!

In June 1992 I began my exchange with the Army as a dentist in Berlin. The situation here was very exciting – many things were changing. The infamous Wall, erected in 1961, which had enclosed the city from the former East, had come down only two years previously.

As a result, the Four Power status, unique to Berlin was diminishing, as the military forces of America, France, Britain and the former USSR began to draw down. Despite this, the influence of the occupying Allies could still be noticed in the different regions of the city, each having their own facilities, such as schools, cinemas, radio and TV stations.

I lived in the Brigade Headquarters Mess, on the site of the notorious 1936 Olympic Village. As well as being the headquarters for the British Army in Berlin, the camp had many facilities: indoor and outdoor swimming pools, numerous running tracks, sports fields and equestrian facilities – in fact it catered for almost any sport imaginable! Surrounding the camp was the Olympic Sports Complex of the Maifeld, Waldbuhne and Equestrian Centre. These not only staged sporting events, often of an international standard, such as American football and polo, but were also prominent cultural venues. Military pageants, such as the Queen's Birthday Parade, as well as opera, orchestral and internationally renowned groups such as U2, Billy Joel etc., performed there. Very convenient when it's on your doorstep!

Further down the road was the Berlin Group Practice, housed in the multi-storey former British Military Hospital. As a hospital, it had previously been fully equipped with surgical and support wards. However, now only the first three floors were routinely used. Downstairs were the medical, X-ray, pharmacy and stores departments. Upstairs, opposite the hairdressers … the dental department!

The department was only a few years old. It was fully furnished with state-of-the-art equipment and units, including fibre-optic and electrosurgery handpieces. There was also a comprehensive intercom system that piped BFBS [British Forces Broadcasting System] throughout the department, to soothe the customers!

As a throwback from the previous problems of materials availability, when the Wall was up, the department also had the luxury of 'local purchase' for materials which were otherwise difficult to obtain from 'the Zone'.

Initially, on my arrival, there was a total of three dentists, with additional visiting oral surgery and orthodontic support. Arrangements for general anaesthesia were made locally with the American Military Hospital or, more rarely, at Rinteln, in 'the Zone'. The clerk and hygienist both served in the RADC, however the DSAs were a mixture of civilian ladies and wives of military personnel. Up until last year, the department also had its own technician. Unfortunately, he was lost with the redundancies. After that all laboratory work was sent to the UK.

In addition to the Brigade Headquarters, there were regiments at Spandau along with engineering and logistical support units. In total, with the families and various personnel connected to the Armed Forces, such as teachers and Embassy staff, we were kept quite busy.

There were quite a few differences I found, working with the Army. The first hurdle was to learn the various regimental job titles [and ranks]. For example: Sappers, Privates, Corporals of the Horse etc.; and then recognising them: never before have I seen so many varieties of green jumper! Also, job titles at the Headquarters were always quite a mystery … What was SO3 G3 anyway?

The Army was well supported in Berlin. A large NAAFI, complete with Burger King, was built on the site of the Spandau Prison where Hess was previously detained. A weekly newspaper, produced for the military, kept everyone up to date with local events. Also, there were many recreational facilities available, such as yacht, golf and saddle clubs and the Army Educational Centre provided day and evening courses in anything from languages to picture framing!

Socially, Berlin was a very busy place. The different Army regiments and units based there, in addition to the RAF at Gatow, meant there was always something happening. Annually, there were large military events such as the Queen's Birthday Parade and the Berlin Tattoo, as well as events organised by the other Allies – for example: the Concours Francais.

And of course, Berlin itself. With its numerous cafes, restaurants, opera houses and theatres, the city was a hive of activity in both the former East and West. The historical legacy of monuments and museums such as the Brandenburg Gate, the Reichstag, and Checkpoint Charlie, in addition to the History of the Wars, the building and destruction of the Wall and the Airlifts, meant there was much to see and explore. Many of the buildings of the former East, such as the Neue Palace at Potsdam, restored after more than thirty years, contrasted greatly with the affluence of the West.

I am very grateful to have had the chance to serve in Berlin with the RADC. It has been a unique opportunity to experience not only the British Army, but also German culture in a large and rapidly changing city of significant historical and political prominence.

These last two years have passed too quickly! ❧

August 1994 saw the Medical Director General (Naval), Surgeon Rear Admiral A L (Tony) Revell QHS, promoted to Surgeon Vice Admiral as the Surgeon General of the Armed Forces. Revell had taken over an unenviable task as Chief of the Armed Forces' Medical and Dental Services at a time of almost unprecedented turmoil. Amongst other measures, it was becoming evident that the closure of all but one of the Service hospitals was in the pipeline. Which was to be the survivor was one out of several causes of inter-Service conflict.

Revell was relieved as MDG(N) by Surgeon Rear Admiral A (Sandy) Craig QHP, a senior medical officer who was to prove to be a good friend of the RNDS during the uncertain times ahead.

The DCS 15 Implementation Team, led by Captain (later Commodore) N (Nicholas) Harris, was quick to arrive in Victory Building.

Amongst many other calls, Harris visited Surgeon Commodore (D) Timothy Hall, who during their discussion called in the Deputy, Surgeon Captain (D) Ted Grant, to introduce him to Harris as his successor.

The following day, Grant received a telephone call from Harris: "When we met yesterday, I understood that you are to be Commodore Hall's successor. Can you clarify for me in what rank you will hold the post?" Grant replied: "In the rank of Surgeon Commodore (D)". "That", riposted Harris, "is not part of my plan for the Dental Agency". "In which case", said Grant, "you will need to take the matter up with the Second Sea Lord. It was he who made the selection and approved the promotion". Nothing more was heard on the matter, but Harris was to prove to have little understanding or sympathy for the Medical and Dental Services as he wielded vigorously his 'DCS 15 axe'.

As the outcomes of Defence Costs Study 15 became clearer, MDG (N), writing in the Journal of the Royal Naval Medical Service announced that in Secondary Care, the Royal Naval Hospital Haslar had been selected as the one and only remaining Service hospital. It would be supported by Military District Hospital Units (MDHU) in several regional NHS district hospitals and managed by a Defence Secondary Care Agency. He went on to state: "Some functions in Primary Dental Care will be rationalised on a tri-Service basis. The ultimate aim would be to achieve agency status[155]".

Shortly after this, it was announced that Air Vice-Marshal J (Jefferson) Mackey, the current Director of Defence Dental Services, had been selected as the Chief Executive of the new Defence Dental Agency.

DCS 15 would, in due course, spawn three agencies: the Defence Dental Agency (DDA), the Defence Secondary Care Agency and the third which would manage medical and dental care for the Armed Forces in Germany. Primary medical care would remain under the control of each of the three Services.

Surgeon Captain (D) J V (John) Holland, Editor of the RNDS Newsletter, summed up well the prospects for the first two of these in his editorial of that time[156]. He also mentioned, in the same editorial, the pending 75th Anniversary of the RNDS and the intention to publish Volume I of this History, to coincide with this event. An extract from the editorial is reproduced below:

> ## 75 Years of Change?
>
> The announcement in Parliament on 14 July 1994 [of the Defence Costs Study], gave only the bare bones of the cost cutting exercise.
>
> Hardnosed financial principals driving the study have accepted that the Defence Dental Services are the most economical way of undertaking an adequate level of dental care for the men and women in the Armed Forces. Considerable work went into getting the facts right and being able to put a figure on the daily cost of dentistry in the Services, per person. [*vide* Robinson's exercise to determine the accurate cost of dental provision within the Royal Navy]. This, which was lower than an organisation such as DENPLAN could offer, must have been impressive.
>
> Also, there is no other organisation which could take on the dental care of the Forces not outlawed by the Dentists' Act [At that time, under the Dentists' Act it was illegal for any corporate body to promote or manage the practice of dentistry in the NHS]. The dentist in the High Street is rather remote from most military bases and is not in a happy state at the moment, so they cannot help either.
>
> This is not to say there will not be cuts. As the Services decline in numbers, so must the Dental Branches. However, the proposed formation of a Defence Dental Agency, to run primary care dentistry, is a big step forward. With proper autonomy and its own budgetary control, the prospect is quite exciting.
>
> Secondary care is not so happy. RNH Haslar will remain as a 'core' hospital, with all three Services represented and an increase in size and beds to accommodate them – the actual number of beds being a matter of journalistic speculation at the moment.
>
> How all this will affect the dental officers of the three Services, employed in secondary care, is not known. Presumably implementation teams will make a pronouncement later in the year. The numbers in secondary care generally, will be reduced quite radically as the hospitals at Aldershot, Halton, Woolwich and Wroughton close. Military District Hospital Units [MDHU] are to be set up in four areas of the country, but so far only Derriford in Plymouth and Catterick are certainties. Other sites have yet to be found, let alone agreed. The next few months will no doubt contain revelations of both a good and bad nature. It is perhaps, supremely optimistic to expect the good news to be in the majority.
>
> [He continued:]
>
> 20 January 1995 will be an important date for all past and present members of the Branch. On this day 75 years ago, the Royal Naval Dental Service was founded by Order in Council. Dentistry in the Navy had progressed slowly from a 'Medical Officer with an interest' basis (some doubly qualified), through ➤

> civilian dentists employed in large establishments, to RNVR dental officers in HM Ships, at sea in the First World War. The story of all this was researched by Surgeon Commander (D) Nick Daws, before he retired. It is hoped that the History up to the formation of the Ministry of Defence in the mid 60s, will be printed in time for the anniversary celebrations.

Volume I of the History of Dentistry in the Royal Navy was indeed published in time for the 75th Anniversary. Ably researched, as stated above by Surgeon Commander (D) Nick Daws, an accomplished amateur naval historian, it was co-authored by him and Surgeon Captain (D) John Holland.

On the evening of 17 November, Timothy Hall, the outgoing Director, was informally dined out by his Board of Management at the Old Lodge Hotel in Alverstoke. A convivial evening was had by all, with tributes paid to Timothy Hall over the port. A more formal 'dining out' would take place at a later date. The next day, it was "business as usual"! On 18 November 1994, Surgeon Commodore (D) Timothy Hall held his last meeting of the DNDS Board of Management. Surgeon Commander (D) G L (Graham) Morrison, who had recently joined the Directorate Staff to run the RNDS personnel desk, acted as secretary to the meeting.

At the meeting, Hall expressed his thanks to Surgeon Captain (D) John Holland and Surgeon Commander (D) Colin Priestland for organising a most successful Wood Lecture and Clinical Day, which had taken place in June.

The main agenda item for the meeting was an update on the progress of DCS 15[157]. The meeting was addressed by both the Director and his Deputy, who outlined progress thus far. The concept of Agency structure was one which was currently preoccupying the Defence Dental Services Policy Board. DNDS had set up his own 'Dental Care Agency Working Group', which had held its first meeting on 22 September. At this meeting concern had been expressed that the 'ring-fencing' of the management cadre within the agency structure, could lead to difficulties with the Branch's relationship with its operational customer – the Fleet. Further problems had arisen at a meeting of the Defence Dental Services Policy Board on 1 November, when it had become apparent that RNDS inputs and concerns had not been fully taken on board.

Subsequent to this, AVM Mackey met with the three single-Service directors in order to thrash out the sensitive issue of the management structure of the embryo agency.

On 14 November, Surgeon Captain (D) Ted Grant, wearing his 'Director Designate' hat, had met again with AVM Mackey. At this meeting the following points were outlined:

- There would be little change to single-Service working arrangements at clinic level.
- There was likely to be continuing debate over the Agency's management structure.
- The Dental Care Agency (as it was then called) would be 'vested' in October 1995. Its 'owner' would be the Surgeon General. 'Shadow' budgets might become operable in April 1995 and should 'go live' in April 1996.
- The location of the Agency Headquarters had yet to be decided, but ideally, it would be situated out of London*.
- The "Regional Dental Officer" system, currently in use in the RAF, would be introduced throughout the UK to manage local clinical services. Regions would be allocated to each of the single-Service Branches, in accordance with Branch size and involvement in each region. This framework would supersede the RNDS Command and Fleet Dental Surgeon structure.
- A small further number of redundancies might be required at Surgeon Commander (D) level.
- A review of Terms of Service (which differed widely between the three single-Service Branches), would be carried out to ensure rationalisation between the three Services. This would address such matters as time promotion, leave allowances and retirement age, in all of which the RNDS was the 'poor cousin'. Due to the sensitivity of these issues, it was predicted that full rationalisation was unlikely to be achieved before 2010.
- Secondary Care would in future be provided by the separate Defence Secondary Care Agency, but officers and staff would remain members of their own single-Service branches.

After some discussion of Grant's statement on the above points, the meeting continued with routine discussions on a number of other administrative matters. DNDS was then able to round off the meeting with the presentation of a cheque for £250.00 to Warrant Officer Dental Surgery Assistant Sally Rowe.

Rowe, who had retired from the Service, a few months previously, bore the distinction of being the first RN Dental Branch rating to achieve the rank of Warrant Officer. Having served with distinction as a Chief Wren DSA in a number of senior appointments, including that of Senior Instructor at the old RN Dental Training School and as manager of the Oral Surgery Department at RNH Haslar, she had reached a 'glass ceiling', there being no provision, at that

---

* It had already been decided that the Defence Medical Agency would be located at *HMS Dolphin*, (to be renamed: Fort Blockhouse), adjacent to the tri-Service hospital at Haslar. It was Grant's suggestion that it would make administrative and operational sense for the Dental Agency to be co-located on the same site. This proposal was not accepted.

time, for a Warrant Officer post within the RNDS. Her talents were, however, recognised by the RN Medical Service and she was selected, over the heads of a number of senior medical ratings, to take up the post of Patient Services Officer at RNH Stonehouse in Plymouth, in the rank of Warrant Officer. The cheque was donated by the officers and ratings of the RNDS and was presented as a symbol of their affection and esteem for Warrant Officer Rowe.

The meeting closed with the readily adopted proposal, by Surgeon Captain (D) Ted Grant, of a vote of thanks to the retiring Director, on behalf of the Board. Commodore Timothy Hall, in turn thanked the Board for their work and support for the Branch, stating that he foresaw difficult and uncertain times ahead, but that he was confident that the 'dark blue' dental service for the Fleet was both required and needed and that the RNDS would weather the storm.

On 26 November 1994, Surgeon Commodore (D) E J (Ted) Grant OStJ QHDS superseded Timothy Hall as Director Naval Dental Services in a time of great turmoil for the Branch. As he himself described it, in his previous role as Deputy Director, he was already running before he hit the ground!

Like most of his predecessors, Grant had had a broad 'training' for this the ultimate appointment as a Royal Navy dentist. Schooled at Epsom College, he had trained for his chosen profession at Guy's Hospital Dental School, emerging in 1962 with a Bachelor of Dental Surgery degree from London University and as a Licentiate in Dental Surgery from the Royal College of Surgeons of England.

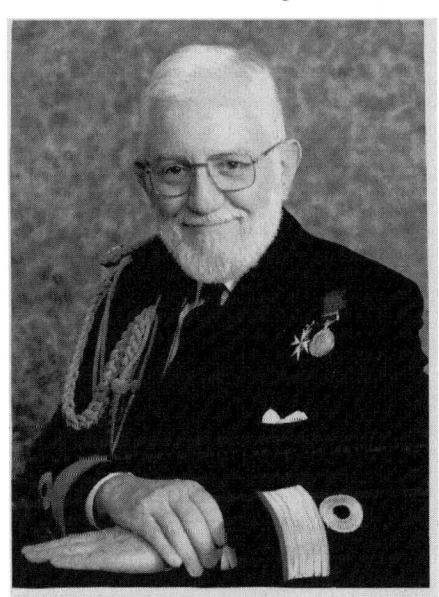

Surgeon Commodore (D)
E J Grant OStJ QHDS

Through the persuasive good offices of Dr Tony Naylor at Guy's, himself an enthusiastic Naval Reserve dental officer, Grant joined the Royal Navy, on a three-year Short Service Commission, in August 1962, after a brief locum house appointment at St. Mary's Hospital in London. He joined in the rank of Surgeon Lieutenant (D).

After a month of New Entry Officer training on the 'Divisional Officers' Course at *HMS Victory* (now *HMS Nelson*), he took up his first appointment at *HMS Ganges*, the 'boys' * training establishment in Suffolk.

---

* At that time, the school leaving age had yet to be raised from 15 to 16 years and two of the RN New Entry Training establishments at *HMS Ganges* and *HMS St Vincent* were dedicated to basic naval training and the continuing education of 15-year-old boy seamen.

In the summer of 1963 Grant joined the Fleet Aircraft Carrier *HMS Victorious*. This appointment was to prove pivotal in aiding his later decision to apply for a permanent commission.

Victorious sailed, at short notice, for the Far East in the autumn of 1963, to relieve the ailing *Ark Royal*. This was at a time when HM Government had ordered that there should be two carrier groups deployed 'East of Suez', which then encompassed most of the then world trouble spots.

With a complement of over 2,500 men, including the embarked air squadrons, Grant was the junior of two dental officers. His boss, the Senior Dental Surgeon was Surgeon Commander (D) A E (Ted) Cadman, who, although their department was always busy, was generous in allowing Grant time for some experiences not usually available to dentists, within or outside the Armed Forces. These ranged from two weeks with a mechanised patrol of the Royal Scots Greys in the Aden Protectorate, to flights off the deck.

Shortly after the ship's arrival in the Far East, Indonesia's President Sukarno attempted to invade Malaysia. This, in the longer term resulted in the ship remaining East of Suez for two years and the ship's company being replaced, for the first time ever, by a massive air trooping operation. Grant was enjoying the 'Eastern Experience' so much that he volunteered to stay on for the second commission. To his surprise, his offer was accepted and he was the only officer from the original complement to return to the UK in the ship in June 1965. It was during the second commission that he met his future wife, Julia, a teacher employed in Singapore to teach in a British Army primary school.

After his return to the UK, it was back to New Entry Training establishments at *HM Ships Fisgard* and *Raleigh* at Torpoint in Cornwall. Whilst serving there he and Julia were married, he transferred to the Permanent List and, in 1967, he was promoted Surgeon Lieutenant Commander (D).

Two years at the Communications School at *HMS Mercury* followed and then, in January 1970, it was back to Singapore, this time to *HMS Triumph* an ex-light fleet carrier, which had been converted to a fleet repair and support ship. This was the best of all worlds. A seagoing appointment based in Singapore, where his wife and family, by now consisting of two boys, lived in a naval married quarter.

Following Prime Minister Wilson's decision to withdraw from Singapore, *Triumph* was the last RN ship to leave the Naval Base, which was handed over to a small UK, Australian and New Zealand contingent – ANZUK.

Back in the UK, Grant was appointed as Staff Dental Surgeon to the Flag Officer Sea Training at *HMS Osprey* at Portland, Dorset. He was promoted Surgeon Commander (D) in June 1974. The following year, he and his family (now with three sons) were off abroad again, this time as the exchange officer with the US Navy at Bethesda, Maryland. The first year was spent undergoing the Comprehensive Dentistry residency in the Navy Graduate Dental School and the second in an honorary fellowship in the Department of Periodontics in Washington Navy Yard.

Back again in the UK, Grant found himself once again a student at Guy's Hospital, whence he emerged in late 1977 with a Master's Degree in Periodontology. From there he was appointed as Officer-in-Charge at the Royal Naval Dental Training School until 1982. Appointments to *HMS Dolphin* on the Staff of Flag Officer Submarines, *HMS Cochrane* on the Staff of Flag Officer Scotland and Northern Ireland and the Naval Dental Clinic at Earl's Court in London, followed. Whilst serving in the latter appointment, Grant was promoted Surgeon Captain (D) in June 1987.

From London, he was appointed to the Institute of Naval Medicine as Director of Dental Training and Research and Head of Training Division. At the end of his time there, it was Grant's sad task to close DDTR's office – victim of the continuing contraction of the Branch and of senior posts within it.

In early 1991, Grant was appointed back to London as Deputy to the Director, Surgeon Commodore (D) Brian Robinson. He also wore a tri-Service hat as 'Dental Management 1'. Ted Grant remained in this appointment when Timothy Hall superseded Robinson and moved with him to Victory Building in HM Naval Base Portsmouth, until his further promotion and appointment as DNDS.

Whilst in the rank of Surgeon Captain (D), Grant was appointed as an Honorary Dental Surgeon to HM the Queen in April 1993 and as an Officer Brother of the Order of St. John of Jerusalem in October 1993.

Most of this chapter has dealt with 'Doom and Gloom', so it is perhaps appropriate to remind ourselves, as the end of this Volume of the Branch History looms into sight, what life in the Royal Naval Dental Services is really all about.

We have met our Welsh colleague Lynford Thomas before. Now bearing the rank of Surgeon Commander (D) and serving as Senior Dental Surgeon in the aircraft carrier *HMS Ark Royal* he has given us yet another glimpse of life at sea in the mid-1990s.

As with his previous articles in the RNDS Newsletter, his account is at times a little jaded and frequently verges on the whimsical[158]! The following is an abridged version.

At Sea – A View from the Valleys!

<u>The Prologue:</u> *Ark Royal* has been my fifth sea-going appointment, but the last one was on Armilla Patrol in 1983. A lot of water has been passed since then. What changes have I noticed and what memories will remain?

<u>Initial Thoughts:</u> Goodness - I feel so old! Other than the Captain and the Master at Arms, I'm about the oldest member of the ship's company. Soon after joining the feeling of excitement is still there, but tempered with the knowledge that long periods during deployment will be tedious and some people are starting to get on my nerves already. It's good to see 'Jack' at sea (i.e. in context) again and something we need to do every so often. Females in boiler suits seem strange at first, but not for long. The strange, empty feeling in the pit of the stomach on sailing from Portsmouth is the same as before. Nearly eight months will be a long time, especially for our families.

Pusser's [Naval slang for anything naval] bunks are ridiculous. The fold-out bunk frame measures 2 feet 4 inches wide. The mattress is two feet wide and about 3 mm thick. I didn't have a decent night's sleep during the whole deployment. What's more [the bunks] fold up in the middle of the night, swallowing the unsuspecting sleeper and frightening him to death!

The food is good. No traffic lights on the menus from the Thought Police of healthy eating. The laundry is hopeless. My clothes seem to be shrinking! I don't believe it – some officers still wear cravats and 'empire-builder' shorts (though not necessarily together) on runs ashore.

<u>Day to Day:</u> I made an effort to see as much as possible of the workings of other departments and it was very worthwhile. Watching the changing of one of the ship's engines or a Harrier rebuild, reminds me of the expertise possessed by many of one's patients, which we sometimes overlook. How do they put up with all that time spent in the Ops. Room? Or the heat in the machinery spaces? Or the cold on the flight deck?

My cabin was spacious and (bunk apart), comfortable. The level of stewarding was exceptional. Dinner was always very civilised and a little wine was taken "for our stomachs' sake". I tried to balance diet and exercise. Exercise lost! The mail delivery was very good and newspaper supplies reasonable. The domestic problems started soon after sailing. Everything works at home until I've gone. Then the washing machine, the central heating, the car etc., play up!

Evening rounds – [and as duty senior officer] a new one on me and I can't say I gained much pleasure from doing them. Nevertheless, a reminder of mess life. It's amazing how many sailors go for weeks at sea without seeing daylight. How do they put up with the lack of space and privacy?

Often surprising how little spare time there can be in the days at sea, after doing all the extra fiddly jobs we are lumbered with. Weekends at sea still felt strange. Still the need to make Saturday nights feel different – quiz nights and fancy ≫

dress. Sundays at sea – cakes after church; curry for lunch; zzzzs pm and film night after dinner. Don't bother seeing a new film for a couple of years before a sea job. You will see them all again!

Work: Nice of you to ask. Yes, there was lots of dental treatment in evidence. The dental department is reasonably spacious by the standards of other ships but, at the end of the day, it is still a small box.

The ME [engineering] side of the ship has huge machinery spaces. About the only compartment smaller than the dental surgery is the welfare fund shop. Now I know my place in the scheme of things!

It is always a pleasure to see one's post-surgical results on a daily basis and to find out how quickly the news of a difficult [wisdom tooth extraction] spreads around the ship. It was a blessing to have a visiting dental hygienist - thank you Leading Wren Hill.

Again, the [dental] challenge of Chinese laundrymen and patients from the Royal Fleet Auxiliary. I think the maximum was 12 'pain cases' in one day. I also saw a few Army patients who were on board from Bosnia. Trauma cases were surprisingly few. The ban on hiring motorbikes on Greek islands helped.

Setting up and exercising the Emergency Operating Theatre and First-Aid teams, was a sobering evolution. The potential for Army casualties, were it all to turn 'pear shaped' in Bosnia, is frightening.

Visits: Due to the timing of the deployment (January to September), the weather was generally good and the visits were mostly new to me: Gib, Bari, Athens, Corfu, Crete, Majorca (twice), Istanbul and Malta. There were family visits to Athens, Majorca and Malta. There were memorable cocktail parties on the flight deck, at anchor off Crete, Istanbul and in Grand Harbour, Malta.

I managed a couple of mini-expeds [sporting or adventurous training activities ashore]. Skiing in Italy and sailing in Corfu. One of the highlights of the trip was getting to Bosnia. Arranging the visit was difficult and necessitated the whole Action Man kit and weapon training. The blue beret definitely suits me! The helo [helicopter] flight into Bosnia was spectacular. It is an amazingly pretty country. On the ground the destruction was much as expected from the TV news reports and just as depressing.

It was interesting to see how the British Army fare. I visited the barracks in Gorny Vakuf and the medical centre was a series of large tents set up in an old factory. The medical facilities were good, but other facilities were very basic. The Army do six month tours. The country experiences extremes of weather, with [both] Summer and Winter being very uncomfortable.

[Back at sea] visits were made with the portable dental unit [PDU] to *HM Ships Coventry, Brilliant* and *Birmingham*. I would like to say what a pleasure it was to work with an old PDU again. It wasn't. Cantankerous, bloody-minded – ≫▸

an unreliable machine from hell. If I'd still had a weapon, I'd have shot it! The frigates were operating nearer the coast and were mostly in defence watches – some very tired people.

Bits and Bobs – memories that will stay with me: The [air] squadrons – definitely very different. The noise of Harriers landing – indescribable when the cabin is directly underneath. The lullaby of Harrier engine ground runs being carried out in the early hours.

Fancy dress evenings – amazing what can be done with cushion covers, cardboard, masking tape, etc. The memorable transit of the Dardanelles at sunset. A full dinner being served on the bridge roof while at anchor – unreal.

Flight-deck sports and 'horse racing'. I will never forget the sight of Leading Wren Hill, dressed in a gash bag and waving her underwear about. (She was actually part of a human fruit machine!). She must have caused untold psychological trauma among the younger sailors.

Women at sea. The media coverage was amazing, as was the time spent entertaining or courting the various news teams. Our coverage was mostly favourable, but there is a surprising naivety in presuming we can 'feed' the media the stories we want them to carry.

I will miss: The sense of purpose on board – the companionship – the excitement (sometimes).

I won't miss: The separation – my bunk – the PDU – Retsina and Ouzo.

One of the reasons that prompted me into writing this article was the fact that the anniversary of my 20th year in the RN has just passed. When I consider what 20 years of NHS dentistry might have done to me, I cannot feel anything but gratitude to the MoD. On a good day, it still feels a privilege to be part of it all.

I joined my first ship in Malta in 1975. My last visit in a ship was to Malta. Spooky or what? Malta is still old and crumbling. Snap!

Back at the Directorate, the process of preparing the three Armed Forces Dental Branches for agency status, continued. It was not an easy process. Following the move of each branch out of London, a small implementation cell remained in London. It was headed by Air Vice Marshal Jefferson Mackey, now named as the Chief Executive designate of the embryo Defence Dental Agency (DDA). It was planned that the DDA would formally launch towards the end of 1995. The RNDS member on the implementation team was Surgeon Captain (D) R S (Dick) Hambly. He bore the title – Deputy Director Defence Dental Services (Personnel and Training).

Whilst his team carried on with the day to day running of the RNDS, ensuring that the Branch continued to meet its operational commitments, Grant was largely involved in negotiating the RN position within and contribution to the new organisation. There were many points of conflict. It had been generally agreed that command and control of Service dentistry at the 'coal face', would be exercised by regional Principal Dental Officers (PDO), in accordance with the existing RAF system. Regions were to be allocated on the basis of the size of each Service Branch and the Service dominance within each region. This was not always as simple as it might seem. For instance, the RN had more men and facilities in Scotland than either of the other two Services. It was therefore agreed, at a meeting with AVM Mackey, that the RNDS would exercise control in Scotland, with the PDO being based at the Clyde Submarine Base in Faslane. The Commanding Officer of RAF Leuchars, however, had other ideas. He would not accept 'his' dentists being under the command of the Navy! Thus, Scotland was divided between two PDOs, one RN and the other RAF.

A huge area of difficulty was that of 'Common Terms of Service'. Terms for promotion, leave allowances, retirement dates and general manning differed widely between the Branches. In the RNDS, as with the 'Big Navy', promotion to Commander and above was by merit. In the Royal Army Dental Corps and in the RAF Dental Branch, although merit could be recognised by earlier promotion, 'Time Promotion' was exercised, with most officers being assured of eventual promotion to Surgeon Captain (D) equivalent.

Rank structures too were different. Within the RNDS, a strict ceiling on the numbers within each rank was imposed by the Director of Naval Manpower Planning (DNMP). There was no pathway within the Branch for senior rates to be promoted to Warrant Officer and for those ratings who were selected for promotion to officer rank, it was necessary for them to transfer to another branch of the Royal Navy, thus leading to a regrettable 'brain drain' out of the Branch.

Within the Royal Navy, the rank of Commodore was 'non-substantive' – that is, it was regarded as an acting rank. On completion of an appointment as Commodore or Surgeon Commodore, the holder of the appointment might advance to Rear Admiral, or revert to Captain. In the case of DNDS, there being no Two Star (Rear Admiral) appointment available within the Branch, he would revert to Surgeon Captain (D) on retirement. In the sister Services, One Star (Commodore/Brigadier/Air Commodore) rank was recognised by an advance in pay and pension scales and the rank was retained on retirement.

This was balanced by Captains in the RN becoming eligible for One Star pension after six years in the rank. However, One Star pay could only be attained ten years after promotion to Captain – thus Grant did not achieve the same pay scale as his opposite numbers in the other two Services, until six months after his promotion to Surgeon Commodore (D).

A veritable Augean Stables! However, most of these anomalies would be ironed out over the next several years, but it would be a slow process.

The RNDS being the smallest branch was very much the 'poor cousin' in most of these issues and DNDS had to fight and negotiate, not only within the tri-Service organisation, but also with the RN in the guise of DNMP over many of them. Early successes, however, included agreement for one extra Surgeon Captain (D) and for the addition of a Warrant Officer billet within the RNDS.

Chief Wren Dental Hygienist Jacquie Watts, the Administration Officer of the Directorate team, was on the point of time retirement from the RN. She had already completed her resettlement courses, including training as a civilian practice manager. She was therefore not a little taken aback when she was sent for by Surgeon Commodore Grant to be asked whether she might consider extending her service in the RNDS – in the rank of Warrant Officer! After a few days of thought and discussion with her husband, she elected to remain in the RNDS, thus becoming the first dental rating to hold the rank of Warrant Officer within the Branch *.

And so, into another New Year. 1995 dawned with Grant's thoughts very much upon the 75th Anniversary celebration of the establishment of the Branch, by Order in Council in January 1920. The celebration was to take the form of a formal dinner to be held in the splendid setting of the Wardroom at *HMS Nelson* among the magnificent murals of William Wylie, depicting the Battle of Trafalgar and other famous sea battles of that era.

Grant was himself much preoccupied with the somewhat lesser skirmishes involved in ensuring the RNDS a reasonable 'slice of the cake' within the embryo Defence Dental Agency. Despite his success over promotions, he was less than happy with the way that planning for the new organisation was progressing.

Admiral Sir Jock Slater GCB LVO was, at that time, Vice Chief of the Defence Staff (VCDS), with tri-Service responsibility for all personnel matters, including Medicine and Dentistry. The proposed medical and dental agencies were therefore very much part of his domain. It had also been recently announced that Admiral Slater was to be the next First Sea Lord. Thus it seemed more than appropriate that he should be invited to the 75th Anniversary Dinner as a Principal Guest.

Other VIP guests were to be Mrs. Margaret Seward CBE, President of the General Dental Council and her husband Professor Gordon Seward CBE, an

---

* As explained previously Warrant Officer Sally Rowe had been promoted out of the RNDS into a Medical Branch billet.

eminent oral surgeon. (It must have been something of a 'first' for a married couple each to hold the CBE!). The family of the Branch founder, Surgeon Rear Admiral (D) E E Fletcher, was also to be represented by his grandson Timothy Fletcher, a civilian marine engineer. The Medical Director General (Naval), Surgeon Rear Admiral Sandy Craig QHP was also present as a guest and one further guest of great importance was to be Surgeon Captain (D) (formerly Commodore) Timothy Hall OBE, the recently retired Director who was to be dined out by the officers of the Royal Naval Dental Services.

As recorded above, the new Director, Surgeon Commodore (D) Ted Grant was far from happy with the progress and direction of planning for the Defence Dental Agency and as President of the Anniversary Dinner he was determined that his speech from the Chair would raise some of his concerns in the presence of VCDS. Having given careful thought to the wording of his speech, he did not wish to embarrass Admiral Slater by springing these problems upon him at the Dinner. He therefore sent him an advanced copy of the relevant extract from his speech.

The 75th Anniversary Dinner was held on Friday 20 January 1995. On that evening 110 past and present members of the Branch and the former Reserve Branch, sat down to a splendid meal. Present at the dinner was the former Surgeon Lieutenant (D) Hugh Brown RNVR who had been serving in the cruiser *HMS Mauritius,* when she fired the opening salvoes of the bombardment which preceded the D-Day landings on the Normandy beaches on 6 June 1944. Also present were a number of newly entered Surgeon Lieutenants (D) and Surgeon Sub-Lieutenants (D) – representing service in the RNDS which covered over 50 years of the Branch's 75.

Once the meal had been cleared from the tables, the port had been passed and the Loyal Toast drunk, Grant rose to his feet. Starting by welcoming their distinguished guests, he then gave a brief *resumé* of the History of the RNDS. He reminded the assembled company that Volume One of the Branch History had just been published, to coincide with the anniversary*. He then went on to give a brief account of the lives and careers of the principal guests, presenting each in turn with a copy of the History.

Having dealt with the past, he next turned to the future of the Branch and its place within the embryo Defence Dental Agency.

He recounted how, under the Directorship of Surgeon Commodore (D) Brian Robinson and in response to the 'Options for Change' defence review, a painstaking cost analysis and restructuring of the Branch had taken place. He then continued:

---

* Volume I of this History, which covered the RNDS from its early beginnings to 1964 was the result of some scholarly research by Surgeon Commander (D) Nick Daws. It was jointly written by him and Surgeon Captain (D) John Holland.

"The new, slimline Branch became extant on April 1 last year, the Directorate having by then moved from London to Second Sea Lord's very pleasant new headquarters, here in Portsmouth Naval Base. Before we moved, we already knew that the 'Front Line First', Defence Costs Study was upon us. It was thus that we were able to give the DCS team accurate facts and figures with such surety that they found that there were "no significant savings to be found" in our organisation.

"Despite this, it was made clear that "*status quo* (did we ever have such a thing?) was not an option" and it was proposed that all three dental branches be examined for tri-Service agency status. This process is currently taking place and, initially, I and my fellow single-Service Directors felt very bullish about the prospect of a stand-alone Armed Forces dental organisation within which, the three branches we believed, could retain their identity and direction, with the Agency exercising budgetary and executive control. Service level agreements could be made with our 'customers' to ensure that an appropriate level of dental care is available to provide the optimum level of dental health for all Service men and women.

"It having already been agreed that our current working and management practices are efficient and cost effective, each Service would be allowed, we assumed, to continue to develop a management system suitable for its particular operational commitments, in order to meet agreed tasking. There would be significant scope for rationalisation in such areas as training and top level management and, once the Agency was up and running, there would undoubtedly be scope to meet the inevitable future demands for further efficiencies. It was stated by the Framework Team, the organisation responsible for setting up Defence Support Agencies, that fundamental to the structure of such an Agency, should be the ability to attract and retain the right sort of people to make the organisation work.

"This then was certainly my vision for the future, shared I know, by my predecessor, Surgeon Commodore (D) Timothy Hall and I believe, by the other Service Directors and the implementation team. Sadly, this rosy vision is rapidly fading. It now appears that the planning of the Agency is not to be allowed to follow the well prescribed course for such projects.

"There are, it seems, hidden agendas.

"Whenever planning seems to be making some progress, it is set aback by a succession of bizarre ideas, generated to our astonishment, principally by those whose directed task is to implement a cost effective and (we had assumed) professionally efficient, tri-Service Dental Care Agency for the Armed Forces.

"These obstructive ideas range from the imposition of common working practices, which are not only untried, but unsuitable, certainly for the management of the delivery of dental care in the Fleet; to redundancy for nearly all ancillary personnel, to be immediately followed by some miraculous recruitment process, which would ensure the immediate support of equally well trained civilians at apparently lower cost!

"Another proposal is for de-enrichment of the ranks of the two-star Chief executive and the one-star Directors. This, apparently with the expectation that the ambitious and talented young dentists who are waiting in the wings to see whether Service life still has something to offer, will not leave for the more tangible rewards of civilian dentistry.

"The process of refuting these ideas takes time and effort which should be applied to constructive planning and I am of the firm belief that should any of these ideas take root, the foetal Agency will be stillborn for want of those prepared to serve in a second rate organisation with little to attract or retain the career minded".

Having been forewarned and having had time to prepare, Admiral Slater's response was robust. Before asking all to rise and to drink to the RNDS and its future within the Defence Dental Agency, he attacked the Director's account of the DDA implementation process, saying, in not so many words: "Put up or shut up!" If, he said, Grant had solid evidence of the process going astray, this was to reach his desk in the Ministry of Defence by the following Friday.

After the dinner and over drinks in the *Nelson* Anteroom, DNDS was approached by several of his officers with the words "You've done it now Sir!" But he was more than happy with Admiral Slater's reaction to his speech. His aim had been to raise awareness to what he considered disturbing trends in the implementation process.

The following day, he tasked Surgeon Captain (D) Geoff Myers to work with him to produce a paper, setting out in detail his concerns and the evidence to support them. As directed, the paper reached Admiral Slater's staff by the following Friday. The consequences of this episode were not to be immediately seen, but, in the event, a number of the more destructive ideas, as spelled out in Grant's speech, were not imposed upon the Defence Dental Agency.

Despite this, the following two years were not to prove easy for the Branch or its Director. However, the 75th Anniversary would seem to be an appropriate point at which to finish this volume of the History of the Royal Naval Dental Services, as they moved towards a 'New Dawn' with a perceptible tinge of purple on the horizon.

*****

Epilogue

The reader of this History will by now, be more than aware that the story has been a mixture of the trials, tribulations, achievements and experiences of those who run and try to ensure the continuation and effectiveness of the RNDS and those who deliver the 'end product' – dental care to the men and women of the Royal Navy and Royal Marines.

If the ending of the final chapter has left the reader with a feeling of uncertainty, be assured – the Branch is currently alive and well and fulfilling its purpose.

What will happen beyond the Coalition Government's October 2010 Strategic Defence Review is not clear at the time of writing. The reader may know the outcome as it affects the RNDS, by the time this History is published. It can only be hoped that those who are responsible for (yet again) reshaping the Defence Medical and Dental Services are fully aware of the huge contribution that the men and women of these Services have made over many years to the Defence of the Realm. Perhaps they should read this book!

The next chapters of the story are for someone else to write, but a brief summary of the 'Story So far', is worth recording here.

In the autumn of 1995, the Headquarters of the embryo Defence Dental Agency formed up in Lacon House in Holborn, London. The DNDS and his team were thus "ripped untimely" from their comfortable offices in Victory Building in the Portsmouth Naval Base to return to the familiar environment of the Ministry of Defence alongside the Surgeon General's department, the SG being the designated 'owner' of the DDA and the other Armed Forces medical agencies.

Back in Holborn, the work continued, as did much of the infighting, as the three Directors and the Chief Executive sought to achieve the right balance for their single-Service Branches within the Agency. After a year of working with a 'shadow budget' the DDA was launched as a semi-independent entity. At the end of 1996, Grant retired as DNDS and was relieved by Surgeon Commodore (D) John Hargraves. In early 1997, the DDA Headquarters moved to the former Institute of Dental Health and Training at RAF Halton. Hargraves remained in post and gave sterling service for nearly five years, steering the Branch with an assured touch through further stormy waters. He was relieved in July 2001 by Surgeon Commodore (D) Geoff Myers. Myers, a hugely talented officer, was the first RN dental officer to have done the Joint Services Defence Course at the Staff College in Greenwich. He had passed this with flying colours and as DNDS, he set about applying his well developed staff skills to both the RNDS and to the DDA. His tenure as DNDS was tragically cut short, when he lost his life in a car accident in October 2004.

Myers was succeeded by Surgeon Commodore (D) G L (Graham) Morrison. Morrison, another officer of great talent and foresight, was to introduce wider career opportunities for his officers, including access to the full range of RN and tri-Service staff courses and to MBA courses as well as to the usual range of dental postgraduate courses.

It was during Morrison's tenure that the Defence Dental Agency was disestablished, the Headquarters structure reverting to that of the 'Defence Dental Services' (DDS). This, in fact, brought about little change other than the DDS no longer having direct control of its budget – *'Plus ça change, plus c'est la meme chose'* *.

In 2008, Morrison was relieved by Surgeon Captain (D) Mark Weston.

Present and past members of the RNDS were saddened by the further de-enrichment of the Director's rank to Surgeon Captain (D). This was, however, inevitable, given the year on year shrinkage of the Royal Navy and thus the Dental Branch which served its men and women.

Weston, in due course, moved with the whole Defence Dental Services Directorate to its new Headquarters in Lichfield, Staffordshire – about as far away from the sea as it is possible to be! After nearly three years of 'keeping the show on the road', Weston was relieved by Surgeon Captain (D) Richard Norris, in February 2011. By this time, the management structure of the DDS had been further de-enriched and Norris found himself wearing two hats; that of DNDS and of Principal Dental Officer South West Region. His office was (and still is at the time of writing) in *HMS Drake* in Devonport, outside the DDS HQ, changing the nature and challenges of leading the RNDS yet again. In some important respects, this puts DNDS closer to his Branch and Service but a future DNDS could find him or herself in any 'medical' post. Our proud history gives us confidence that whatever the future holds, the RNDS will make a success of it.

So much for the Directors and management staff. At the 'coal face' the officers and ratings of the DNDS continued to provide the excellent service for which they were noted and much appreciated. The new regional command structure, after the dust had settled, worked well and continues to do so to this day.

The operational demands upon the Royal Navy and Royal Marines have increased greatly since the turn of the Century, resulting in more sea time for the men and women of the Branch. With Operation Telic in Southern Iraq and Operation Herrick in Afghanistan, many young dental officers have also been involved in increasingly hazardous operations, particularly those attached to Royal Marines units.

At a clinical level, RNDS personnel continue to provide a high level of up to date care, with most dental officers sitting and passing a progression of postgraduate qualifications.

To whosoever undertakes the task of writing the next phase of this History, there is plenty of good material here and it is a story worth telling. Good luck!

Ted Grant
Alverstoke
April 2012

---

* "The more things change, the more they are the same." – Alphonse Karr 1808–90

Appendix 1

Hospital Dentistry

Preface

Hospital Dentistry within the Royal Naval Dental Services forms an important part of the services which RN dental personnel provide to the Royal Navy and the Royal Marines.

The History of the Naval Hospitals is a long one but the practice of surgical, hospital dentistry in its modern form is much shorter and has evolved to become, of necessity, a separate specialty to that of general dental practice. Those dental officers who have, over the years, developed the required skills and who have met the ever increasing requirements for additional qualifications have lived and worked to a large extent in a parallel environment to their general dental practitioner colleagues. Having said that, they have all started their professional careers in the general dental services of the RNDS and many, as recounted below, have returned to the 'main body' of our Service, from time to time, to practice general dentistry or to take up senior administrative appointments.

I am greatly indebted to my former boss and my predecessor as Director of Naval Dental Services, Surgeon Captain (D) (formerly Commodore) Timothy Hall OBE OStJ Royal Navy, for the following fascinating account of the trials, tribulations and triumphs of those RNDS officers and ratings who chose the challenge of Hospital Dentistry. He has been greatly assisted in compiling and writing this account by Surgeon Captains (D) John Holland, Stewart Bussell and other colleagues from the RNDS cadre of Oral and Maxillofacial Surgeons.

E J G

A BRIEF HISTORY OF THE EVOLUTION AND DEVELOPMENT OF HOSPITAL DENTISTRY WITHIN THE RNDS

By T J C Hall

PART 1

Specialists and Consultants

Introduction

Dental Officers served in Royal Naval Hospitals from the earliest days of the Royal Naval Dental Service. In 1965 there were well established Dental Clinics in the home Hospitals at Haslar in Gosport, and Stonehouse in Plymouth and overseas in Malta at Bighi and later Mtarfa and also in Gibraltar. Each of these Hospitals had its own character and ambiance and between them they formed the core, if not the front line, of the Royal Naval Medical Service. They supported a worldwide Navy and the Royal Marines.

However, by the end of the thirty year period covered by this book really only RNH Haslar remained and even that great naval establishment which had served the Navy, the Royal Marines, the Army and Royal Air Force and the people of Gosport for 254 years would finally be closed by the Ministry of Defence on 30 March 2007.

When the Royal Hospital Haslar, as it was by then called, was finally decommissioned it had given 25 years more service than had *HMS Victory*! How this retreat of the Naval Hospitals came about is perhaps more a political than a medical subject and it is beyond the scope of these few pages.

This appendix to the History of the Royal Naval Dental Services is about some of the RNDS hospital personnel and the dental clinics in which they worked. Importantly, it outlines the changes that occurred in the hospital officers' training and in the scope of their practice over some thirty years. It also briefly describes the unique contribution of two hospital dental specialists to the UK Atomic Energy Authority Radiation Survey during the nineteen sixties and seventies.

The years covered by this volume, 1964-1995, saw many thousands of Naval, Royal Marine and Army personnel plus their dependants and countless civilians receive high standard hospital dental and oral surgery care in the

Royal Naval Hospitals. It was provided by an increasingly highly trained cadre of RNDS officers, dental nurses, hygienists, and dental technicians.

These staff provided not only specialist hospital care, but also general dentistry for their ships' companies [those other personnel who served in the hospitals]. They also gave instruction in the management of dental emergencies to generations of new entry RN Medical Officers, Nurses and Medical Assistants. In turn the RN Hospital Anaesthetists and Surgeons provided general duties dental officers with hands-on training in the techniques of emergency fluid replacement and endotracheal intubation needed for their war roles.

The primary role of a Naval Hospital was to train medical and dental personnel for war. Several Oral Surgery Consultants were deployed in the South Atlantic Campaign in 1982 and in the Gulf Wars of 1991 and 2003. Two of these operational deployments have been described in other chapters of this History, so the comments here are few.

Dental Specialists and the Civilian Consultants

For many years before 1965 the Navy's Medical and Dental Services had two grades of Specialist Officer serving in the Naval Hospitals. They were appointed as Specialists or Senior Specialists. This system had served the Armed Forces well. But by the early 1960s, it became recognised that the wider demands of duties in the Armed Forces were making it difficult for an officer to become and then remain, as proficient in a specialty as his civilian NHS counterparts. The latter, increasingly tended to work in one specialist discipline and in a static appointment with a stable patient base.

Service specialists however had long benefited by being easily able to seek advice from civilian consultants about difficult cases. Such Consultants were usually distinguished and influential members of their professions with national reputations. The Navy formally recognised them by appointing them as 'Civilian Consultants to the Royal Navy'. Their names and specialities were listed in the annual Navy List. Both the Medical and Dental Branches were fortunate that these gentlemen freely gave their expertise and advice. Importantly many also willingly offered their training facilities to Armed Forces trainees.

The Navy List records that in 1965, there were some 14 or so Civilian Dental Consultants. This list reflected the geographical spread of the Navy within UK and it included such prominent names in Oral Surgery as Sir Robert Bradlaw, Sir Terence Ward, Sir Paul Bramley, B W Fickling and Norman Rowe. Over the coming years, the numbers of such consultants were reduced and fewer patients were actually referred to them, but others came forward to offer the Navy training and career guidance for its aspiring oral surgeons.

Derek Henderson and Professors Tony Naylor, Khursheed Moos, Brian Cooke, Roy Duckworth, Jack Tulley, and Messrs. Frank Hasleden, David Barnard, Gordon Dickson, David Birnie, Tom Crewe, Roy Whitlock and others freely gave the RNDS such support over later years.

Without this the RNDS would never have been able to train the Consultants and Specialists it needed for the care of the Fleet and Royal Marines in the 1970s, 80s and 90s. Good friendships were made in these NHS units and many dental officers felt a sincere debt of gratitude for the training they received. They were fortunate to have studied in stimulating and respected departments.

The Introduction of Service Consultants and Armed Service Consultant Selection Boards

In 1962, the Medical Director General (Naval), Surgeon Vice Admiral W R S Panckridge, announced that a further specialist grade in addition to that of Specialist and Senior Specialist was to be made, namely that of Consultant. This was a major milestone. This Consultant grade was to be common to the Medical and Dental Branches of all three Services.

It was clearly established from the start that all officers who wished to attain Consultant status, would have to hold a higher qualification and pass the scrutiny of a civilian selection board. Every applicant would be required to demonstrate training and experience equivalent to that expected of a civilian applicant for an NHS Consultant post. These Armed Service Consultant Approval Boards were soon held in great respect. Known as 'ASCABs', they have stood the test of time. They reported to the Medical Directors General and advised whether an applicant was adequately trained and professionally ready for appointment to Consultant status. If he was not, he was not appointed.

In the case of Dental Surgery soon to be known as 'Oral Surgery and Oral Medicine' and later to evolve into 'Oral and Maxillofacial Surgery', ASCABs were normally chaired by the Dean of the Faculty of Dental Surgery of the Royal College of Surgeons of England. He was assisted by two or three eminent civilian oral surgery consultants and often by the Chief Dental Officer from the Department of Health. The Boards traditionally sat in the Council Room of the Royal College of Surgeons of England. The appropriate Service Advisors to the Medical Director General (Navy) were present when a

Board was held, but they were not part of the Board and had no vote. Though they had mentored the candidate through his higher specialist training they were only present at the Board to assist its members if required, and then perhaps buy the candidate a drink afterwards if he had been successful!

Over the years the ASCABs scrutinised an applicant's experience and training in ever increasing depth. MDGs(N) ensured that all Consultant Advisors 'marched together' and that the Royal Colleges' training schedules were properly fulfilled. By the mid 1980s, applications from all the surgical disciplines including oral surgery were circulated to all the RN Advisors for comment before any candidate was presented to an ASCAB. Additionally, the Professors of Naval Surgery commented in writing on the adequacy of the training. This was to avoid any individual specialty presenting an unprepared candidate. It could be sobering for an Oral Surgery Advisor to see how many research papers candidates in other specialties published during their training! All this ensured that professional parity was maintained with civilian NHS appointments.

Over the years the standing of the Royal Naval Medical Service became enhanced in civilian circles, but by the 1990s this parity resulted in the medical branch losing a number of highly trained mid-career consultants to the NHS.

This did not occur in the Dental Branch perhaps because of the increasing requirement within a very competitive field for a medical degree and a full surgical fellowship.

As the Consultant training pathway became formally established in the late 1960s and 1970s, the scene was set for the extension of clinical practice within the Naval Hospitals. Training times were lengthened and the home hospitals' patient bases were expanded. Both steps aided new entry medical officer recruitment but had less effect on the dental branch, which is essentially a primary care service.

Widening the Hospital Patient Training Base

Good surgical specialist training requires busy clinical practice. This was why when MDG(N) announced the introduction of the new Consultant grade in 1962, he also announced that the Naval Hospitals were to expand to take referred National Health Service patients.

His successor, Surgeon Vice Admiral Caldwell, returned to this same point five years later. He noted that "the so called reciprocal agreement" with the NHS had resulted in over 2,000 more NHS patients being treated during

1967 in Naval Hospitals than vice versa. He added, "that this is good … but we must go further". That process was to continue for many years and by 1980 the Oral Surgery Department in RNH Haslar had doubled its 1965 total annual New Patient Referral rate to just over one thousand new referrals a year. Half of these were civilians, the level of Service patient referrals having changed little.

This policy of increasing the hospital patient base made great sense for secondary medical and dental care, but at times it sat somewhat uncomfortably within the RN Dental Service. The Dental Branch as already noted, is essentially a primary care service for the Royal Navy and Royal Marines. It is only complemented to treat dependants and a limited number of entitled civilians when they are overseas. There was no 'fat' in Branch numbers to undertake much additional secondary care civilian work. Nor was it easy to support lengthy specialist training requirements. Moreover the primary care dental specialties of for example, Restorative Dentistry and Periodontology, started to use the Branch's Training Margin* as well, once the value of secondment for MSc Degree training, became recognised. In the 1970s, Dental Branch Appointers had to balance the increasing demands of the Royal College's requirements for Oral Surgery training with the Branch's primary duty of keeping the Fleet dentally fit.

Understandably, questions were sometimes asked as to why a dental officer was spending his time undertaking oral surgery for civilians. It was easy to think that, if a specialist had not got enough sailors needing secondary care on his list, then perhaps he should be working part time in a Naval Barracks where there was always work to be done. However, the Oral Surgery higher training bodies and the ASCABs did not recognise general dental practice experience. Indeed they did not wish even to know that primary care, albeit for hospital staff, was being undertaken by trainees or consultants in Service hospitals.

The Navy's War Plan spelt out exactly the number of sea-going and hospital billets that were to be filled by Consultant Oral Surgeons in war, and by the 1990s it was the War Role that justified every one of the Branch's uniformed primary or secondary care personnel.

RNDS Directors and their appointers had to plan increasingly far ahead to ensure the specialist war requirement could be met. Long-term manpower planning in a small specialty like oral surgery, with a complicated and ever lengthening training pathway could be tricky.

---

* The Training Margin was a small additional number allowed to the Branch Scheme of Complement, to compensate for those personnel undergoing training 'out of Branch' or not in clinical posts.

Experience from earlier wars, including that of the United States Navy in Vietnam, indicated that any major conflict could well result in a large number of serious facial injuries. And expert clinical opinion was clear that unless the casualty evacuation route to UK was very short, the skill with which the first surgical procedure for a major facial injury was undertaken would play a significant part in the patient's final outcome. Obviously an injured Royal Marine or sailor deserves the very best care that can be provided within the prevailing circumstances and this may require fully trained personnel near the operational front. Moreover, experienced operators work more quickly and might assess more realistically what required doing immediately, and what could wait until after evacuation. This would perhaps be important should limited facilities become overloaded with multiple casualties. Maxillofacial trauma surgery can be time consuming.

The Specialist's Role

The prime reason for the RNDS to have Oral Surgery Consultants is as just noted, the War Role requirement, but in practice the secondary purpose of providing support to general duties dental officers and the Fleet in peacetime, occupied nearly all the work undertaken in the Naval Hospitals over this thirty year period.

In general, dental undergraduate training only gives limited experience in exodontia* and dento-alveolar surgery† and many new entry officers recognised their limitations in this field and were happy to refer their patients. Moreover the RNDS probably has a higher proportion of young and newly qualified personnel than does the profession as a whole, and before Dental Vocational Training was established these recently qualified dentists were often required to practice alone in remote situations.

However it was well recognised that if hospital dental surgery was required for a sailor or Royal Marine every effort should be made to make it available quickly. There was no place for long waiting lists. 'Keep the Fleet fit, and keep it at sea' was the order of the day. The less the interruption to the Navy's operational duties and its associated training the better. Ships large and small have many key personnel who are essential to their activities. Often one highly trained individual is not easily interchangeable with another and the loss of one

---

* Tooth removal.

† Surgery involving the bone surrounding the teeth. The other area in which the hospital clinics could frequently help general practice dental officers, was in providing access to general anaesthesia. General anaesthesia had rightly been withdrawn from all dental clinics in the early 1960s. The RNDS was several years ahead of the civilian world when it introduced this policy. So by 1965 any general anaesthesia required for dental purposes was undertaken in a hospital by a trained medical anaesthetist.

individual from a twenty-four-hour, seven-days-a-week watch bill immediately puts an additional load on others. Ships do not carry spare replacement personnel. Thus sailors always had priority over civilians in the RN Hospitals and sea-going sailors always came first. Consultation or operation dates weeks or months ahead were simply not what the Navy required.

In practice this meant that all procedures needing general anaesthesia however simple were undertaken in either an Anaesthetic Room or an Operating Theatre. At times that could appear a rather heavy handed way of dealing with a simple extraction, especially when the additional administration and paperwork involved was considered. In later years this problem was largely overcome by the introduction of a day-case ward enabling the facility of short, light anaesthetics from which patients recovered rapidly, to be used. For service personnel from outlying areas this would mean staying overnight in a reception ward from which they would be returned to duty the following day. Eventually, most dento-alveolar cases would be treated in this way.

Those dental officers who worked in the hospitals were very fortunate in the cooperative and skilled way they were assisted by many excellent RNMS anaesthetists. They were also aided by highly efficient operating theatre staff. These well trained and motivated teams could turn patients around on an operating list at a speed not often seen in the NHS. Many a civilian consultant, who visited a Royal Naval Hospital, perhaps while on RNR recall duty, commented on our good fortune. It was also a helpful feature of working in a Royal Naval Hospital, that when one wished to discuss a problem with a consultant of another specialty it was very easy just to walk around the hospital and do so. The Radiologists, Surgeons, ENT colleagues and Pathologists were invariably most willing to help and once they knew that the 'toothie' was interested in this or that they might refer their own patients for an opinion. The Navy's "all of one company" attitude could be a valuable adjunct to a day's work in a hospital. This was again envied by some civilian colleagues. The RNHs were happy places to work.

As the home hospitals expanded and developed their Accident and Emergency Departments, so the intake of trauma rose. Road accidents and the like cause multiple injuries and a case with say, a fractured femur or traumatised abdomen might well require urgent operation soon after injury. If a facial fracture had been sustained as well, it would often be best for that to be treated at the same time even though it might not in its self be so urgent. This was just one of the reasons why the RN oral surgeons went to great lengths to try to provide twenty-four hour casualty cover. If the Hospital was providing a full A&E service, it was right that the oral surgeons played their part. This could at times be difficult for a single-handed consultant who found himself with no junior staff. Later on, 'Joint on Call' rosters were established with the local NHS Hospital Units, much to the benefit of both parties. Perhaps such arrangements formed the very beginnings of what was eventually to become a full integration of oral surgery care within the NHS under the Armed Forces Secondary Care Agency. This major development is mentioned later.

The RNDS Consultants and Specialists

In 1965 the RNDS had two Consultants in Dental Surgery. They were Surgeon Captains (D) Alistair Macdonald-Watson and Derek Goodridge.

Soon to follow were Surgeon Commanders (D) Alec Smith, Brian Cliff, Roy Travis, and "Hoppy" Boyd. In the seventies Surgeon Commanders (D) Geoff Sharpe, Timothy Hall, Stewart Bussell and Geoff Keeble followed.

Surgeon Commanders (D) John Holland and George Rudge were appointed in the nineteen eighties and Surgeon Commander (D) Chris Sanderson in the early nineties. Also, in the early nineties Surgeon Lieutenant Commander (D) Keith Riden joined the Branch having served as a medical Officer in the RNMS. He had gained his medical degree as a medical cadet after qualification and following experience in general dental practice. Sadly he was soon to die from a malignancy while in an Oral Surgery post serving with the Royal Air Force in Cyprus.

Surgeon Lieutenant Commander (D) Steve Liggins gained his dental fellowship and a medical qualification, followed by pre-registration appointments in the RN Medical Service, but he left the Service at his own request.

Many other officers served in the Naval Hospitals over these years for various periods of time and at various levels. They contributed much to the hospitals' daily work but are too numerous to name individually. Mention should though be made of two officers who held the Fellowship of the Royal College of Surgeons and served as Senior Specialists. They are Surgeon Commander (D) Clive Langan and Surgeon Lieutenant Commander (D) Stephen Day. Both served in RNH Gibraltar and Clive Langan undertook a hospital appointment at RAF Akrotiri in Cyprus.

Although partly outside the period covered by this History, recognition must also be made of the specialist work and achievements of Surgeon Commander (D) Stephen Taylor who manned RNH Gibraltar for several years and who served at sea in the Falklands War, and of Surgeon Commander (D) Richard Hayward. Both of them obtained Master of Science degrees in Oral Surgery from the University of London while serving in the Navy and both took premature voluntary retirement when the RNDS required redundancies during a period of contraction. Moreover both these officers were later awarded the singular honour of Fellowships in Dental Surgery, without examination, by Royal Colleges. Richard Hayward also became Dean of the Faculty of General Dental Practitioners from 2006-2009 and gave the Wood Lecture in 2009. Stephen Taylor became an examiner for the Royal College of Surgeons of Edinburgh's Diploma in Implantology when it was first held in 2009.

The Royal Naval Reserve Dental Branch played an important part in the RN Hospital oral surgery world. During the years 1964-95 five officers in particular undertook frequent recall 'training' appointments in the RN Hospitals. They were, Surgeon Captain (D) Hugh Cannell RNR, Consultant Oral and Maxillofacial Surgeon at the Royal London Hospital who also became the Principal Dental Officer (Reserves); Surgeon Commander (D) Geoffrey Cheney RNR, who was a Consultant Oral and Maxillofacial Surgeon at Norwich and who had also served as a Seaman Officer in the Royal Navy in his earlier years; Surgeon Commander (D) Anthony Peebles RNR, who was the Consultant at St Peter's and Kingston Hospital, Surrey; Surgeon Commander (D) David MacIntyre RNR, Consultant at Inverness Hospital; Surgeon Commander (D) Gordon Irvine RNR, Consultant at Southmead Hospital, Bristol and Surgeon Commander (D) Christopher Howell RNR, from the Queen Victoria Hospital East Grinstead.

Their recalls were always eagerly anticipated. These officers not only provided extra mural clinical stimulus, but they were also excellent friends to their colleagues in the regular Service. Additionally, their secondments often enabled single-handed RN personnel at home and overseas to take annual leave! The disbandment of the RNR Dental Branch in March 1992 was a great loss.

The Increasing Scope of Oral Surgery

The last decades of the twentieth century saw major changes in the status and surgical boundaries of NHS Oral and Maxillofacial Surgery. What had initially been basically a dento-alveolar and simple mandibular fracture discipline in the early 1960s, soon advanced in NHS Regional Hospitals to include the full range of maxillary, zygomatic * and orbital† trauma surgery. Temporomandibular joint‡ and submandibular salivary gland surgery were also regularly practised by the mid 1970s. Elective bimaxillary orthognathic surgery•

---

* Cheek bone.

† Eye socket.

‡ The joint of the jaw.

• Corrective surgery to realign the jaws.

became routine and iliac crest [hip] bone grafting was practised in most oral surgery departments. The RNDS worked hard to keep up with this progress and by the nineteen eighties this range of care was available in house to the Navy. As has already been mentioned the RN Consultants had been fortunate from the 1970s onwards in their civilian higher training secondments and they began to introduce these advancing techniques into the Royal Naval Hospitals when they returned.

Case Reports in the Journal of the Royal Naval Medical Service from 1975 onwards reflected this progress. For example Surgeon Commander (D) Geoff Sharpe was able to report in 1976, that the surgical correction of jaw deformity was now well established in the Service. However, there were always to be two areas of advanced maxillofacial surgery, which did not fit well within Naval Hospital practice. These were surgery for malignant disease and cleft lip and palate surgery. Both require a high case load to achieve clinical competence and long term care by one consultant over several years within a multidisciplinary team is highly desirable for cleft lip management. Thus these sub specialties were not practised in the RN hospitals.

The Royal Colleges had established Joint Committees for Higher Training in Dentistry early on and those bodies set out the mandatory training requirements. These were revised from time to time to reflect the expansion of oral surgery practice. It became the role of the ASCABs to enforce such changes. Their requirements increased over the years. Thus Hall, who sat his Consultant Board in 1975 only had four months' civilian secondment time, but Holland and Rudge in the 1980s had twelve months and in the 1990s, Sanderson had a full three years working in a busy Senior Registrar post exactly in line with his civilian counterparts. All this was before the addition of a medical degree, let alone the full Surgical Fellowship which was to become commonplace and later virtually essential for an NHS Maxillofacial Consultant appointment.

In 1985 Oral and Maxillofacial Surgery became recognised by the Royal College of Surgeons as a Surgical Specialty of Medicine. This meant that a medical qualification in addition to a higher dental qualification was sooner or later to become mandatory. Such a lengthy consultant training pathway from say entry to the Royal Navy as a Surgeon Lieutenant (D) with just the basic dental qualification, then became an unrealistic target for the Branch. This was to bring problems for MoD manpower planning in the late 1990s and after.

However, internal branch recruitment for specialist training was buoyant in the 1960s, 1970s and 1980s. Indeed, there were periods after the closure of the RN Hospital in Malta, when there were too many consultants or trainees for the hospital posts available.

The Naval Consultant Career

Given all the expense and effort that went into establishing and maintaining the consultant cadre from 1964-95, it is perhaps surprising to find that of the 11 officers who were appointed to consultant posts in oral surgery from 1964 onwards, a mere five continued to work in that capacity up to normal retirement age. Only Smith, Travis, Rudge, Holland and Sanderson stuck the course! The remaining five moved into senior RNDS administrative posts. This pattern did not occur in the RADC or the RAF Dental Services, but it was in line with the RN Medical Service career pattern.

Orthodontics

Perhaps mention should be made of the specialty of Orthodontics, although the RNDS has never had any Consultant Orthodontists, its overall tasking having never justified them. However, at the very end of the period covered by this History, Surgeon Lieutenant Commander (D) Nick Turnbull RN commenced higher training to consultant level in Orthodontics as a tri-service trainee within the tri-Service Defence Dental Agency.

It was in 1968 that the RNDS Director Surgeon Rear Admiral (D) Bill Forrest accepted a suggestion from Surgeon Lieutenant Commander (D) Stewart Bussell, that the RNDS should put an officer up for the Royal College of Surgeons' Diploma in Orthodontics. Providing the Fellowship in Dental Surgery was already held, that then only required a one-year full-time course. Surgeon Lieutenant Commander (D) Timothy Hall was appointed first for this training, since that fitted best into the overall appointing plot. Hall acquired the Royal College of Surgeons of England Diploma in 1970 and Stewart Bussell followed immediately after, completing in 1971. Both were Specialists working towards a consultant grading in oral surgery and the orthodontic diploma was then regarded as an "add on".

At this time the Army which had extensive family commitments in the Far East and in BAOR *, had already put several officers through the Diploma in Orthodontics. The RADC regarded both specialties as hospital based and suitable to be practised by one individual working primarily as a Consultant in Oral Surgery. The RAF Dental Services policy was different. They provided orthodontics for their large overseas commitments with fully trained orthodontists, but these officers were not trained as surgical

---

* British Army of the Rhine.

consultants. Orthodontics was then mainly practised during childhood and the early teenage years and thus the RNDS's requirement was only where it had dependant family commitments abroad in Malta and Gibraltar. The Navy's orthodontic requirement was much the smallest of the three Services.

Bussell and Hall provided this service when they were serving in these overseas bases and they continued it afterwards for many years on a visiting basis from the UK. However, by the 1990s, the regular use of fixed appliances over an eighteen month to two years period made treatments harder to manage on a visiting basis. More and more often, diagnosis and advice alone seemed best for a child overseas rather than actual treatment. Fixed appliances require frequent and regular specialist maintenance. Certainly the RADC had long recognised the difficulty of treatment continuity with families returning to the UK and they ran a Central Orthodontic Registry at Royal Army Medical College, Millbank. This system worked well with removable techniques, especially if the family knew when and where they were going!

By the 1990s, the number of naval overseas families had decreased considerably. But by then orthodontic cases began to be referred for tooth movement in adult serving personnel prior to advanced restorative work. The specialties of Restorative Dentistry, Prosthodontics† and Endodontics‡ had come fully of age since the 1960s and patients were increasingly loath to lose a key tooth. It had become an achievable objective for most people to maintain most teeth, if not their full dentitions, for life. A few decades earlier such patients would have moved progressively towards full dentures.

So by the 1990s orthodontic techniques were beginning to be used to move teeth into more favourable positions for complex restorations or periodontal management. At the same time pre-surgical orthodontics had become firmly established prior to orthognathic surgery. Bussell and Hall continued to meet these needs for selected naval personnel. But this was not always as easy as it sounds. Adult orthodontics and orthognathic surgery when mixed with Service turbulence are not easy bed-fellows! Some felt that such complex elective work was not suitable for service personnel. But when it was the 'best practice' approach to assure the longevity of a dentition why should a serviceman be denied it by virtue of his employment?

In the early 1990s, the clinic at RNH Haslar was able to help the RADC to train an officer to Consultant status in Orthodontics. Mr David Birnie Consultant Orthodontist at the Queen Alexandra's Hospital (QAH), Cosham, arranged an approved training programme for Lieutenant Colonel Philip Sims RADC at the MoD's request. This involved three chairside days

---

† Fixed & removable dentures.

‡ Root canal treatment.

a week at Haslar. NHS patients on the QAH waiting list post diagnosis, who lived in the local area, were offered treatment at RNH Haslar to enhance the patient base. This was much appreciated by a number of families based on the Gosport side of Portsmouth Harbour. Surgeon Captain (D) Timothy Hall was approved as a supervisor for Sims' training while he worked at Haslar under David Birnie's guidance. For the record Sims passed his ASCAB first time!

Also by the 1990s, the 1960's one year Diploma in Orthodontics had been replaced by a three year Royal College Membership in Orthodontics. A mandatory further three years of supervised higher training was then required in addition before Consultant accreditation could be achieved or an ASCAB sat. "Six years' training to move a tooth six millimetres", as one officer once put it!

Thus the training for both oral surgery and orthodontics became extended by many years and their pathways increasingly diverged. Obviously the 1960's days of the Armed Forces giving an oral surgeon a one year course in orthodontics had long gone.

Nevertheless Bussell's suggestion to Admiral Forrest back in 1967, that an officer be sent on a one year Diploma Course had proved to be a rewarding investment for the RNDS over some twenty five years. Albeit one that would never be repeated. Bussell continued to practice the specialty as a civilian for the Armed Forces in Hong Kong following his retirement from the RN and Hall also practised the specialty for the NHS at Queen Alexandra Hospital, Cosham when he retired. So their skills were not lost to the profession.

The Strontium 90 Assay Project at the Royal Naval Medical School

Before we turn to the hospitals themselves, mention should be made of two Senior Specialists in Dental Surgery who had served in Naval Hospitals in the 1950s and subsequently worked at the RN Medical School in Alverstoke (later to become the Institute of Naval Medicine).

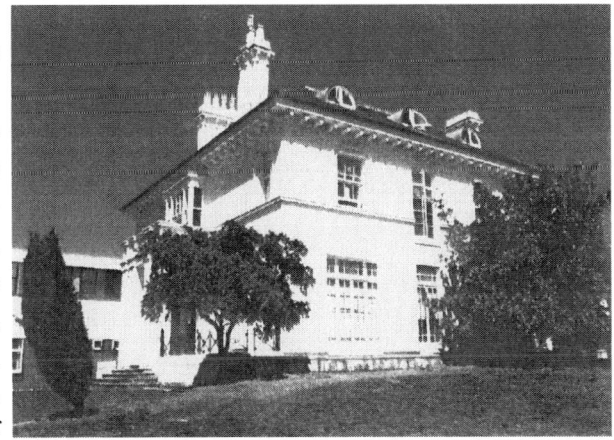

The Royal Naval Medical School – later the Institute of Naval Medicine

The Strontium 90 Assay Project has been briefly referred to in Chapter 9, when Admiral Holgate's career was covered. It does however deserve a further note here.

It was a National project undertaken by RNDS hospital specialists which contributed significantly to the science of radiation as a whole. It was original work and based on a simple premise already well established in dentistry. Namely that unlike bone the hard dental tissues once formed are not subject to physiological structural remodelling.

Surgeon Captain (D), later Surgeon Rear Admiral (D), W Holgate originated this work in 1959, but it fell to Surgeon Captain (D) W E Starkey to carry it through the 1960s to completion in 1971. When Starkey retired from the Navy, he continued the investigations at the Medical Research Council's Dental Research Unit in Bristol where he was supported by a personal MRC grant.

The Strontium 90 Assay Project was an ongoing survey sponsored by the Royal Navy in conjunction with the United Kingdom Atomic Energy Authority. Its aim was to demonstrate and measure the radioactive strontium 90 accumulations that occurred in developing UK human dental tissues following the nuclear fall-outs that were the result of the major atmospheric nuclear weapon testing programmes of the 1950s and 1960s.

Four papers were published; one in the British Dental Journal, one in the International Dental Journal and two in the Journal of the Royal Naval Medical Service. A further paper was presented at the Second Symposium on Naval Medicine at the Royal College of Physicians in London in 1969.

Premolars and third molars were collected from all parts of the country by 70 dental practitioners and various RNDS clinics. These teeth were chosen as they were frequently removed, undiseased and unrestored, as part of routine care for orthodontic or impaction problems. Their crowns and roots were divided and the incremental Strontium 90 growth patterns laid down in the hard tissues were studied to demonstrate the fluctuating conditions of nuclear contamination that occurred from atmospheric fallout.

The years between 1955 and 1962, when the major powers had undertaken weapon tests and fallout had occurred were well known, as was the age of the subjects. By 1965, over 10,000 teeth had been examined.

It is important to appreciate that developing dental tissues unlike bone or soft tissues are never remodelled. Thus Strontium 90, if ingested, is incorporated as an irreversible deposit in dental structures. It has a radioactive half life of 28 years. Starkey concluded that the levels of the radioactive deposits he found were not of immediate clinical relevance.

He went on to suggest that if nuclear weapons were ever to be used directly on human populations, the fallout ingestion levels would be tens of thousands of times higher and would last over many days.

He concluded that any dental tissues developing at such a time would provide a detailed record of the radiation received in a community or by any individual for many years after. This technique neatly and scientifically demonstrated that the teeth can provide information on the levels of internal radiation received from ingested fallout, up to several years after the event.

Those who knew 'Podge' Starkey will recall that he had an amusing turn of phrase and it is easy to imagine him quietly chuckling when he finished a presentation on this subject with the words: "so the teeth are living fossils!"

Inter-Service Co-operation

The sectarian problems in Northern Ireland required an on-going presence at Musgrave Park Hospital, Belfast for a consultant maxillofacial surgeon, which the RADC was finding increasingly onerous and therefore requested the help of the other two services. Consequently, RNDS consultants joined a roster and visited for a month at a time carrying out routine oral surgery and trauma care. By this time the level of trauma had greatly reduced and was much more of the civilian kind experienced in mainland hospitals, much as the result of drunkenness between soldiers and relatively simply treated.

However, this set a precedence for inter-service co-operation which was to serve well in the momentous changes to service hospitals from 1994 onwards. A shortage of RADC consultants resulted in Surgeon Commander (D) John Holland spending two years in BMH Hanover (1986-1988) in exchange for a general-duties RADC dental officer. This, along with attendance at RADC meetings and courses, resulted in a fair understanding between the three consultant advisors. An announcement was made in July 1994 that Haslar had been selected as the Tri-service hospital with the closure of the other service hospitals. Lessons learned from the closure of RNH Stonehouse and the opening of the MDHU at Derriford enabled a workable plan to be drawn up in a short time to use the limited space in the department at Haslar to incorporate the other two services. This relied very much on the good relationship between the individual consultant advisors. The plan relied on consultants making peripatetic visits to the larger bases such as Tidworth, Brize Norton and Lossiemouth from where inpatient treatment was arranged at Haslar or out-patient treatment carried out on site. This all required great dedication from the consultants with much mileage travelled by car over the years.

Tri-Service camaraderie was further enhanced by annual symposia at which papers were read by trainees in the relatively benign atmosphere of their peers and consultants.

Keynote lectures would be given by invited experts on a variety of topics and visits made to local sites of interest. The meetings would begin with interviews of the trainees by the consultant advisers, when their progress could be monitored and any of their worries assuaged. These meetings were hosted by each service in turn and were enjoyed and appreciated by everyone, helping to cement inter-service friendships and reminding those trainees in civilian secondments that their service still existed and was interested in their progress.

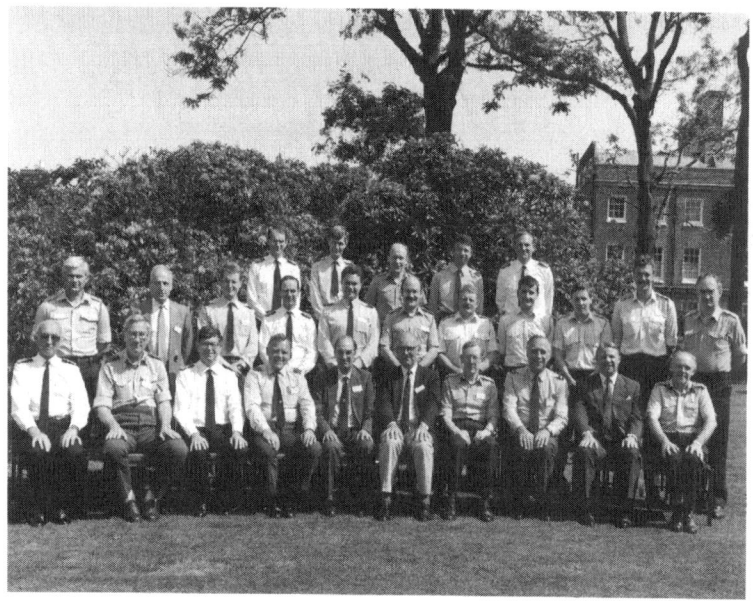

Tri-Service Oral Surgery Symposium – RNH Haslar – 1992

*****

PART 2

The Royal Naval Hospitals and their Dental Clinics

"We shape our buildings and afterwards our buildings shape us"
(Winston Churchill 1944)

ROYAL NAVAL HOSPITAL HASLAR

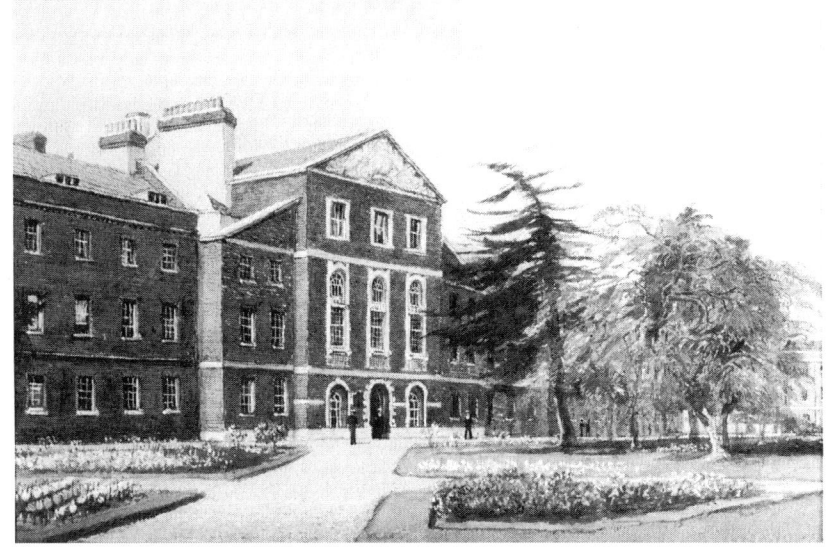

The Royal Naval Hospital Haslar showing the 1965 Dental Department on the first floor immediately to the left of the Main Entrance.

(From a watercolour by Kevin Holmes.
Reproduced by permission of the Haslar Heritage Group)

Much has been written elsewhere about the history of RN Hospital Haslar. The hospital was conceived along with RNH Plymouth and RNH Chatham in 1744 when a Memorial was presented in Council to His Majesty King George the Second. The first patients entered in 1753. Any readers seeking a fuller account of Haslar's buildings and long history are referred to the writings of Surgeon Rear Admiral Gordon Pugh, Surgeon Vice Admiral A L Revell and the Haslar Heritage Group.

Suffice to say here that the years 1964-1997 saw the Dental Department in RNH Haslar move between four locations and change its name from the Dental Department, to the Oral Surgery Department , and then to the Department of Oral and Maxillofacial Surgery.

The Centre Block and E Block Dental Clinics 1965-1983

In 1964 a two-surgery Dental Clinic was already well established in a fine location on the first floor of the main front block of the Hospital, more or less above the Main Arcade. The surgeries looked north-eastwards directly down on to the original and at that time only, Main Gate. Further on lay the Haslar Jetty and Portsmouth Harbour.

1964 was still very much the era of 'upright' chairside dentistry and any dental officer waiting in that clinic for an impression to set would easily observe a pair of straight iron rails set into the small road below him, leading away down to the Haslar Jetty. RNH Haslar had been built to care for His Majesty's sick and injured seamen and traditionally these patients were landed at the jetty by boat from the Fleet at Spithead after which they were hauled into the hospital in wagons along these rails. But by 1964 this particular transport to Hospital Admissions was no longer in use!

Nevertheless it was probable that the majority of walking patients and most hospital staff still arrived each day at the same jetty, having crossed from HM Dockyard or one of the naval establishments around the harbour by boat.

Of course there had always been land access to Haslar by road through Alverstoke or Gosport, but in the mid 1960s not many patients or staff owned a private car and those who came by road around the harbour had to face a journey of some 17 miles. On rare but memorable occasions, badly injured patients were brought from ships at sea by helicopter. The aircraft landed on playing fields in *HMS Dolphin* adjacent to the main gate. Such evolutions were easily observed from the 1964 Dental Clinic.

In 1964 both surgeries had the standard dark green 'RNDS' Rathbone dental unit and the matching upright dental chairs of the day. They also had open gas fires. Laboratory work was undertaken in the RN Barracks across the harbour. In the early 1960s operating sessions were held on the same floor in a small theatre close to the Department. This overlooked the main central gardens. Soon this changed to Theatre No 3, which was on the top floor of the northeast corner of the frontage in B Block. There were two operating lists a week, one on a Monday morning and one on a Thursday afternoon.

In the sixties there was something of a pattern to these operating lists.

Fully intubated* general anaesthesia was used and, subject to clinical appraisal, third molar contralateral impactions† were removed at the same time to avoid further problems occurring in far off parts [of the world!]. Frequently, there were six or so cases of third molar surgery on the Monday morning and four or five dental clearances on a Thursday afternoon, often with immediate dentures being fitted. Emergency abscesses or trauma cases might be added to the list at short notice.

By the late 1970s, the dental clearances had thankfully decreased as the dental health of the men in the Fleet improved and periodontal management‡ advanced. That improvement was underpinned by the newly introduced WRNS Dental Hygienists.

Rating inpatients were accommodated in wards near the Dental Department, but officer patients went to a separate Officers' Block, which was some two hundred yards away. They travelled to and from the operating theatre by 'tilly'§. First to the Main Arcade and then by a rather ponderous lift which took them to the floors above.

This Officers' Block was closed after a few years and it was replaced by an Officers' Ward situated within the main hospital. It eventually became the School of Naval Medical Staff Training where, in 1987 Surgeon Captain (D) S N Bussell, an Oral Surgery Consultant, became its Officer-in-Charge as the Director of Medical Staff Training.

Much later, when the Defence Secondary Care Agency became established in 1996 the old Officers' Block became the main administration block for the hospital's Commanding Officer's staff. At that time the newly named department of Oral and Maxillofacial Surgery moved into Haslar's old administration corridor in what had originally been 'A' block adjacent to the Main Arcade. Surgeon Captain (D) John Holland appreciated the irony of sitting on the exact point from where distinguished Admirals and Medical Officers-in-Charge had run the whole Hospital for at least a century or more!

But back in 1964, the Dental Department was complemented for two officers. One billet was for a Consultant and one for a trainee of varying seniority. They were supported by two WRNS Dental Surgery Assistants.

The Dental Department moved on 6 June 1966 to the ground floor of what was then 'E' Block. This was on the ground floor of the north-western wing of the main ward area of the hospital. It was regarded as a 'temporary' move at the time but the Clinic remained there for 16 years until the central

---

* An anaesthetic tube passed through the nose and throat.
† Impacted wisdom teeth, both sides of the jaw.
‡ The management of gum disease.
§ Naval slang for a 'utilicon' minibus/ambulance.

Cross Link complex was finally built in 1983. There was nothing unusual in departments moving around in Haslar Hospital. It had long been recognised that the modernisation of RNH Haslar actually began as soon as the hospital was completed in 1762 … and it never really stopped afterwards.

John Holland a long time Haslar hand used to observe that all the hospital departments, wards and offices instinctively tended to demonstrate a slow innate amoeba like movement. This ensured that if staff moved away for more than a month or two, they would need to undergo a period of reorientation upon return. It kept one on one's toes! At one time all the blocks were re-lettered to run alphabetically from the northwest corner so 'E' Block became 'A' Block and 'A' Block became 'D' Block etc. – chaos reigned!

The move into the new 'E' Block Clinic was welcome. It enhanced the Department considerably. New facilities included a good sized dental laboratory, an X-ray room for an Orthopantomograph Machine*, a dark room, a seminar room, a DSA changing room and a small office for the Senior Dental Surgeon. Importantly, the clinic also went from two to four surgeries, with updated equipment in each. This gave the potential for a general duties dental officer to be borne for routine staff care if one could ever be spared from the RNDS' overall bearing. A WRNS Dental Hygienist could also be borne. The Leading Wren hygienists worked on the wards and treated fracture and orthognathic patients. They also assisted disabled long-stay medical and surgical patients on the hospital wards with their oral hygiene care, in addition to more routine duties for hospital staff.

RNH Haslar was a large hospital in the mid and late sixties with around six to seven hundred beds and perhaps further capacity for expansion. Whilst it was easy in those years to find a bed and admit a service patient, it was rather harder for junior staff to discharge them. All the necessary paper work, case summary and diagnosis, medical category, after care management, medication etc., had to be written up and correct 24 hours in advance, ready for submission to the Senior Medical Officer (Surgical) prior to discharge via a formal naval routine. Smart juniors could have case summaries written before extubation† had taken place…….after all they could always be crossed out later if circumstances changed. But if they were not ready in time discharge would be delayed by a day!

It has to be appreciated that once a sailor was discharged from an RN Hospital the Navy would automatically return him and his kit to his Ship for full duty. The hospital had a Baggage Kit Store for sea going sailors. But obviously a minesweeper in an Atlantic gale is no place for even a couple of days

---

* A specialised X-ray machine, which produces a 'panoramic' view of the jaws.
† Removal of anaesthetic tubes.

of convalescence. Thus use was often made of 'Hospital Sick Leave' even for straightforward third molar surgery. This gave the patient a few days recovery time with his family and provided a rail warrant for the journey. Even so, going from Portsmouth Harbour to say the north of England by train, was not that easy with brand new immediate full dentures or intermaxillary fixation!*

But sailors who did not wish to 'go home', or were not ready to travel long distances were able to stay in the hospital. Beds could usually be found for this during the seventies. Such convalescing patients might be granted 'afternoon shore leave'. Dire warnings on the perils of the Gosport taverns were stressed if intermaxillary fixation was in place, or when a fracas ashore had been relevant to the original admission!

Although the uniformed staff in the Dental Department changed every couple of years or so in typical naval fashion one stalwart civilian Mr Charles Milne MBE, provided extraordinary continuity in the Department from the 1950s, into the 1960s and on to the mid 1970's. He ran the Office and managed the appointments, paperwork, Reports and Returns, the shipping of laboratory work and the ordering of stores. Nobody arrived in the clinic for duty before Mr Milne did, and nobody left later. One summer afternoon a year Charlie Milne would leave his desk and go to the Hospital's annual Sports Day which was held on the *HMS Dolphin* playing Fields. There, every year right up to his retirement, he would invariably win the Veterans' 100 yard sprint! When he finally retired in 1975, Surgeon Captain (D) Alec Smith arranged a suitable presentation to acknowledge Charlie Milne's 58 years of service to the Crown. He had completed 34 years with the Royal Marines and 24 years with the Dental Branch – surely something of a record.

It should be noted that the RNDS received similar lengthy loyal service from many other 'retired' service personnel in a number of dental clinics and various shore establishments around the country. In those years that generation of ex-servicemen was part of the Royal Navy's tested and trusted support. They had seen active service in the Second World War, they kept the 'engines running' and they knew 'how things worked' and 'how they were done'. They were utterly reliable, never sick and worked very long hours.

When Mr Milne retired RNH Haslar's Dental Department's good fortune with staff continued. Senior WRNS Dental Surgery Assistants who had been trained in the RN Dental Training School, were drafted to the Hospital.

They gave excellent service and became the Clinic Managers. Although their training had been in general dentistry, those sent to the hospitals rapidly had to master the techniques of assisting in an operating theatre environment.

---

* The wiring together of teeth in both jaws, following fracture of the jaw.

They attended all the regular operating sessions managing the instruments and frequently assisting the operator with suction and retraction. The QARNNS* operating theatre sisters generally only took a case if an extra-oral approach or similar was being undertaken. Theatre sisters did however assist with out of hours emergencies, since they were already available in the theatres and had an 'on-call' roster.

Not only did the WRNS DSAs rapidly become efficient at surgical assisting, but several additionally came to master the mysteries of orthodontic chairside nursing, where there was an array of individual orthodontic brackets for every tooth and a bewildering range of different arch wires. By the 1990s, every orthodontic bracket and every arch wire used in the Straight Wire Technique had a different, sixteen-digit NATO stock number! No sooner had this orthodontic inventory been mastered, than the management of facial fractures delivered another array of complexity in the form of titanium plates with their special screws and special instruments.

Whenever 'drafty' insisted on moving a competent Wren DSA to another establishment, usually after eighteen months or two years in post, one's spirits would sink, but their replacements nearly always rose quickly up the steep learning curve and rapidly became as competent as their predecessors.

The WRNS Dental Senior Rates who organised everything, were often outstanding and worked hard integrating quickly not only into a new clinical environment but also mastering the strange, complex, hospital administration and record system and acquired an uncanny ability to find records misfiled by the resident staff.

As already mentioned the years in 'E' Block saw a doubling of the secondary care patients referred to the department. The majority of this increase was referred by local civilian general dental practitioners from the increasingly populated Gosport peninsular. The variety of pathology seen expanded and all patients referred were treated, apart from cases of malignancy. These were few and were rapidly referred to an appropriate centre.

In addition and by way of a contrast some very senior retired officers still chose to attend Haslar for their general dental care. RNDS Regulations did not normally entitle any retired personnel to primary dental care, but other regulations stated that Admirals of the Fleet remained on the 'Permanent List'! Thus, one day the Clinic in E Block was privileged to treat Admirals of the Fleet Earl Mountbatten of Burma and Lord Fraser of North Cape. At their request, they met together after their appointments for coffee in a cabin on the Officers Ward, and the Medical Mess provided its best silver pot and

---

* Queen Alexandra's Royal Naval Nursing Service.

china cups. Although there were no flies on the wall, Admiral Fraser had told the SDS that he intended "to remind Dickie, that while he had indeed served under him, Dickie had himself also served under Fraser!"

Not long afterwards, tragedy struck. At the end of a routine dental visit in early August 1979 Admiral Mountbatten turned to Surgeon Commander (D) Timothy Hall, then the SDS and announced as he left the clinic, that he would not be available for another appointment for a few weeks as he was off to Ireland for a summer break. As he walked to his car he turned round and added the words "…….the safe part". Earl Mountbatten was assassinated at Mullaghmore, County Sligo on 27 August 1979.

A few months later, a Memorial Service was held at Romsey Abbey to which those various Haslar Officers who had recently attended him were invited along with their wives. It was a sad impressive occasion on a grey wintery afternoon. Several badly injured members of Earl Mountbatten's close family were present.

The Crosslink Block* at Haslar Hospital became functional in January 1984 and it was formally opened by Admiral Sir John Fieldhouse that April.

Around this time RNH Haslar was regarded as being a 435 bedded hospital. 'Crosslink' added a single story fourth block across the open Quadrangle. This major build was rather similar in concept, though perhaps less elegant, to that initially planned by Theodore Jacobsen FRS, Haslar's Architect in 1746. The impetus for this project was that there was a requirement for more space and co-location of the outpatient departments. The Crosslink contained an expanded Accident and Emergency Department, an enlarged X-ray or Imaging Department, a new ENT Department, five fully up to date new operating theatres and a new more spacious Oral Surgery Department. The latter's four surgeries overlooked the Hospital's now rather smaller enclosed lawned Quadrangle. The accommodation was fitted out to a high standard and this gave a much more welcoming and brighter feel to the Clinic than had been achievable in 'E' block. Surgeon Captain (D) John Holland persuaded the Patients' Welfare Fund to provide and stock a good sized aquarium, which soothed the worries of both patients and the Senior Dental Surgeon alike!

The Oral Surgery Department continued to flourish in Crosslink throughout the 1980s and into the early 1990s. The department's expansion of the 1970s was built upon and the clinic's equipment enhanced. The Orthopantomagraph machine was moved to the X-ray Department which now had space for it and a Cephalostat† was added. This move was an improvement and not before time given the advancing radiological legislation. It also spared the WRNS

---

* A new, modern outpatients and operating theatre complex.

† An X-ray apparatus for measurement of the parameters of the skull.

DSAs from having to become 'radiographers' as well as 'theatre sisters', when they arrived at Haslar.

The X-ray Department soon also acquired a Computer Axial Tomograph (CAT scanner) and a Magnetic Resonance Imaging (MRI) machine. The latter was opened by HRH the Prince of Wales in 1994. Funding was also achieved in the early 90s for some sessions for a civilian practitioner to be employed solely for the primary dental care of the hospital staff.

However by 1994, ominous clouds were rapidly developing which would result in yet another move for the Department and which would much more importantly have the profoundest of major implications and cause fundamental changes for the Armed Forces Medical and Dental Services. The Defence Costs Study, Group 15 (Medical) announced in 1994, that there was to be only one joint tri-Service Hospital, albeit at Haslar. It was directed that this was to be supported by four Military District Hospital Units. Army and Royal Air Force Hospitals were to close and their staff move to Haslar. The hospital was to be renamed the Royal Hospital Haslar and was to be 'owned' by a new body called the Defence Secondary Care Agency. A separate Defence Dental Agency was to be established for the Services' primary dental care. These sweeping changes are described elsewhere. Initially, the tri-service unit was accommodated in the Crosslink clinic but this was too small to take the increased numbers. A new, much larger clinic was planned in D Block, which was to be redeveloped with a new day-case unit, wards and postgraduate centre.

The new clinic, sited in the previous administration corridor had five surgeries, a double surgery for orthodontics, four offices for clinical staff and a staff rest room.

Equipment was rescued from closing RAF Hospitals, which permitted a very modern and effective set-up. With the day-case unit one floor above and the in-patient ward and children's ward on the top floor, this was the ultimate geographical efficiency. The support staff increased three-fold to twenty-one and became a mixture of the three services who managed to live and work in harmony. Multifactorial clinics involving surgeons, orthodontists, periodontists and restorative specialists were set up to promote solutions to the dental problems of service personnel.

These clinics concentrated on orthodontics/surgical orthodontics and the treatment of missing teeth with osseointegrated implants followed by advanced restorative work. Funding for all this was cunningly hidden in the medical budget where it was negligible amongst the costs of orthopaedic implants.

All this was too good to last: Nemesis struck and in due course the whole thing closed.

Admiral Sir Michael Boyce Second Sea Lord took the Salute at a "Beat Retreat and Sunset Ceremony" on 1 April 1996 marking the transfer of the Royal Naval Hospital Haslar to the Defence Secondary Care Agency with the name of the Royal Hospital Haslar. This would later be transferred to the NHS Portsmouth Hospitals Trust, which would then finally close the hospital in 2009.

The Royal Hospital Haslar was the United Kingdom's last Military Hospital.

*****

ROYAL NAVAL HOSPITAL STONEHOUSE

The 'Memorial' to King George the Second in 1744 which successfully resulted in the building of the Royal Naval Hospital at Haslar had also made the case for Naval Hospitals at Plymouth and Chatham. Thus a Royal Naval Hospital came to be built at Stonehouse in Plymouth. Its first Governor was appointed in 1795.

Stonehouse Hospital was not as close to the harbour's edge as was Haslar, but it could be approached by boat along Stonehouse Creek. The Stonehouse District of Plymouth with its Royal Marine Barracks, the large Naval Dockyard and the Royal Naval Barracks at Devonport are all on the east side of Plymouth Harbour. So the hospital was well placed to serve the Fleet and the Royal Marines.

While Haslar was built of red brick RNH Stonehouse was built of Devon granite. The general layout of the ward blocks, gardens, and other buildings had a certain similarity to Haslar and both their churches, St Luke's in Haslar and the Church of the Good Shepherd at Stonehouse, stood in prominent positions. There was also a separate Officers Block, Medical Mess and Surgeon Rear Admiral's Residence at Stonehouse. But all that said the two hospitals were far from being identical.

In the 1960s and 1970s, Stonehouse Hospital had a delightfully relaxed and pleasant but efficient ambiance. This was no doubt, partly due to the way the staff conducted themselves and to the high standard at which the lawns, gardens and wards were kept, but there was also something much more subtle at work.

Stonehouse was always regarded as a friendly hospital. Two passages from the Journal of the Royal Naval Medical Service, written several years later and quite separately refer, albeit obliquely to this. When in 1986, Surgeon Rear

Admiral Dudley Gurd was reminiscing in retirement about his years of service in the West Country, he wrote:

> "There is something magical in the feeling of relaxation experienced, when one travels west of Exeter and it is a therapy which should be repeated as often as possible".

Also in 1995, when Surgeon Rear Admiral Sandy Craig, Medical Director General (Naval), was writing of the official closing ceremony for RNH Plymouth he commented:

> "…… that it marked the end of a Naval Hospital whose buildings and fabric were imbued with the warmth and friendliness for which it was renowned. Even the sternest of individuals seemed to mellow as they took up their Plymouth appointments and drafts".

The Dental and Oral Surgery Clinics

In 1964 the Dental Department was housed on the first floor of a small separate building close to the southern wall of the Hospital, somewhat away from the main ward blocks and operating theatres. There were two surgeries, the larger with a small side office for the Senior Dental Surgeon. There was also a small waiting area and a department office. Laboratory work was undertaken in the Command Dental Laboratory in the Royal Naval Barracks, Devonport at *HMS Drake*. The Department was complemented for one Consultant and a junior. Two operating sessions were available per week and not surprisingly, the work pattern was very similar to that at Haslar. Retired Wardmaster Lieutenant Charles Bastable RN ran the Office.

At that time, patients were referred from the many ships and submarines based at Plymouth and from a number of shore establishments, including Royal Naval Air Station at Culdrose in Cornwall. The RN Barracks at *HMS Drake* was a major nearby establishment and source of work. It supported the surface Fleet, while the SM2 [Second Submarine Squadron] clinic in the Dockyard was responsible for the Devonport based nuclear submarines. *HMS Raleigh* is the Navy's only New Entry Training Establishment for rating recruits and this was nearby at Torpoint in Cornwall, so it also looked to RNH Stonehouse for support; as did the Britannia Royal Naval College at Dartmouth, the RN Engineering College at Manadon, the Royal Marine Training Establishment at Lympstone, the Royal Marine Barracks in Stonehouse and 40 Commando at Bickleigh. Patients also came from RNAS Yeovilton in Somerset and sometimes from *HMS Osprey*, the Naval Base at Portland in Dorset. It was a large parish.

Mention was made earlier in this chapter of the support that the RNDS received from Civilian Consultants to the Royal Navy. Trainees at RNH Stonehouse were fortunate in that an excellent relationship that had been established with the Oral Surgery Department at Greenbank Hospital Plymouth. Mr Paul Bramley (later Sir Paul, and Dean of Charles Clifford Dental School Sheffield) had been appointed there as the sole oral surgery consultant for the South West region in the late 1950s. He was later joined in that geographically large area by Mr Tom Crewe.

RN trainees were made welcome in Greenbank's busy unit and much was learnt at the outpatient clinics and their frequent 'out of hours' trauma operating sessions. This department's cooperation with RNH Stonehouse continued long after Paul Bramley and Tom Crewe had moved on with their successors such as Sandy Davies and others. Two of the RNR Dental Branch consultants named earlier, Geoffrey Cheney and Hugh Cannell, undertook their Senior House Officer posts at Greenbank Hospital in the late 1960s.

The 1979 move to the new Oral Surgery Clinic

In 1979 the Stonehouse Dental Department moved into new accommodation. A modern style, single-story building had been designed and built on a vacant site close by the old clinic, which had once been designated the lunatics' recreation ground! The building was of the portacabin-type construction with 3 Surgeries, a Recovery Room, Staff Offices and a Dental Laboratory, which was manned by Mr Ed Hannaford. It was named the Department of Oral Surgery.

The one drawback was its lack of insulation making it very hot in the summer and freezing in the winter. This was made worse by a survey at night with an infrared camera, which showed the building to be leaking heat at an alarming rate. No more insulation was added but the heating turned off over-night making the place even colder on winter mornings. One Senior Dental Surgeon spent much time illegally tweaking the heating controls in an attempt to mitigate this early green initiative. He failed!

As referred to in the main text of this History, Roy Travis retired in November 1982, from the Royal Naval Hospital Plymouth. His contribution to hospital dentistry and Naval oral surgery had been immense. As well as serving in all the RN Hospitals and some Army hospitals, he guided many dental officers through their Fellowships and higher training years during the 1970s. He was a very skilled and experienced operator, who could move effortlessly between complex restorative dentistry, skilled prosthetics and major oral surgery.

In the mid 1980s, there was some concern over the future of the hospital at Stonehouse. But in 1986, the Medical Director General (Naval) was able to announce that RNH Plymouth would be retained on site at its current size. The Falklands campaign had shown the need for medical and dental support for the Fleet and Royal Marines in war. 104 Medical and Dental Officers and a large number of medical and nursing personnel had been deployed to the South Atlantic at very short notice for Operation Corporate * and it was not known when they might be needed again. Also, by the mid 1980s, the hospital was contributing significantly to the NHS hospital work in Plymouth. It provided Accident and Emergency care for a large area of Devon and East Cornwall taking its turn with the civilian hospitals by doing a weekly surgical 'take day'.

On the basis of this stay of execution a new clinic was planned in one of the hospital blocks and architect's plans were drawn up for a new super-clinic similar in concept to that eventually built at Haslar. Despite this in 1994 it became inevitable that RNH Plymouth's days were numbered when the already mentioned Defence Costs Study 15 (Medical) was published that year. This, as already noted, directed that all but one Service Hospital were to close and that four Military District Hospital Units (MDHU), were to be established in their place.

Thus the Royal Naval Hospital Stonehouse officially closed on 15 March 1995 and a Military District Hospital Unit opened on 12 April 1995 at Derriford Hospital on the northern outskirts of the City of Plymouth, some five or six miles from the Naval Base.

Although outside the period covered by this volume, it is sad to note that by 2007 when the tri-Service Secondary Care Agency finally closed at the Royal Hospital Haslar, the RNDS had no Oral Surgery Consultants at Derriford nor indeed in the West Country. Nor even at the Agency's centre at Selly Oak Hospital Birmingham. Only Surgeon Captain (D) Chris Sanderson RN remained as Consultant Oral and Maxillofacial Surgeon for the Royal Navy. He was based in the MDHU at Queen Alexandra Hospital at Cosham near Portsmouth and had served as Medical Officer in Charge of the Navy's casualty receiving ship *RFA Argus* during the second Gulf War.

---

* The Falklands Conflict.

THE ROYAL NAVAL HOSPITALS at BIGHI and MTARFA, MALTA

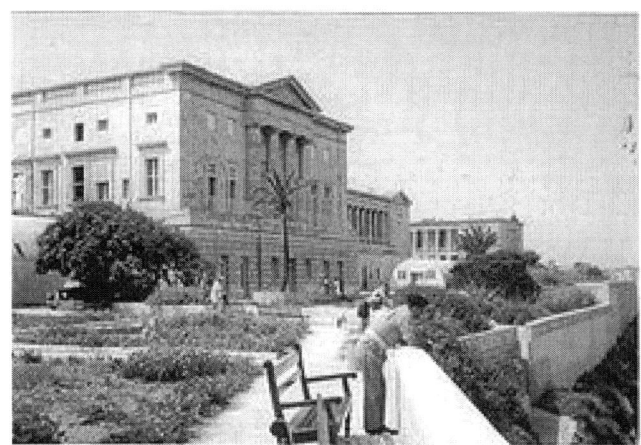

Royal Naval Hospital Bighi – Malta

Malta had been a principal overseas base for the Royal Navy and the Mediterranean Fleet for very many years. The Royal Naval Hospital at Bighi stood on a high promontory overlooking the Grand Harbour at Valletta. The site was said to have been identified by Admiral Lord Nelson in 1797 as suitable for a naval hospital. Bighi Hospital opened around 1832 and by 1964 it had completed many years of valuable service, which included seeing action in two World Wars.

The Dental Clinic at Bighi was in a good position on the west side of the hospital looking over the magnificent harbour towards Valletta. There was a balcony off the department from which a fine view could be enjoyed. Surgeon Captain (D) 'Podge' Starkey once claimed that this was the perfect stage on which to train one's operatic voice by projecting Oratorios across the water to Valetta! It was certainly ideal for the staff to watch the fleet enter harbour and moor up opposite Bighi.

The clinic, next to the chapel (which had been condemned as unsafe due to war damage), had two surgeries and a laboratory with a large waiting room. It never had the benefit of air-conditioning so some filling materials were tricky to use in high summer. It was run by a Chief Petty Officer who was helped by two Maltese civilians, one of whom made tea of such concentration that spoons were at risk of dissolving.

As with RNHs Haslar and Stonehouse, the hospital had been built primarily for sailors arriving from the Fleet. Entry from the harbour had been initially up the promontory by a broad stone staircase from a pontoon on the rocks below – said to be built for knights in armour, with very shallow steps.

Later, a mechanical lift was built which went directly down to the harbour edge. From there, an efficient harbour service criss-crossed the harbour. The delights of Valletta were a few minutes away by water or half an hour by car through narrow streets and risking the somewhat carefree driving style of the locals. When the Malta government took over the hospital to use as a school the first thing they did was build a new road of decent access.

RNH Bighi closed on 22 September 1970, its layout no longer being considered ideal for a hospital and it had been damaged by bombs and cannon shells during the war so large parts were deemed unsafe. The staff and patients were then transferred to what had been the Military Hospital at Mtarfa. Mtarfa lay some miles inland, on top of a hill, and although this hospital had been closed as an Army hospital in 1962 it had later been rebuilt and brought up to date before Bighi closed.

The David Bruce Royal Naval Hospital at Mtarfa, Malta formally opened on 2 October 1970. General Sir David Bruce had been a distinguished RAMC Officer who was remembered not least for his work on Malta Fever and Sleeping Sickness and also for his work on Brucellosis.

Several dignitaries attended the opening ceremony, including the Director Naval Dental Services Surgeon Rear Admiral (D) W I N Forrest CB. The hospital had all the expected In and Out Patient Departments and a large Medical Store. It supplied the Armed Forces Medical and Dental centres in Malta and also those then in Libya, as well as the ships at sea.

The purpose built clinic was situated under the operating theatres in what had been an entrance hall. It had two surgeries and a dental laboratory. This clinic did have air-conditioning, greatly improving working conditions, but all the surgery waste went out into one drain, which collected a large number of snails, which from time to time were harvested by one of the locals. Outside was a garden with paths, palms and a profusion of Bougainvillea which was always cool even in the hottest summer.

In 1972 the British were forced to leave Malta during protracted negotiations with Prime Minister Mintoff. Sadly, a 'scorched earth' policy was adopted prior to leaving and when negotiations came to a successful conclusion and the British returned, there was much damage to be repaired before normal service could be resumed. Mtarfa then closed in March 1978 when the British finally withdrew with much of the equipment being made over to the Malta Dental School presided over by Professor George Camilleri, civilian consultant at the Malta Dental School, who had always been a great friend to the department.

ROYAL NAVAL HOSPITAL GIBRALTAR

The original Naval Hospital in Gibraltar that was known as the 'Old Naval Hospital' had been closed in 1922, prior to conversion into Married Officer Quarters. After that hospital care for Service personnel was provided at the British Military Hospital rather higher up the Rock. The Royal Navy took over this British Military Hospital from the Army on April Fool's Day 1963 and it then became the Royal Naval Hospital Gibraltar. RNH Hong Kong was passed to the Army at about the same time.

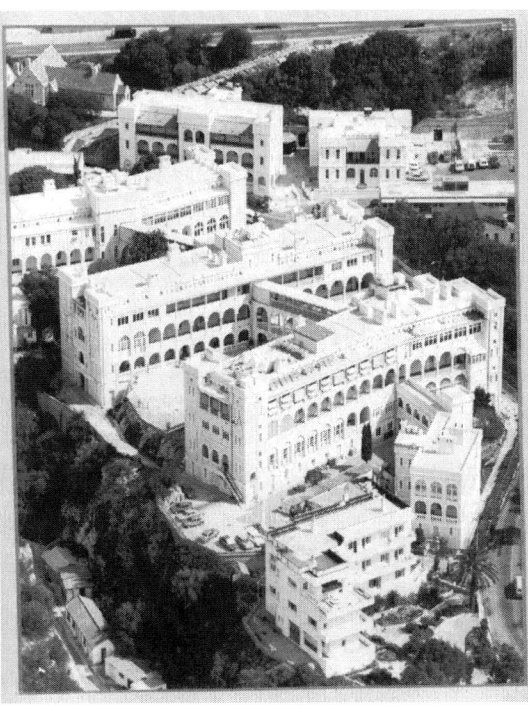

Royal Naval Hospital Gibraltar - previously British Military Hospital

RNH Gibraltar stood on the Europa Road towards the southern end of the Rock. It consisted of three main blocks. Each block had three floors and these were interconnected at all levels by open arcades. It was considered to be a 40-bedded hospital at that time and it had Medical and Surgical wards as well as a busy Maternity Unit.

The stonework of the Edwardian building was painted a light blue grey, which gave an open and airy feeling during the hot summer months. Separate outpatient clinic buildings, which were soon to be modernised, stood immediately across the Europa Road. Also a much smaller disused 'bomb proof hospital' was to be found nearby, tunnelled into the Rock.

This was named Gorts Hospital after the Second World War Governor of Gibraltar, Field Marshal Lord Gort VC.

Like Bighi Hospital in Malta, RNH Gibraltar enjoyed fine views to the west extending around the Bay of Algeciras and onwards up into the hills of Andalucia. Gibraltar Harbour with its three shipping moles and large dry docks could be seen to the North. To the south lay Europa Point and beyond that, the Straits of Gibraltar. Morocco was clearly visible on a clear day across the Straits. And the Jebel Musa massive, which together with the Rock of

Gibraltar had formed the original classical 'Pillars of Hercules' could easily be seen.

The Dental Department was situated in a small separate building on the northern side of the Hospital. It was said to have once been a stable block for RAMC Officer's horses. But by 1963 it had been well converted into a pleasant, self-contained and fully functional dental clinic.

There were two good-sized surgeries and a smaller third one, a largish waiting room, and a general office. A sizeable storeroom and a dark room were easily accommodated in the loft above the waiting room. There was also an adjacent dental laboratory. This was initially equipped for routine acrylic work but later chrome cobalt casting and a porcelain crown furnace were added. This laboratory served the other two Service dental clinics on the Rock as well as all the passing ships.

In 1964 the clinic was complemented for a Senior Specialist in Dental Surgery and a junior officer. Sometime later a part-time Dental Hygienist was added to the complement.

RNH Gibraltar was commanded during its 'first commission' by a Medical Officer in Charge, Surgeon Captain Forbes Guild RN. The first naval Senior Dental Specialist was Surgeon Captain (D) E B Mackenzie and the first junior dental officer was Surgeon Lieutenant (D) Stewart Bussell.

Most of the RNDS Specialists and Consultants named previously worked in Gibraltar over the next thirty years, albeit for varying periods of time. Also most of the RNR specialists made their way to Gibraltar at one time or another for their annual 'training' appointments. Some RNDS specialist personnel were indeed able to enjoy two married accompanied overseas tours at RNH Gibraltar, during their careers. They were fortunate, as overseas opportunities became much less available to the Branch as a whole when the UK's overseas defence commitments in the Far East and Malta steadily reduced between 1965 and 1996.

In 1964 all three Services had a substantial presence on the Rock. The tri-Service total of uniformed personnel, UK civilians and dependants and the Gibraltar Regiment was perhaps in excess of ten thousand. There was a large HM Dockyard and Naval Base, supported by *HMS Rooke* (the Gibraltar RN shore establishment), an operational Royal Air Force airfield at North Front and a sizeable Army Barracks supporting a complete UK battalion and a Royal Engineers' 'tunnelling troop'. In addition, the Gibraltar Regiment had its own locally entered personnel and Barracks. The numbers returned for the clinic always included some 33 rock apes which from time to time required treatment after fights. Other animals to be treated included the Admiral's dog with a tumour and the tiger skin of one resident battalion band, which had lost its canine teeth; their replacement being a triumph for the technician, Mr Ken Clark.

In 1964 both *HMS Rooke* and RAF North Front had established Dental Centres staffed by the Royal Naval and Royal Air Force Dental Branches. But when the Royal Army Dental Corps withdrew from BMH Gibraltar, it fell to the Naval Hospital dental staff to undertake all the primary dental care required for Army personnel and their families on the Rock in addition to their specialist duties.

This pragmatic arrangement worked well, although it increasingly precluded any recognition of a junior's time in Gibraltar counting towards consultant grading or of Gibraltar justifying a Consultant post.

In the late 1960s and the early 1970s, the routine specialist work consisted of a small but steady flow of third molar and dento-alveolar surgery and a much larger number of paediatric cases, requiring multiple extractions under general outpatient anaesthesia. Time consuming conservation of the deciduous and mixed dentition was routinely practised in the clinic, but in many cases, extraction was the only option when faced with multiple 'gum boils', unrestorable crowns and distraught mothers who had suffered weeks of sleepless nights. One gained the impression that the Army families bore the brunt of this rampant disease.

A regular school visit 'Fluoride Mouthwash' routine had been introduced on the Rock by Surgeon Captain (D) Tony Naylor RNR Professor of Preventive Dentistry at Guy's Hospital. This was fully established in all the Defence Service Schools by 1970. But unfortunately at that time many children were still arriving in Gibraltar having not had the benefit of such preventive measures years before in the UK. These school fluoride mouthwash and oral hygiene sessions were supervised by WRNS Dental Hygienists.

While facial trauma was not over frequent there were certainly quite a few cases in Gibraltar each year. There were plenty of opportunities to fall down on the Rock – sometimes quite dramatically! Parades and sporting activities accounted for some cases, but also the dry docks in the Dockyard were deep and the decorative pond at the bottom of the three story Casino foyer was shallow! No doubt the bars of Main Street played a part as well. However, the incidence of serious road traffic accidents was low. Gibraltar measures only two and a half miles in length and half a mile in width and with but 37 miles of road above the ground.

Nevertheless around 1970 one young soldier confounded the odds and turned his Land Rover upside down on a bend in Europa Road directly outside Beaulieu House, Surgeon Captain (D) 'Mac' Mackenzie's residence. At the time he was the hospital's Senior Dental Surgeon. The vehicle went through the scullery wall and into the kitchen. Mac's usually unfailing sense of humour was sorely tested by this. Not only was he was abruptly woken in the middle of the night but he then had to go and fix the driver's fractured mandible. Worse still, the next day he found he had to replace his wife's recently purchased new washing machine!

Although the Service patient commitment on the Rock was small by UK standards, pre-consultant level clinicians of all the acute specialties could find themselves tested on occasions. In the sixties and seventies Gibraltar seemed far from home. There was no regular, easy telephone communication with UK with which just to 'talk over' a problem case. Telemedicine was still well into the future. Certainly casualty evacuation by a civil airline was possible for a seated and stabilised patient, and a more serious case could be flown to the UK under the care of a fully manned medical team onboard an RAF CASEVAC aircraft. This had to fly out especially from UK and was a weighty option, normally only used in very urgent serious medical situations.

Back in 1965 four civilian general dental practitioners in Gibraltar formally approached the Medical Officer in Charge, then Surgeon Captain Murchison, to request that the hospital's dental officers be allowed to treat referred Gibraltarian patients requiring hospital dental care at St Bernard's Civilian Government Hospital. There were not many such patients and usually they only required a straightforward dento-alveolar procedure that had been judged to be unsuitable for local anaesthesia in general practice. That said, three civilian cases from around this time are still remembered.

One was an alveolar carcinoma in a 20-year-old Gibraltarian woman, and one a diffuse mass in the neck, which proved to be a lymphosarcoma. The Gibraltar Government funded both these patients' management in UK. The third was a case of 'Ludwig's Angina'. It presented with sublingual swelling which was as 'hard as wood' to palpation in accordance with the text book descriptions of this unpleasant, dangerous infection. It was associated with an untreated mandibular fracture in a patient suffering from underlying psychiatric illness. It was managed over several difficult weeks in St Bernard's Hospital.

Mention has already been made to the extensive views enjoyed around Gibraltar from the hospital and no department had a better view of the harbour moles and the Dockyard than the Dental Clinic. One Sunday evening in the early seventies the duty dentist was telephoned to be told that a submarine passing on passage through the Straits had sent a RADEN [request for dental treatment] signal "Immediate treatment" was requested. The hospital dental surgery was opened up and the dental officer was able to observe the submarine berth alongside the South Mole. Transport was already waiting. Minutes later, an inferior dental nerve block* coupled with a little wrist action had relieved a key submariner of his misery and even while the instruments were still being tidied up the dental officer was able to observe his patient, by then already far below him return on board the boat. Moments later it slipped and immediately disappeared rapidly beneath the waters to continue its patrol…… upon 'Her Majesty's Business'. Two long-standing adages well known in the Dental Branch had been witnessed within the hour from the clinic's fine view point that evening. 'Never let the Sun set on Surgical Pus' and always 'Keep the Fleet at Sea'!

The dental staff were not the only ones to appreciate the view from the clinic. The Rock enjoyed a constant round of important visitors, one or two of whom, inevitably required emergency dental treatment whilst there. One such visitor was Lord Avon, who as Sir Anthony Eden was a former Prime Minister and a member of Winston Churchill's war cabinet. After treatment, the former PM lingered for some time, enjoying the splendid view from the surgery. The Senior Dental Surgeon, Surgeon Captain (D) Stewart Bussell naturally declined the offer of a professional fee and a month later an appropriately annotated copy of the Eden memoirs arrived.

Much more useful work was to be done for all three Services in RNH Gibraltar over the next twenty years. But by the mid 1990s as with the other Royal Naval Hospitals RNH Gibraltar's days were drawing to a close. The Service population on the Rock had by then reduced very considerably and the hospital was no longer required. Moreover maintenance demands had steadily increased as the fabric of the buildings had weathered.

In 1996 the Medical Director General (Naval) directed that RNH Gibraltar was to close. All medical secondary care requirements were then concentrated in Devil's Tower Road close to RAF North Front. Yet another rewarding era was over.

*****

---

* Local anaesthetic.

Appendix 2

Recipients of the Harvey-Fletcher Medal and Prize

Date	Name	Basis for Award
1980	Surgeon Lieutenant Commander (D) G W Myers	Management
1883	Surgeon Captain (D) B Robinson	Training
1985	Surgeon Lieutenant Commander (D) A M Prosser	Operational
1988	Surgeon Commander (D) A J Woodman	Training
1991	Surgeon Commander (D) D C C Alexander	Research
1994	Surgeon Commander (D) S Lambert Humble	Management (IT)
2001	Surgeon Lieutenant Commander (D) T B Elmer	Operational
2004	Surgeon Captain (D) R C Sanderson	Operational

N.B At the time of going to press there have been no awards since 2004

*****

Appendix 3

Royal Navy Dental Officers Deployed on Operation Corporate – The Falklands Conflict 1982

Surgn Lieut (D) R E Brown – *RFA Resource*

Surgn Cdr (D) N Harkness – *HMS Invincible*

Surgn Lieut (D) P Hodgson – 42 Cdo RM

Surgn Cdr (D) J V Holland – Naval Party 1710 (*SS Canberra*)

Surgn Cdr (D) G B Keeble – *SS Uganda*

Surgn Lieut (D) A M Prosser – 40 Cdo RM

Surgn Lieut (D) S I Reeves – *HMS Glamorgan*

Surgn Lieut Cdr (D) G H Rhimes – *HMS Antrim*

Surgn Lieut Cdr (D) J D Roberts-James – *HMS Bristol*

Surgn Cdr (D) G H Rudge – Surgical Support Team 2 – (*SS Canberra/Ajax Bay*)

Surgn Lieut Cdr (D) R C Sanderson – *HMS Fearless*

Surgn Lieut (D) N R Sturgeon – 45 Cdo RM

Surgn Lieut Cdr (D) S D B Taylor – *HMS Hermes*

Surgn Lieut Cdr (D) P L Titchen – *HMS Intrepid*

*****

REFERENCES

Chapter 1

1. DCI 464/64 Comnd 2097 – July 1963.
2. JRNMS 1964; 50: 180 RNMC Dinner – Address by MDG.
3. JRNMS 1964; 50: 210-11 A Portable Dental Surgery for Frigates and other Small Ships – KA Johnson.
4. JRNMS 1966; 52: 97 RNMC Dinner – Address by MDG.
5. BDJ; 1964; 116:101-2 Dental Volunteers in Hong Kong – F R B Mathias
6. JRNMS; 1969: 55: 70 Hong Kong Dental Penetration Squad – P Moorhouse
7. DCI 277/66
8. DCI 641/66
9. DCI 1017/66
10. CMND 2903 Quoted in BDJ: 1967;122:81-2
11. JRNMS 1967; 53:91 RNMC Dinner – Address by MDG
12. JRNMS 1966; 52:187 Obituary of Surg Capt (D) J T Wood RN
13. DCI 499/67
14. DCI 395/68
15. DCI 1268/69
16. JRNMS 1968; 54:93 Obituary of Surg Rear Adm (D) E E Fletcher
17. N/MDG 303/1/68/C RNDS Archive
    N/MDG/ PERSL/312 MSC2/70 RNDS Archive

Chapter 2

18. JRNMS 1970; 56: 294 RNMC Dinner – Address by MDG
19. JRNMS 1971; 57: 155 Operation Burlap
20. JRNMS 1971; 57: 162 'SKUA'D'
21. Personal Account – Chap 38 A Glimpse of the Cold War – B Robinson
22. JRNMS 1971, 57: 150 RNMC Dinner – Address by MDG
23. Report of DMS Inquiry Committee
    HMSO 1973: 17-19 Chap IV; Dentists & Dental Supporting Services
24. Report of DMS Inquiry Committee
    HMSO 1973: 44 Chap VII; Training Establishments
25. JRNMS 1972; 58:9-11 Hearts and Minds in the Philippines
26. N/MDG/492/1/73/D 6/8/73 Copy held by late N G Daws
27. JRNMS 1978; 64: 22 A New Mobile dental Clinic – A A Davies
28. JRNMS 1972; 58: 56-58 Moroccan Boar Hunt

29   JRNMS 1975; 59: 165 RNMC Dinner – Address by MDG
30   Letter held in archive of late N G Daws Sir R Swiss, 22/03/77
31   Letter held in archive of late N G Daws A E P Duffy, 04/05/77
32   N/US 166/77 A E P Duffy, 05/09/77
33   DCI 644/78
34   DCI 392/79

Chapter 3
35   RNDS Newsletter 1980; 1; 2: 5 Harvey-Fletcher Prize Award
36   RNDS Newsletter 1980; 1; 1: 17 Film preview – "Toothie RN"
37   RNDS Newsletter 1980; 1; 2: 6 Film Stars RN (G W Myers)
38   RNDS Newsletter 1980; 1; 1: 24 Mass Casualty Treatment Training (B Robinson)
39   Operation Corporate: Dental Report – (J V Holland)
40   RNDS Newsletter 1980; 1; 2: 2 Serving in Tomorrow's Navy Today (K Pendrill)
41   RNDS Newsletter 1981; 2; 1: 12 Clinical Day, Wood Lecture & Director's Dinner – 20 March 1981
42   RNDS Newsletter 1980; 1; 3; 2 Shanghai Visit – September 1980 (R Leworthy)
43   RNDS Newsletter 1981; 2; 2; 28 The Haute Route – Easter 1981 (M D Hocking)
44   RNDS Newsletter 1981; 2; 3; 2 To Russia with Love! (C E C S White)
45   RNDS Newsletter 1981; 2; 2; 14 Diploma in dental Health Education
46   RNDS Newsletter 1981; 2; 3; 13 The Royal Navy Visited (J Aitken)

Chapter 4
47   Personal Communication. N. Barker – CO *HMS Endurance*/Author
48   RNDS Newsletter 1982; 3; 2; 'Falklands Issue'
49   JRNMS 1983; 69;1 'Falklands Issue'
50   RNDS Newsletter 1982; 3; 12-14 *HMS Antrim*: Deployment to South Atlantic – April–July 1982 – G H Rhimes
52   Deployment Report – July 1982 RE Brown to Fleet Dental Surgeon
53   RNDS Newsletter 1982; 3; 12-14 *HMS* Antrim: Deployment to South Atlantic – April–July 1982 – G H Rhimes
54   SDS *Invincible* Annual Report N Harkness
55   JRNMS 1983; 69;1; 36-37 'Falklands Issue'
56   RNDS Newsletter 1982; 3; 2 N R Sturgeon – From San Carlos to Stanley in 200,000 Easy Steps
57   RNDS Newsletter 1982; 3; 20 A M Prosser – Extracts from Report.

58	Operation Corporate: Dental Report 1982 – Paras 11 – 14 J V Holland	
59	Operation Corporate: Dental Report 1982 – Paras 34 – 51 J V Holland – "Specialist Employment"	

Chapter 5

60	RNDS Newsletter 1982; 3;3;2 C White & A M Prosser – Exercise Andes Rover
61	JRNMS 1983; 69;2;118 Obituary – P Hodgson
62	RNDS Newsletter 1983; 4; 2; 14 Full of Eastern Promise – S J Robey
63	RNDS Newsletter 1983; 4; 2; 24 An attempt at the London Marathon – C Howell
64	RNDS Newsletter 1983; 4; 2; 29 Carribtrain 83 with *Invincible* – N Harkness
65	RNDS Newsletter 1983; 4;1;3 Appointment of F R B Mathias as DNDS
66	RNDS Newsletter 1983; 4;25 Letter from America – J Hargraves
67	JRNMS 1986; 72; 1; 3 Editorial
68	RNDS Newsletter 1983; 4; 5; 3 Director's Message – F R B Mathias
69	RNDS Newsletter 1984; 5; 3; 6 A A Davies – Obituary
70	RNDS Newsletter 1984; 5; 3; 53 Senior Rates Refresher Course No. 1
71	RNDS Newsletter 1984; 5; 3; 51 Dental Hygienist Refresher Course No. 1
72	RNDS Newsletter 1984; 5; 3; 13 An Accident at Sea – G Lumley
73	JRNMS 1985; 71; 2; 131 Service Notes
74	RNDS Newsletter 1985; 6; 1; 10-18 The Wood Lecture & Clinical Day
75	RNDS Newsletter 1985; 6; 1; 21-22 The Harvey-Fletcher Prize
76	D/SG(DDS)/959/1/4/5 – 2 April 1985
77	Personal Communication B Robinson – January 2008
78	RNDS Newsletter 1985; 6; 1; 28-31 'Coldfinger' or 'What Goes Up Must Come Down, Only Faster!' – E J Grant
79	RNDS Newsletter 1985; 6; 2; 7 A Message From the Director – D A Coppock
80	Minutes – 10 Oct 1985 RNDS Managers' Meeting
81	RNDS Newsletter 1985; 6; 2; 24 A Hong Kong Experience – S Lambert Humble

Chapter 6

82	RNDS Newsletter 1986; 7; 1; 1 Editorial
83	Minutes – 12 Feb 1986 RNDS Managers' Meeting
84	JRNMS 1986; 72; 2; 87 Caries Activity in a sample of 25 year olds – Sugars or Dentistry? – D C C Alexander
85	RNDS Newsletter 1986; 7; 1; 15 Should We Dress Up Like Spacemen and Avoid Public Lavatories – Y Evans

86 RNDS Newsletter 1986; 7; 2; 24-28 Did the Earth Move for You Too? – D L Thomas

87 JRNMS 1987; 73; 2; 158-159 Obituary – J B Inverdale – R L Travis

88 JRNMS 1987; 73; 3; 213 Obituary – K E J Fletcher – W I N Forrest

89 JRNMS 1987; 73; 3; 213 Obituary – K A Johnson – J A Page

90 RNDS Newsletter 1987; 8; 1; 5-7 The Royal Naval Reserves – T J C Hall

91 RNDS Newsletter 1987; 8; 1; 10-14 The Royal Naval Reserve Dental Branch – H Cannell

92 RNDS Newsletter 1987; 8; 1; 35-36 What's Next? – M R C Gall

93 D/SG(DDS)999/1/4 – 16 Mar 87 Minutes of DNDS Managers' Meeting 1/87

94 D/SG(DDS)952/5/23 – 23 May 89

95 RNDS Newsletter 1988;9;1;4 Death Announcement: A Prosser
    RNDS Newsletter 1988; 9; 2; 3-4 Obituary: A Prosser

96 RNDS Newsletter 1988;9;1;11-13 Mobiles, Prime Movers & PDUs, the Past, Present & Future – B Robinson

97 D/SG(DDS)999/1/4B – 10 Nov 88 Minutes of DNDS Managers' Meeting 3/88 – 4 Nov 88

98 RNDS Newsletter 1988; 9; 1; 26-32 Exercise Annapurna Pitstop – Nepal – February 1988

99 RNDS Newsletter 1989; 10; 1; 77-80 Obituary SRA(D) Osborne – W I N Forrest

100 RNDS Newsletter 1989; 1; 10; 94 Editor's Note

101 RNDS Newsletter 1989; 1; 10; 1 Editorial

102 RNDS Newsletter 1989; 1; 10; 3 The Alan Acton Davies Memorial Prize (Announcement)

103 RNDS Newsletter 1989; 1; 19; 8-13 A Walk in the New Forest – P G Edwards

104 RNDS Newsletter 1990; 1; 11; 22 *HMS Heron*'s Sports News

105 RNDS Newsletter 1990; 1; 11; 10 Obituary – P R J Duly

Chapter 7

106 D/SG(DDS) 952/5/23 – 27 Nov 89 Man S. Org Study

107 D/Man S(Org)10/682 – Apr 90 Review of Defence Dental Services – Man S(Org) Report No. 682

108 D/Med(F&S2)/4/17/GJG/150/90 – 8 Jun 90 Letter to DUS(PL)

109 RNDS Newsletter 11;1; 1- 4 – 1990 Editorial – Progress or Change? – E J Grant

110 JRNMS 1990; 76; 1; 67 – Feb 90 Editorial

111 D/SG(DDS) 999/1/4 – 9 Apr 90 Minutes of DDS(N) Managers' Meeting 1/90

112 RNDS Newsletter 11; 2; 27-28 – 1990 Views of West & East Berlin – S Wolstencroft

113 RNDS Newsletter 11; ; 7-8 – 1990 Kenneth Peter Charles Pritchard – An Appreciation – A J Woodman

114 RNDS Newsletter 11; 1; 83-87 1990 Dai Pan or How green was my (Happy) Valley –L Thomas

115 RNDS Newsletter 11; 1; 43; – 1990 Postscript by Consultant Adviser – J Holland

116 RNDS Newsletter 11; 1; 51-53 – 1990 The Royal Marines 'Dental Branch' – M Hocking

117 RNDS Newsletter 11; 1; 90-96; 1990 Caries Risk Assessment Study {The Occurrence of Dental Pain at Sea } Royal Marines Arduous Training Project} – D C C Alexander

118 Personal Communication – April 2008 The End of the Cold War – B Robinson

119 RNDS Newsletter 11; 1; 57-58; 1990 Training Matters – A J Woodman – Also see Editor's Footnote

120 RNDS Newsletter 11; 1; 97-98; 1990 Obituary – Mr Ron Coote BEM – E J Grant

121 JRNMS 1990; 76; 3; 178 – Winter 90 The RN Medical Club Dinner – Address by MDG(N)

122 D/SG(DDS) 995/1/42 – 19 Oct 90 Redistribution of DDTR Tasks

Chapter 8

123 RNDS Newsletter 11; 2; 9-11; 1990 RFA Argus – E J Grant

124 JRNMS 1991; 77; 233 The RN Medical Club Dinner 1991 – Address by MDG(N)

125 RNDS Newsletter 12; 1; 5-10; 1991 2nd August and all that … – N P Mallon

126 RNDS Newsletter 12; 1; 3-5; 1991 Argus Experience – R Burnside

127 JRNMS 1992; 78; 81-86 No Safe Haven? Kurdish Relief Operation. April-July 1991 – A R O Miller

128 RNDS Newsletter12; 1; 13-14 1991 Letter From Northern Iraq – C D J Redman

129 JRNMS 1992; 78; 103-105 Operation Haven – One Year On – M Norris

130 JRNMS 1992; 78; 107-108 Operation Haven – C L Freeman

Chapter 9

131 D/SG(DDS) 999/1/4 July 91 Minutes of DDS(N) Managers Meeting – 12 July 1991

132 RNDS Newsletter 1992; 13; 1; 12 The Dental Guard – S Stone

133 RNDS Newsletter 1992; 13; 1; 25 Easter in Hong Kong – N Turnbull

134 RNDS Newsletter 1992; 13; 1; 23 Report on *HMS Fearless* Trekking Expedition – Nepal '91 – G Sidoli

135 RNDS Newsletter 1992; 13; 1; 20 Operation Pisang 91 – S Howe
136 RNDS Newsletter 1992; 13; 1; 5 Royal Naval Reserve Dental Branch (1915-1992) – Anon
137 D/SG(DDS) 999/14/9 Dec 91 Minutes of DDS(N) Managers Meeting – 9 Dec 1991
138 RNDS Newsletter 1992; 13; 2; 1 Editorial – J V Holland
139 RNDS Newsletter 1992; 13; 2; 15 Royal Naval Hospital Haslar – J V Holland
140 D/SG(DDS) 999/1/4 March 92 Minutes of DDS(N) Managers' Meeting – 20 Mar 1992
141 RNDS Newsletter 1992; 13; 2; 26 Commander Dental Training (Report)
142 FDS Pre- Meeting Report/16 Jun 92 Command & Staff dental Advisers Meeting – Fleet Input
143 2SL 761/7/23 June 92 Review of the Royal Naval Dental Services – Loose Minute
144 DBH/17/11 Notes for Meeting With COS CINCNAVHOME 17th Dec 1992
145 JRNMS 1993; 79; 1; 51 RNMC Report – D A Lammiman
146 RNDS Newsletter 1993;14; 1; 4 Surgeon Commodore (D) Brian Robinson – An Appreciation
147 D/SG(DDS) 999/1/4 19 Aug 93 Minutes of DDS(N) Board of Management – 8 Jul 93
148 RNDS Newsletter 1993; 14; 1; 15-17 6000 Feet to 16000 Feet in Less Than 72 Hours…? But I'm Not a Marine!!! – B Jamieson
149 JRNMS 1993; 79; 3; 162-163 Obituary – SRA(D) W Holgate
150 RNDS Newsletter 1993; 14; 2; 14-15 Sea Time? – Armilla group 5 report – M F Thomas
151 RNDS Newsletter 1993; 14;2; 25-26 Mount Kinabalu – RNDS Expedition 7th/8th March 1993 – T B Elmer

Chapter 10
152 D/MDG(N)/DNDS/1500/8/68/A; June 1994 Minutes of DNDS Board of Management – 9 Jun 94
153 RNDS Newsletter 1994; 15; 1; 6-7 The Wood Memorial Lecture and Clinical Meeting 1994.
154 RNDS Newsletter 1994; 15; 1; 12-13 British Army of the Rhine Exchange: Berlin 1992-1994 – J Fenwick
155 JRNMS 1994; 80; 2; 48-49 Our Way Ahead – A Craig
157 D/MDG(N)/1500/8/68/A; Dec 1994 Minutes of DNDS Board of Management – 18 Nov 94
158 RNDS Newsletter 1995; 16; 1; 30-34 *HMS Ark Royal* – Grey Funnel Line Cruises – From Club 18-30 to Saga Holidays – D L Thomas

*****

INDEX

Addy, Professor Martin, 214
Aitken, Major John RADC, 51
Ajax Bay, 54, 58, 59, 63, 66, 67, 71, 72, 75, 76, 271
Alan Acton Davies Memorial Medal and Prize, 97, 114, 135
Alexander, D C C (David), 97, 114, 147, 153, 182, 270
All Arms Commando Course (AACC), 152, 153
Anniversary, 75th Anniversary Dinner, 228
ANZUK, 19, 222
Armilla Patrol, 52, 59, 84, 165, 166, 204, 206, 224
ASCAB: Armed Services Consultant Approval Board, 237, 238, 239, 244, 247
Ashdown, Rt Hon. Paddy, 181
Atlantic Conveyor, 64, 71
Australia Antigen, 25

Barker, Captain Nick, 53
Barnard, David, 237
Barraclough – Gober Report, 91
Bastable, Charles, 260
Becket, Sue (L/Wren), 189
Bennett, Morris, 10

Bethesda: US Navy Hospital, 20, 87, 223
Bighi: see RNH Bighi
Birnie, David, 237, 246, 247
Black, Captain J J, 85
Bluff Cove, 62, 69, 72
BMH Hanover: British Military Hospital, 249
Boswell, Gillian, 139
Boyce, Admiral Sir Michael, 259
Boyd, "Hoppy", 242
Bradbeer, Jonathan, 2, 3
Bradbury, Surgeon Vice Admiral Sir Eric, 12, 22
Bradlaw, Sir Robert, 236
Bramley, Sir Paul, 101, 236, 261
Bravyy: Kotlin Class Soviet Destroyer, 17, 18
Britannia Royal Naval College (BRNC), 206, 260
British Dental Association, 4, 25
British Dental Journal (BDJ), 5, 13, 248
British Joint Services Hovercraft Expedition to Peru: Exercise Andes Rover, 78, 79
British Military Hospital, Stanley, 99
Brown, Hugh, 229
Brown, R E (Rupert), 59, 271
Burnside, Rita, 164, 165, 168, 171
Bussell, S N, 103, 109, 119, 133, 161, 234, 242, 245, 246, 247, 253, 266, 269

Cadman, Surgeon Rear Admiral (D) A E (Ted), 29, 30, 31, 32, 222
Calderbank, Karen, 165
Caldwell, Surgeon Vice Admiral, 238
Camilleri, Professor George, 264
Campion, Bernard, 33
Canadian Armed Forces, 213
Canberra, SS, 16, 53, 54, 55, 57, 58, 60, 63, 66, 71, 72, 74, 75, 76, 271
Cannell, Hugh, 119, 243, 261
Canniesburn Hospital, 189, 199
Caribtrain, 84
Caries Risk Assessment Study (CRAS), 153
Central Examining Board for Dental Hygienists, 38, 139
Certificate of Proficiency in Dental Hygiene, 8, 38
Cheney, Geoffrey, 243, 261
CHOTS: Corporate HQ Office Technology System, 212
Clark, Ken, 267
Clayton, Admiral Sir Richard, 34, 37
Cliff, Brian, 242
Clinical Profile Monitoring System

(CPMS), 104, 157
Colbeck, Richard, 172
Combat Casualty Care Course: "C4", 44, 62, 83, 100, 102, 103, 109, 136, 145, 146, 161
Command Dental Laboratory, 21, 187, 260
Commander Dental Training (CDT), 112, 129, 149, 158, 161, 192, 199, 207

Commando:
3 Commando Brigade Royal Marines, 13, 66, 172, 199
40 Commando Royal Marines, 23, 57, 58, 71, 73, 78, 101, 172, 179, 260
42 Commando Royal Marines, 58, 67, 83
45 Commando Royal Marines, 3, 58, 67, 70, 172, 177
Commando Logistics Regiment, 172, 177
Commando Training Centre Royal Marines (CTCRM), 83, 123, 192

Compton, Sir Edmund, 22
Compton Committee, 22, 90
Cooke, Professor Brian, 237
Coote, Ron, 74, 158, 159, 160
Coppock, D A (David), 20, 39, 87, 101, 103, 107, 108, 109, 111, 126, 133, 145, 148, 149, 158, 199
Coward, Vice Admiral John DSO, 181
Craig, Surgeon Rear Admiral Sandy, 168, 217, 229, 260
Crewe, Tom, 237, 261
Crump, Kay (Wren), 190

David Bruce Royal Naval Hospital: see RNH Mtarfa
Davies, A A, 25, 96, 97, 114, 128
Davies, Sandy, 261
Daws, Nick, iii, vii, ix, 214, 219, 229
Day, Stephen, 242
Defence Costs Study: "DCS 15", 212, 217, 218, 219, 230, 258, 262
Defence Dental Agency (DDA), 158, 217, 218, 226, 228, 229, 231, 232, 233, 245, 258
Defence Medical Equipment Depot (DMED), 8, 74
Defence Secondary Care Agency, 217, 220, 253, 258, 259
Dentaims, 146, 147
Dental Caravan, 24, 25, 128, 129
Dental Envelope: F Med 271, 8, 103

Dental Strategy Review Group, 111
Dental Surgery Design Steering Committee, 114
Dental technicians, 22, 38, 89, 94, 113, 125, 126, 186
Dental Treatment Form: M, 8, 9
"Dentists with a Difference": (Recruiting Film), 192
Derriford: District General Hospital, 218, 249, 262
Dewar, Surgeon Commander Paxton, 163
Dickson, Gordon, 237
Diploma in Orthodontics: Dip Orth, 198, 245, 247
DNMP: Director of Naval Manpower Planning, 200, 227, 228
Drouet, Paula, 130, 133
Duckworth, Professor Roy, 237
Duffy, Patrick MP, 31, 32
Duly, P R J, 7, 8, 37, 38, 83, 86, 112, 139, 140, 155

Eastman Dental Institute, 3, 122, 142, 145
Edwards, Liz, 172, 173
Edwards, P G (Peter), 136
Elmer, T B (Tim), 137,

208, 210, 270
Elrick, Crawford, 172
Emslie, Professor R D, 104
Evans, Yvonne, 114
Evans, Karin, 110
Exercise SUBOK, 23

Faculty of Dental Surgery, 123, 237
Faculty of General Dental Practice (UK), 123, 243
Falkland Islands, 16, 53, 55, 58, 66, 141
Falklands Conflict, vii, 7, 44, 53, 54, 56, 59, 65, 78, 83, 84, 90, 123, 127, 140, 141, 152, 154, 159, 162, 164, 262, 271
Fenwick, Julie, 214
Fickling, B W, 236
Field Hospital: 32 Field Hospital RAMC, 165
Fieldhouse, Admiral Sir John, 257
Finnegan, Surgeon Rear Admiral (D) C J, 10
First Avenue House, 94, 109, 199, 210, 212
Flanagan, D V (Dominic), 165
Fletcher, Surgeon Rear Admiral (D) E E, 6, 9, 20, 29, 118, 229
Fletcher, K E J (Ken), 29, 118
Fletcher, Timothy, 229
Form F Med 271: Dental Record Folder, 8, 103
Forrest, Surgeon Rear Admiral (D) W I N,
9, 10, 11, 12, 20, 21, 199, 245, 247, 264
Fraser, Admiral of the Fleet Lord Fraser of North Cape, 256, 257
Freeman, Charlotte (L/Wren), 172, 173, 177
Frigate Portable Dental Unit (FPDU), 3, 4, 31, 46, 74, 76, 127, 128, 165, 204

Gall, M R C, 123
Galtieri, General Leopoldo, 53, 68, 84
Gellatley, P S J (Peter), 16, 18
General Belgrano (Argentinian Cruiser), 57, 63
General Dental Council (GDC), 1, 7, 8, 31, 38, 109, 115, 139, 158, 228
General Medical Council (GMC), i
Gill, Janet, 106
Goodridge, D L (Derek), 10, 242
Gorts Hospital, 265
Graham, Steve (Sgt), 190
Grant, E J (Ted), vii, 9, 13, 14, 19, 34, 35, 37, 43, 87, 106, 119, 161, 180, 181, 194, 196, 197, 200, 212, 213, 217, 219, 220, 221, 222, 223, 226, 227, 228, 229, 231, 232
Greenbank Hospital Plymouth, 261
Guild, Surgeon Captain Forbes, 266
Gurd, Surgeon Rear Admiral Dudley, 260
Guy's Hospital, 7, 12, 29, 86, 103, 104, 118, 133, 198, 221, 223, 267

Haig, Alexander (US Secretary of State), 53
Hall, T J C (Timothy), iv, v, 4, 5, 42, 103, 117, 190, 196, 197, 198, 199, 200, 207, 210, 211, 213, 217, 219, 221, 223, 229, 230, 234, 235, 242, 244, 245, 246, 247, 257
Hambly, R S (Dick, 42, 161, 187, 226
Handbook for Royal Navy Dental Surgery Assistants: BR 888D, 140
Hannaford, Ed, 261
Hargraves, John, iii, 87, 89, 158, 182, 192, 232
Harkness, Neil, 63, 84, 271
Harris, Nicholas, 217
Harvey, Staff Surgeon Christopher, 20
Harvey-Fletcher Medal and Prize, 20, 21, 38, 39, 83, 101, 127, 129, 130, 146, 181, 270
Haslar: see Royal Naval Hospitals
Hasleden, Frank, 237
Hayward, Richard, 242, 243
Head of Management Services

(Organisation): Man S Org, 127, 142
Henderson, Derek, 214, 237
Hepatitis B, 25, 114, 151
Heseltine, Rt Hon. Michael MP (Secretary of State for Defence), 91
Higgs, D M, 186
Hill, Caroline, 214

HM Ships
HMS Alacrity, 46, 64
HMS Alliance, 189
HMS Antelope, 60, 61, 64
HMS Antrim, 46, 56, 57, 61, 62, 64, 271
HMS Ardent, 57, 59, 60, 61, 64
HMS Argus, 28
HMS Ark Royal, xi, 16, 17, 18, 30, 47, 104, 145, 205, 222, 223, 224
HMS Arrow, 31
HMS Avenger, 65, 84
HMS Birmingham, 99, 225
HMS Blake, 40
HMS Brazen, 166, 167, 168
HMS Brilliant, 64, 204, 225
HMS Bristol, 271
HMS Broadsword, 64, 71, 99, 100
HMS Cambrian, 3
HMS Cardiff, 51
HMS Centaur, xi, xii, 3, 82, 86
HMS Centurion, 200

HMS Ceres, 30
HMS Cochrane, 105, 107, 110, 126, 158, 223
HMS Collingwood, 29, 148
HMS Condor, 124
HMS Conqueror, 57
HMS Cornwall, 206
HMS Coventry, 46, 64, 71, 204, 205, 206, 225
HMS Cumberland, 29, 118
HMS Devonshire, 2, 43
HMS Daedalus, 28, 30, 145
HMS Dolphin, 37, 101, 125, 134, 139, 181, 199, 214, 220, 223, 252, 255
HMS Drake, 95, 97, 182, 187, 233, 260
HMS Eagle, 10, 32, 103
HMS Endurance, 53, 54, 56
HMS Europa, 28
HMS Fearless, 47, 57, 64, 72, 74, 186, 271
HMS Forth, 11
HMS Fulmar: RN Air Station, Lossiemouth, 96
HMS Gambia, 96
HMS Ganges, 118, 221
HMS Glamorgan, 19, 54, 271
HMS Glasgow, 57
HMS Glendower, 128
HMS Hampshire, 2
HMS Hartland Point, 11
HMS Hermes, 37, 55, 64,

103, 139, 271
HMS Heron: RN Air Station Yeovilton, 30, 204, 260
HMS Howe, 21
HMS Hydra, 13, 14
HMS Intrepid, 13, 14, 23, 47, 58, 64, 72, 73, 271
HMS Invincible, 45, 47, 63, 64, 65, 84, 85, 90, 104, 186, 271
HMS Jamaica, 96
HMS Jufair, 198
HMS Kenya, 21
HMS Leander, 4
HMS London, 2, 3, 166, 167
HMS Mercury, 51, 222
HMS Maidstone, 118
HMS Mauritius, 229
HMS Nelson, 7, 34, 36, 40, 45, 51, 78, 95, 97, 112, 129, 133, 192, 197, 204, 207, 214, 221, 228, 231, 263
HMS Neptune: Clyde Submarine Base, 134, 227
HMS Ocean, 28, 32
HMS Osprey, 204, 222, 260
HMS Pembroke, 28
HMS Phoenicia, 145
HMS Phoenix, 166
HMS Plymouth, 72
HMS Protector, 15, 16
HMS Raleigh, 9, 48, 86, 145, 169, 192, 222
HMS Rodney, 133
HMS Rooke 266, 267
HMS Saker, 28

HMS Seahawk: RNAS Culdrose, 28, 136, 260
HMS Sheffield, 57, 60, 63, 64
HMS Simbang, 11, 13
HMS Southampton, 206
HMS Sultan, 39, 198, 201
HMS Tamar, 4, 5, 11, 86, 109, 110, 130, 149, 150, 151, 183
HMS Tenby, 145
HMS Terror, 11, 19, 28, 203
HMS Triumph, ix, 11, 13, 19, 222
HMS Urchin, 4
HMS Venus, 4, 198
HMS Vernon, 35
HMS Victorious, 3, 9, 30, 222
HMS Victory, 189, 221, 235
HMS Warrior, 189
HMS Yarmouth, 18, 60, 61, 62
Hocking, Malcolm, 48, 152
Hodgson, Peter, 58, 67, 69, 82, 83, 271
Holgate, Surgeon Rear Admiral (D) Bill, 96, 203, 204, 248
Holland, J V (John), iii, vii, ix, 15, 16, 53, 58, 66, 74, 75, 187, 188, 197, 217, 219, 229, 234, 242, 244, 245, 249, 253, 254, 257, 271
Home, Sir Alec Douglas, x
Howe, Sarah, 183

Howell, Chris, 84, 243
Hunter, Surgeon Rear Admiral (D) John, 21, 22, 28, 29, 30
Hussein, Saddam, 147, 161, 166, 171

Iles, J G, 97
Indonesian Confrontation, x, 9
Institute of Dental Health and Training (IDHT), 7, 112, 232
Institute of Dental Surgery: see The Eastman Dental Institute
Institute of Naval Medicine (INM), iii, 42, 96, 101, 102, 114, 119, 125, 140, 146, 153, 161, 181, 199, 203, 214, 223, 247
International Dental Journal, 248
Inverdale, J B, 117, 118
Irvine, Gordon, 243

James, David, 4
Jamieson, Barbie, 201
Jarrett, Sir Clifford, 22, 90, 91
Jarrett Report, 22
Johnson, K A, 4, 118, 119
Joint Services Defence Course (JSDC), 134, 158, 232
Jolly, R T (Rick), 59, 61, 163
Jones, Air Vice Marshal John, 93, 94, 125, 126, 142

Journal of the Royal Naval Medical Service (JRNMS), iv, 5, 13, 26, 54, 217, 244, 248, 259

Keeble, G B (Geoff), 54, 76, 102, 242, 271
Kelly, I L (Ian), 147
Killick, Charlie, 164, 167, 170
King, Rt Hon. Tom MP, Secretary of State for Defence, 173, 179, 181
Kings College Hospital Dental School, 82
King-Turner, Bill, 21

Lacon House, 232
Lakonia, SS, xi, xii, 86
Lambert Humble, Stephen, 109, 113, 130, 161, 207, 213, 270
Lammiman, David, 157, 194, 195, 197
Langan, L C (Clive), 104, 242
Layard, Admiral Sir Michael, 194
Liggins, Steven, 106, 190, 242
Lindsay, David, 48
London & Haslar Gold Medal, 20, 203
London Hospital, 37, 139, 243
Lumley, G (Graeme), 97, 100
Lympstone: see Commando training

Centre Royal Marines

Macdonald-Watson, Alistair, 242
Mach, Steve, 20
MacIntyre, David, 243
Mackenzie, E B 'Mack', 25, 266, 268
Mackey, Air Vice Marshal Jefferson, 217, 219, 226, 227
Mallon, N P (Nigel), 165, 166, 168, 170
Malta, 10, 16, 19, 21, 24, 32, 37, 82, 87, 95, 139, 145, 203, 225, 226, 235, 244, 246, 264, 265, 266
Malta George Cross Fiftieth Anniversary Medal, 21
Man S. Org: Management Services Organisation, 127, 142
Manadon: RN Engineering College, 260
Martin, I R (L/MA(D)), 204
Mathias, F R B (Frank), 94, 95, 101, 103, 107
Maxwell, Alan, 208, 209, 210
May, D L (David), 22
McLean, Dr John, 125
MDHU: Military District Hospital Unit, 217, 218, 249, 262
Medical Research Council (MRC), 96, 203, 248
Milford, Jo, 150
Milne, Charles MBE, 255
Minor Dental Valise 3
Mintoff, Dom, Prime Minister of Malta, 87, 264
Moffat, Lieutenant General Sir Cameron, 93
Moore, Alan, 119
Moore, Major General J J, 72
Moore, Nicki (L/Wren), 182
Moorhouse, Peter, 5
Moos, Professor Khursheed, 189, 237
Morse, Rear Admiral Ron DC USN, 213, 314
Mountain, Surgeon Rear Admiral (D) W L, 2, 3, 9, 30, 45
Mountbatten, Admiral of the Fleet Earl Mountbatten of Burma, 256, 257
Mtarfa: RNH Mtarfa, 235, 264
Murchison, Surgeon Captain, 268
Musgrave Park Hospital, Belfast, 124, 249
MV Norland, 58
Myers, G W, 38, 39, 78, 134, 156, 158, 165, 171, 182, 192, 212, 231, 232, 270

Naples: NATO Base, 38, 115, 116, 117, 149
Naval Dental Clinic (NDC), 114, 115, 223
Navy Graduate Dental School (NGDS), 20, 87, 223
Navy News, 33
Naylor, Professor M N (Tony), 7, 12, 214, 221, 237, 267
New Management Strategy (NMS), 160, 191
Norris, Mary, 172, 173, 174, 176, 177
Norris, Richard, viii, 233
Nott, Rt. Hon. John MP, Secretary of State for Defence, 47, 51, 53, 74, 78, 91, 112

Odstock Hospital, 199
Operation Burlap, 13, 15
Operation Corporate, 54, 59, 66, 74, 141, 262, 271
Operation Granby, vii, 164, 165, 168, 171, 181, 182
Operation (Safe) Haven, 172, 174, 177, 179
Options for Change, 147, 154, 180, 182, 191, 194, 210, 229
Order of St John of Jerusalem, 87, 101, 146, 223
Osborne, Surgeon Rear Admiral (D), L B (Ginger), 133
Owen, Suzanne (PO Wren), 189

Panckridge, Surgeon Vice Admiral W R S, 237
Pan's People, 19, 20

Pavitt, Laurie MP, 143
Peake, Debra, 135
Peebles, Anthony, 243
Pidgeon, J (John), 15,
Poppelwell, Nick, 106
Popham, B F S (Ben) 28
Prime Mover, 25, 128, 129
Principal Dental Officer (Reserves), 243
Pritchard, Ken, 149
Prosser, A M (Andy), 58, 71, 78, 101, 102, 127, 270, 271
Pugh, Surgeon Rear Admiral Gordon, 251

QE2: Queen Elizabeth II, 55, 62, 75
Queen Alexandra's Hospital (QAH), 246, 247

RAF Akrotiri, 242
RAF Halton, 7, 112, 232
RAF Leuchars, 227
RAF North Front, 267, 269
RAF Dental Branch, 93, 108, 157, 186, 187, 191, 227, 245
Raffetto, Ed, 20
Read, Netty (Wren), 190
Reagan, President Ronald, 53
Red and Green Life Machine, see SST2
Redman, C D J (Chris), 172
Reeves, S I (Steve), 271
Revell, Surgeon Vice Admiral Tony, 216, 217, 251

RFAs
RFA Argus, 162, 163, 164, 165, 167, 168, 169, 170, 171, 262
RFA Brambleleaf, 206
RFA Diligence, 166, 167
RFA Fort Grange, 167
RFA Olna, 100
RFA Olwen, 97
RFA Pearleaf, 84
RFA Resource, 271
RFA Sir Galahad, 13, 65, 69, 72
RFA Sir Tristram, 65, 69, 72
RFA Stromness, 58
RFA Tidespring, 19

Rhimes, G H (Godfrey), 56, 61, 62, 271
Riden, Keith, 242
Rimini, Freda, 7
RN Medical School: see Institute of Naval Medicine
RN Medical Staff School, 119
RN Staff Course, 158

Royal Naval Hospitals
RNH Bermuda, 10
RNH Bighi, 10, 95, 235, 263, 264, 265
RNH Gibraltar, 25, 242, 265, 266, 269
RNH Haslar, 258, 259, 260, 262, 263
RNH Hong Kong, 265
RNH Mtarfa, 235, 264
RNH Plymouth: (RNH Stonehouse), 118, 221, 249, 251, 259, 260, 261, 262

Roberts-James, J D, 271
Robey, S J (Steve), 84
Robinson, B (Brian), iii, iv, v, 9, 16, 38, 39, 42, 83, 93, 102, 103, 104, 114, 117, 126, 127, 129, 144, 145, 147, 154, 158, 160, 161, 180, 181, 186, 187, 191, 192, 193, 194, 195, 196, 197, 218, 223, 229, 270
Rogers, B F (Brian), 31, 32, 37
Rowe, Norman, 45, 236,
Rowe, Sally, 113, 220, 221, 228
Royal Army Dental Corps (RADC), 51, 90, 108, 112, 124, 149, 150, 190, 208, 214, 215, 216, 227, 245, 246, 249, 267
Royal College of Physicians, 248
Royal College of Surgeons of Edinburgh, 243
Royal College of Surgeons of England, 96, 123, 134, 198, 221, 237, 245
Royal Fleet Auxiliary: see: RFAs
Royal Hospital Haslar, 235, 258, 259, 262
Royal Marines School of Music, 115
Royal Naval Barracks, Portsmouth, 5
Royal Naval College, Greenwich, 115

Royal Naval Dental Training School (RNDTS), 7, 8, 32, 34, 35, 36, 97, 111, 112, 122, 129, 139, 140, 223
Royal Naval Reserve (RNR), 7, 10, 12, 119, 180, 181, 186, 197, 241, 243, 261, 266, 267
Royal Naval Reserve Dental Branch: see RNR (above)
Rudge, G H (George), 53, 58, 59, 66, 75, 76, 101, 164, 167, 169, 181, 242, 244, 245, 271
Rule, David, 213,
Rust, Helen (Wren), 182

San Carlos, 57, 58, 59, 60, 66, 67, 71, 72, 73, 75
Sanderson, R C (Chris), 57, 165, 242, 244, 245, 262, 270, 271
Santa Fe: Argentinian Submarine, 57, 63
Saxonia, MV, 60
Second Submarine Squadron (SM2), 260
Seward, Margaret CBE, 228
Seward, Gordon CBE; 228
Sharpe, G D (Geoff), 7, 189, 242, 244
Sheiham, Professor Aubrey, 181
Shepherd, Tony, 41
Sidoli, Gio, 183, 186

Sims, L/Col Philip, 190, 246, 247
Singapore, 11, 13, 14, 19, 28, 82, 84, 90, 118, 126, 203, 222
Slater, Admiral Sir Jock GCB LVO, 228, 229, 231
Small Systems Group (SSG), 130
Smith, Alec, 242, 245, 255
Speight, Alex (MA(D)), 164, 173
SST2: see Surgical Support Team 2
St Bernard's Hospital, 268
Stacey, C T (Clem), 84, 101
Starkey, W E ('Podge'), 95, 96, 248, 249, 263
Steele-Perkins, Surgeon Vice Admiral D D, 1
Stephens Report, 91
Stone, Sara (Wren), 182
Stonehouse: see RNH Plymouth
Strategy Review Group, 111, 125
Strontium 90 (Assay Project), 96, 203, 247, 248
STUFT: "Ships Taken up from Trade", 53, 55
Sturgeon, N R (Nigel), 58, 67, 71, 271
Sukarno, President of Indonesia, 222
Surgical Support Team 2 (SST2), 58, 59, 66, 75, 76, 271
Swann, M J (Mike), 13, 14
Swiss, Sir Rodney, 31, 32

Taylor, S D B (Stephen), 205, 242, 243, 271
Taylor, Ann (Wren), 182
Thatcher, Margaret, Prime Minister, 47, 53
The Eastman: see Institute of Dental Surgery
Thomas, D L (Lynford), 115, 149, 223
Thomas, M F (Mike), 204
Titchen P (Peter), 58, 271
Toms, Kim, 78
"*Toothie RN*": Recruiting Film, 39
Travis, R L (Roy), 82, 242, 245, 261
Trefgarne, Lord, Under Secretary of State for the Armed Forces, 95
Tulley, Professor Jack, 237
Turnbull, Nick Turnbull, 183, 245
Turner, Surgeon Rear Admiral (D) P S 'Titch', 2, 21
Turner Dental School, Manchester, 28, 96

Uganda, SS, 54, 55, 57, 63, 66, 72, 74, 75, 76, 102, 271
United Kingdom Atomic Energy Authority, 248
University of Birmingham, 211
US Navy Dental Corps, 10, 20, 87, 103, 213, 214
USS Hewitt, 205
USS Carl Vinson, 88, 89

285

Victory Building, 207, 210, 212, 213, 217, 223, 232
Vocational Training, 109, 122, 123, 129, 134, 206, 207, 213, 240

Wallace, L M A, 165, 166
Ward, Sir Terence, 236
Watt, Surgeon Vice Admiral Sir James, 30
Watts, Jacquie, 207, 212, 228
Waverly Committee, 22
Weston, M W (Mark), 114, 129, 233
White, Catherine, 48, 78
White, Eleanor, 106, 126
Whitlock, Roy, 237
Wickens, G L (Graham), 23, 24
Wilkinson, C J (Kit), 10
Wilson, Harold, Prime Minister, x, 10, 12, 222
Wilson, Dave (POMA), 106
Winter, Professor G B, 142
Wolstencroft, Simon, 147
Wood, Surgeon Captain (D) J T, 6, 45, 198
Wood Lecture and Clinical Day, 6, 45, 101, 125, 181, 213, 214, 219, 243
Woodman, A J (Alan), 36, 112, 129, 161, 270
Woodward, Rear Admiral Sandy, 54, 55,
Wrigley, P C (Peter), 6, 134

Yellowlees, Sir Henry, 22, 90, 91, 92, 93, 94, 101

Zuckerman, Sir Solly Zuckerman, Chief Scientific Adviser to HMG, 25